THE *BEST* of

The Whole Pediatrician Catalogs I–III

JULIA A. McMILLAN, M.D.
FRANK A. OSKI, M.D.
both from the
Department of Pediatrics
State University of New York,
Upstate Medical Center at Syracuse

JAMES A. STOCKMAN, III, M.D.
Department of Pediatrics
Northwestern University
School of Medicine

and
PHILLIP I. NIEBURG, M.D.
Centers for Disease Control

W. B. SAUNDERS COMPANY   1984
Philadelphia • London • Toronto • Mexico City • Rio de Janeiro • Sydney • Tokyo

W. B. Saunders Company: West Washington Square
Philadelphia, PA 19105

1 St. Anne's Road
Eastbourne, East Sussex BN21 3UN, England

1 Goldthorne Avenue
Toronto, Ontario M8Z 5T9, Canada

Apartado 26370–Cedro 512
Mexico 4, D.F., Mexico

Rua Coronel Cabrita, 8
Sao Cristovao Caixa Postal 21176
Rio de Janeiro, Brazil

9 Waltham Street
Artarmon, N.S.W. 2064, Australia

Ichibancho, Central Bldg., 22-1 Ichibancho
Chiyoda-Ku, Tokyo 102, Japan

Library of Congress Cataloging in Publication Data

McMillan, Julia A.
　The best of the Whole pediatrician catalogs I-III.

　Includes indexes.
　1. Pediatrics–Handbooks, manuals, etc. I. Title.
II. Title: Whole pediatrician catalog. [DNLM: 1.
Pediatrics–handbooks. WS 39 M478w]
RJ48.M325 1984　　　618.92　　　84-10503
ISBN 0-7216-1216-4

The Best of the Whole Pediatrician Catalogs I-III　　　　　　　　　　　　　ISBN 0-7216-1216-4

Last digit is the print number:　9　8　7　6　5　4　3　2　1

INTRODUCTION

The first volume of *The Whole Pediatrician Catalog* was published in 1976. At that time we did not know there would be any successors. Volumes 2 and 3 were a continuation of our attempt to compile some more of the useful information concerning the diagnosis and management of problems in pediatric patients.

The Best of The Whole Pediatrician Catalogs is a collection of entries from Volumes 1, 2, and 3 that we felt were the most useful and most difficult to find in other easily available references.

We recommend, just as we did in introducing Volumes 1, 2, and 3, that the reader briefly review the contents of the entire book so items may be recalled when the need arises.

We hope that you find this compendium both helpful and enjoyable.

Julia A. McMillan

Frank A. Oski

James A. Stockman, III

Phillip I. Nieburg

CONTENTS

1
THE HISTORY AND PHYSICAL EXAMINATION

FONTANELS

An abnormality in size of the anterior fontanel may be a tip-off to abnormality in the infant. Figure 1–1 displays the fontanel size, defined as $\frac{\text{length} + \text{width}}{2}$, as measured with a steel tape in 201 normal infants.

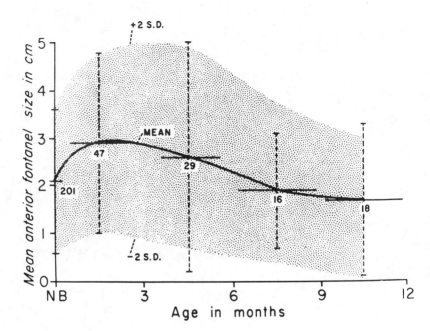

FIG. 1–1

The tables below list conditions associated with an unusually small (or prematurely closed) fontanel or with an unusually large fontanel.

*Disorders in which Premature Closure or Small Fontanel for Age
May Be a Feature*

       Microcephaly

       High Ca++/vitamin D ratio in pregnancy

       Craniosynostosis

       Hyperthyroidism

       Normal variant

> *Fontanel*—From the French word *fontanelle*, which is the diminutive for *fontaine*, the word for fountain.

Disorders in which Large Fontanel for Age May Be a Feature

SKELETAL DISORDERS	CHROMOSOMAL ABNORMALITIES	OTHER CONDITIONS
Achondroplasia	Down's syndrome	Athyrotic hypothyroidism
Aminopterin-induced syndrome	13 Trisomy syndrome	Hallermann-Streiff syndrome
Apert's syndrome	18 Trisomy syndrome	Malnutrition
Cleidocranial dysostosis		Progeria
Hypophosphatasia		Rubella syndrome
Kenny's syndrome		Russell-Silver syndrome
Osteogenesis imperfecta		
Pyknodysostosis		
Vitamin D deficiency rickets		

References: Popich, G.A., and Smith, D.W.: J. Pediatr., *80*:749, 1972. Barness, L.A.: Manual of Pediatric Physical Diagnosis. 3rd Ed. Chicago, Year Book Medical Publishers, Inc., 1966, pp. 49–50.

HEAD CIRCUMFERENCE IN PREMATURE INFANTS

Patterns of head growth in premature infants seem to be a function of gestational age as well as of the infant's health. Mean head circumference increments for healthy premature infants are as follows:

GESTATIONAL AGE	WEEKLY HEAD CIRCUMFERENCE INCREMENTS (CM/WEEK)		TOTAL INCREMENT (FIRST 16 WEEKS OF LIFE)
	Weeks 1–8 of Life	*Weeks 9–16 of Life*	
30–33 weeks	1.1	0.5	13.2 cm
34–37 weeks	0.8	0.4	9.8 cm

In sick premature infants, the head circumference increases at a slower rate. This increase averages 0.25 cm per week during the first 16 weeks of life. "Sick" premature infants are those requiring artificial ventilation and/or intravenous feedings for periods of two weeks or longer.

Premature infants should be suspected of having intracranial pathologic changes if:

1. They are apparently healthy but their head circumference increments do not approach these data.

2. They are sick yet have a rate of head growth approaching that of a healthy infant of the same gestational and postnatal age.

Reference: Sher, P.K., and Brown, S.B.: Dev. Med. Child Neurol., *17*:705, 1975.

HEAD CIRCUMFERENCE IN TERM INFANTS

Expected head circumference (HC) during infancy can be estimated by remembering that the average full-term infant will show the following increments in head growth:

PERIOD	HC INCREMENTS
First 3 months	2 cm/month = 6 cm
4–6 months	1 cm/month = 3 cm
6–12 months	0.5 cm/month = 3 cm
First year	12 cm

TRANSILLUMINATION — NORMAL VALUES

Transillumination of the skull is a valuable procedure in the diagnosis of a variety of central nervous system anomalies of infants. The results of transillumination can be difficult to interpret because of variation in intensity of light source and lack of reliable standards for transillumination in normal children.

The introduction of the "Chun Gun" has helped to resolve these problems of interpretation. The "Chun Gun" is named in honor of Dr. Ray Chun, a pediatric neurologist who was instrumental in its development. Light is provided by a focused projection lamp, which emits a constant bright light. Heat is dissipated by two absorbing filters and five cooling fans. The instrument has a two-position switch. The first position activates a weak red lamp that allows the operator to view the infant in a dark room; the second position turns off the red lamp and activates the projection lamp.

Normal values for transillumination of normal infants are listed below. Note that values are reported as distance from center of light beam. The radius of the Chun gun's outlet is 2 cm. Thus if values are recorded from the edge of the beam they will be 2 cm less. It will be noted that the transillumination distance, as measured from the center of the beam, was about 5 cm in all areas and in all ages, with a standard deviation of less than 1 cm. Values in excess of 7 cm should therefore always be viewed with suspicion. Possible diagnoses include hydrocephalus, subdural effusions or hematoma, porencephaly, cerebral atrophy, or hydranencephaly.

Transillumination Distance as Measured from Center of Light Beam

	NUMBER OF SUBJECTS	FRONTAL		PARIETAL		OCCIPITAL	
		cm	*1 SD*	*cm*	*1 SD*	*cm*	*1 SD*
Newborn	50	5.4	0.4	4.8	0.4	4.5	0.5
Two months	50	5.6	0.6	5.1	0.5	5.4	0.7
Four months	50	5.7	0.7	5.0	0.3	5.1	0.5
Six months	50	5.5	0.6	5.0	0.5	5.1	0.5
Nine months	50	5.7	0.7	5.0	0.7	5.0	0.5
Twelve months	25	5.7	0.3	5.1	0.4	5.2	0.5
Eighteen months	25	5.4	0.4	4.9	0.5	4.7	0.5

The figures below provide normal values for premature infants of varying gestational ages. The upper figure in each graph describes the total length of the transillumination, while the lower figure indicates the total width of the transillumination. Note that with increasing gestational age the area of normal transillumination increases.

References: Cheldelin, L. V., Davis, P. C., Jr., and Grant, W. W.: J. Pediatr., *55:*937, 1975. Swick, H. M., Cunningham, D., and Shield, L. K.: Pediatrics, *58:*658, 1976.

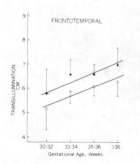 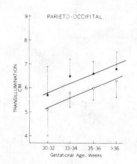 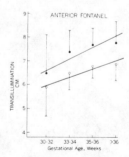

FIG. 1–2

SIMPLE FORMULAS FOR APPROXIMATING HEIGHT AND WEIGHT OF CHILDREN

Not infrequently the information on the height and weight of your patient is available but you cannot find a growth grid to determine whether or not the information is normal. This is particularly true for the child from 1 to 12 years of age. The simple formulas below will enable you to calculate quickly what the 50th percentile should be.

For Weight (in pounds)

Ages 1 to 6 years = (age in years X 5) plus 17.
Ages 6 to 12 years = (age in years X 7) plus 5.

For Length (in inches)

Ages 2 to 14 years = (age in years X 2.5) plus 30.

Reference: Weech, A.: Am. J. Dis. Child., *88*:452, 1954 (as modified by Vaughan, V.C., III, and McKay, R.J. (Eds.): Nelson Textbook of Pediatrics. 10th Ed. Philadelphia, W.B. Saunders Co., 1975, p. 25).

STRABISMUS

Strabismus, or squint, is a result of one of three major pathologic processes:

1. An imbalance in the ocular muscles of the two eyes as a result of maldevelopment or innervation.
2. A difference in the refraction of the two eyes.
3. A visual defect in one eye.

Strabismus may be either paralytic or nonparalytic. Nonparalytic strabismus is seen frequently in infants during the first 6 months of life. After this age strabismus requires an explanation and treatment in order to avoid amblyopia. A paralytic squint is abnormal at any age.

When the squint is of the nonparalytic type (concomitant), all muscles move the eye normally, but they do not work in conjunction with each other. The two eyes are in the same position relative to each other, whatever the direction of gaze. The nonparalytic squint is not associated with diplopia. In young infants the presence of strabismus can easily be confirmed by shining a light at the eyes from directly in front of the patient. The reflection of the light should normally be in the center of the pupil or at a corresponding point on both corneas.

When the squint is of the paralytic type (nonconcomitant) owing to muscle paralysis, the eyes are straight except when moved in the direction of the paralyzed muscle. If full ocular movements are elicited in one eye when the other is covered, then a paralytic strabismus can be excluded.

Nonparalytic squint is seen in children with hydrocephalus, cerebral palsy, retinoblastoma, corneal opacities, and refractive errors.

Paralytic squint should suggest the presence of a brain stem lesion and increased intracranial pressure.

CONGENITAL LACRIMAL STENOSIS

Obstruction of the lacrimal ducts (dacryostenosis), often in association with purulent dacryocystitis, is relatively common in infancy. It should be suspected in an infant with a purulent discharge from the eye whose corresponding conjunctiva appears normal. Another presentation may be recurrence of purulent discharge soon after cessation of ophthalmic antibiotic therapy for what had been thought to be conjunctivitis. The diagnosis is confirmed if pressure over the lacrimal sac produces an outpouring of mucopurulent material from the lacrimal punctum.

The goal of open passage of tears can be accomplished by an ophthalmologist using probing of the lacrimal tract, a procedure requiring general anesthesia. The goal may also be reached by a nonoperative technique easily taught to parents.

The technique is based on forcing the fluid collected in the lacrimal sac through the obstructed lacrimal drainage tract. This is accomplished by placing the tip of the thumb above the sac at the medial angle of the eye and slowly and steadily rolling the thumb caudad, thereby increasing the pressure in a downward direction (Fig. 1–3).

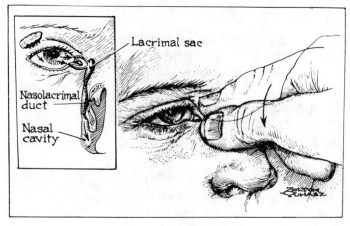

FIG. 1–3

The problem of reflux of fluid – and thus pressure – into the conjunctival sac, caused by a momentary release of thumb pressure, is easily avoidable with some practice. Care should be taken to avoid inadvertent contact between the baby's skin and the thumbnail. This technique should be used three to four times daily for a month before you decide that no improvement has occurred and referral to an ophthalmologist is made. Because the pressure generated by the thumb depends on the presence of fluid in the lacrimal sac, it can be applied only once each time; the sac takes several hours to refill. Ophthalmic antibiotics may be used to control infection caused by the obstructed tract.

Reference: Riffenburgh, R.S., and Yubasz, Z.: Pediatr. Digest, June 1971, p. 21.

WHITE PUPILLARY REFLEX

Sometimes it is not possible to visualize the fundus of the eye. This is especially true in the nursery setting. Normally, the ophthalmoscope will elicit a red pupillary reflex, the reflection of a vascular retina and choroid through a clear lens and anterior and posterior chambers. When it is not possible to clearly visualize the fundus, the least that should be done is to observe this red reflex. Obtaining a white pupillary reflex signifies that a lenticular opacity (cataract) is present or that some other intraocular pathogenesis is present. Disorders associated with white pupillary reflexes include:

1. Cataracts
2. Colobomas
3. Retrolental fibroplasia
4. Chorioretinitis
5. Organized vitreous hemorrhage
6. Congenital retinal fold
7. Intraocular foreign body
8. Retinal detachment
9. Metastatic retinitis and endophthalmitis
10. External exudative retinitis of Coats
11. Larval agranulomatosis (toxocara canis or cati)
12. Persistent primary vitreous

Reference: Robb, R. M.: Hosp. Pract., *12:*107, 1977.

THE VISUAL ACUITY OF NORMAL CHILDREN

A friend of yours tells you that her 1 year old child has been examined by her pediatrician and is said to have "perfect 20/20" vision. Your child, who is also 1, has 20/200 vision. Who should get a new physician?

Visual acuity at birth is poorer than at any other time of life and only gradually improves to the 20/20 range at the time of entrance to kindergarten. The accompanying table indicates the expected average acuity of preschool children. An acuity of 5/200 should not be misinterpreted to mean that the newborn is practically blind. Just stick your tongue out at a newborn and see what he does back to you!

AGE	AVERAGE UNCORRECTED ACUITY
Birth	5/200
1 year	20/200
2 years	20/40
3 years	20/30
4 years	20/25
5 years	20/20

Reference: McCrary, J. A.: J.A.M.A., *208:*1195, 1969.

PHOTOPHOBIA

Although the illnesses associated with photophobia are often obvious and relatively easily diagnosed (e.g., viral conjunctivitis, measles, or bacterial meningitis), there are other, more subtle conditions that must be considered when the primary diagnosis is not so obvious. Some of these associations are listed below.

More Common Associated Infections

Measles
Coxsackie B infection
Lymphocytic choriomeningitis
Viral conjunctivitis
Arbovirus infection
Bacterial meningitis

Less Common Associated Infections

Phlyctenular conjunctivitis
Yellow fever
Psittacosis infections
Rickettsial infections

Noninfectious Associations

Infantile glaucoma
Albinism
Vitamin A deficiency
Keratitis (e.g., Reiter's
   syndrome)
Erythropoietic porphyria
Acute cerebellar ataxia
Chédiak-Higashi syndrome
Aniridia
Cystinosis
Migraine
Corneal ulcer
Hysteria (in older child)
Arsenic poisoning
Mercury poisoning
Drug toxicity
   Trimethadione
   Ethosuccimide
   PAS

References: Wintrobe, M.M., Thorn, G.W., Adams, R.D., et al. (Eds.): Harrison's Principles of Internal Medicine. 7th Ed. New York, McGraw Hill Book Company, 1974. Illingworth, R.S.: Common Symptoms of Disease in Children. 5th Ed. Oxford, Blackwell Scientific Publications, 1975, p. 184. Barnett, H.L. (Ed.): Pediatrics. 15th Ed. New York, Appleton-Century-Crofts, 1972.

THE EYELASH SYNDROME

All adults appreciate the fact that a foreign body in the eye is both annoying and painful. The most common foreign body to produce such discomfort indoors is the eyelash. We frequently forget that eyelashes may get into the eyes of infants as well. The next time you are confronted with an irritable, crying baby for which you cannot find a suitable explanation, be sure to check the eyes for a foreign body. If you find it, you can produce an instant cure.

DETECTION OF HEARING PROBLEMS IN INFANCY

Impaired hearing during the first year of life has profound effects on language and emotional, social, and intellectual development. Detection of hearing losses during this time is important because:

1. More severe and more prolonged impairments cause greater reductions in speech and language development.
2. It is desirable to initiate therapy for hearing loss by 6 months, and it is practical to do so by 6 to 12 months.
3. Adequate hearing assessment is possible by 4 to 8 months.
4. When hearing loss is not restorable, various measures are available and indicated to promote language and speech development and to minimize the effects on emotional and social development.

Impaired hearing has been associated with several sets of perinatal circumstances, the occurrence of any of which is an indication for early (by 4 months) audiologic evaluation and for long-term follow-up.

Conditions Associated with High Risk of Hearing Loss

1. Family history of hearing loss before approximately 50 years of age without obvious cause.
2. Maternal viral infection during pregnancy (especially rubella).
3. Defects of ears (including pinnae), nose, lips or palate.
4. Birth weight under 1500 gm.
5. Bilirubin above 20 mg/dl.
6. Prenatal treatment of mother or postnatal treatment of infant with ototoxic drugs (including kanamycin or gentamicin).
7. Multiple congenital anomalies of any kind.

Suspicion of hearing loss should be raised beyond the perinatal period in several circumstances:

AGE	CLUE
Any time	Failure of infant to respond to loud environmental sounds.
Any time	Failure to awaken or move about in response to speech or noise when asleep in quiet room.
By 4–5 months	Failure to turn head or eyes toward sound source.
By 6 months	Failure to turn purposefully toward sound source.
By 8 months	No attempt to imitate sounds made by parents.
By 8–12 months	Lack of variety in melody and sounds during babbling.
By 12 months	No apparent understanding of simple phrases.
By 24 months	Little or no spontaneous speech.

Occurrence of any of these clues is an indication for audiologic and otologic evaluation.

Reference: Goodman, A.C., and Chasin, W.D.: *In* Gellis, S.S., and Kagan, B.M. (Eds.): Current Pediatric Therapy. 7th Ed. W.B. Saunders Company, Philadelphia, 1976, p. 518.

CAUSES OF DEAFNESS

Middle ear disease is the most common cause of acquired deafness in children. Congenital deafness, however, is often part of a more significant syndrome or disease state, the signs of which may or may not precede the deafness. Certain of these disorders are treatable; all are of great prognostic significance.

Reference: Chasin, W. D.: Hosp. Pract., *12:*103, 1977.

Inborn Causes of Deafness

WITHOUT ASSOCIATED ANOMALIES
 Congenital severe, both dominant and recessive
 High-frequency hearing loss, both dominant and recessive
 Midfrequency hearing loss, recessive

ASSOCIATED WITH RETINITIS PIGMENTOSA
 Usher's syndrome
 Cockayne's syndrome (mental retardation and dwarfism)
 Alström's syndrome (obesity)

ASSOCIATED WITH HEREDITARY NEPHRITIS
 Alport's syndrome
 Herrmann's syndrome (mental retardation, diabetes, and epilepsy)
 Muckle-Well's syndrome (urticaria and amyloidosis)

ASSOCIATED WITH CONGENITAL HEART DISEASE
 Jervell and Lange-Nielsen syndrome (prolonged Q-T interval, Stokes-Adams attacks)
 Lewis' syndrome (congenital pulmonic stenosis)

ASSOCIATED WITH SKELETAL DISEASE
 Crouzon's disease (mixed hearing loss)
 Treacher-Collins syndrome
 Mohr syndrome—oral-facial-digital syndrome II (conductive hearing loss)
 Albers-Schönberg disease
 Pyle's disease (progressive childhood deafness)
 Van der Hoeve's disease (conductive hearing loss)

ERRORS OF METABOLISM
  Morquio's disease
  Tay-Sachs disease
  Hurler's syndrome
  Wilson's disease
  Waardenburg's syndrome

ENDOCRINE SYSTEM DISORDERS
  Pendred's syndrome (severe congenital sensorineural hearing loss)

ASSOCIATED WITH NERVOUS SYSTEM DISORDER
  Von Recklinghausen's disease
  Huntington's chorea
  Friedreich's ataxia
  Richards Ruudel disease (severe progressive deafness)

ASSOCIATED WITH OTHER ANOMALIES
  Auricular anomalies (microtia, aural atresia, preauricular fistulas)
  Congenital syphilis
  Congenital rubella

LOW-SET EARS

Low-set ears can be a finding of extreme importance. There is a controversy over what constitutes low-set ears. We prefer a method of evaluation suggested by Dr. Murray Feingold. In Figure 1–4, the face has a sheet of x-ray film held over it. On the margins of the film are measurement scales, and the center of the film is bisected by a horizontal line that is aligned with the medial canthi of the eyes. The amount of the ear lying above the line is measured as well as the overall length of the ear. If the ear is below the center line, the ear is low set. If 10 per cent or less of the overall length of the ear is above the line, the ears are said to be low set. If low-set ears are found, look carefully for other physical abnormalities.

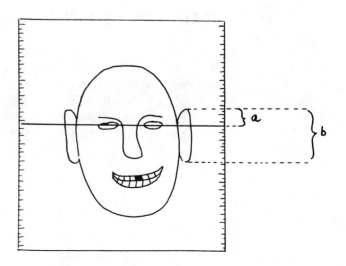

FIG. 1–4

If $\frac{a}{b} \times 100 \leqslant 10$, the ears are low set.

Some Syndromes Associated with Low-set Ears

> Apert's syndrome
> Camptomelic syndrome
> Carpenter's syndrome
> Cri-du-chat syndrome

LOUDNESS

The extent of hearing loss is measured in terms of how loud a sound must be at any given pitch before an individual can hear it. You can roughly gauge the degree of hearing loss by using the scale below.

THRESHOLD OF HEARING (db)

Faint whisper	10	Quiet breeze
Whisper	20	
Soft speech	30	Quiet house
	40	
Average conversation	50	Quiet automobile
	60	
Loud voice	70	Very noisy office or restaurant
	80	Heavy street traffic
	90	
Beginning discomfort for pure tones	100	Riveter at 40 ft
	110	
	120	Propeller aircraft at 20 ft
Tickle sensation	130	
Pain	140	Jet afterburner at 40 ft

Reference: Valadian, I., and Porter, D.: *In* Physical Growth and Development. Boston, Little, Brown & Company, 1977, p. 20.

TEETH AND GUMS

While examining the mouth, the physician often looks past the teeth and gums directly to the pharynx. Proper oral hygiene is an essential part of preventive medicine, and it is the duty of the pediatrician, as well as the dentist, to advise the parent and child about dental care. The pediatrician should be able to recognize gingival disease that is common to the infant and child. A list of these problems, along with their clinical features and treatment, is presented on following page.

DISEASE	CLINICAL FEATURES	TREATMENT
Gingivitis Early	There is slight edema of gingival margin with color change from pale pink to reddish or bluish red.	Gingivitis is caused by bacteria which form dental plaque. Treatment involves removal of that plaque. Regular tooth brushing is a necessary component of plaque removal. The type of brush used is not important nor is one particular brushing technique better than another. Brushing does not remove plaque between the teeth, however, and dental floss should be used along with brushing for this purpose. The gingivitis should resolve within several days of the institution of the above regimen. Fibrous enlargement of the gingiva due to gingivitis must be surgically removed.
Moderate	Inflammation is present. The gingiva is red and glazy and bleeds with manipulation.	
Severe	The gingiva is red and enlarged, so that it covers more of the tooth than is normal. It may bleed spontaneously, and ulcerations may be present.	
Juvenile periodontitis	The gingiva may appear normal, and the only symptom is increased tooth mobility. The permanent first molars and lower incisors are primarily affected. There is extensive bone loss evident on radiologic examination.	Periodontitis may be prevented by strict attention to proper dental care. Recognition of the disease by the pediatrician is an indication for referral to a dentist.
Gingival hyperplasia	This is noted particularly in patients with acute myeloblastic and acute monocytic leukemia and in those treated with diphenylhydantoin. The earliest signs are beadlike enlargements on marginal and interdental areas that coalesce to form large tissue masses. These masses may cover the teeth completely in some areas. The tissue is pink and firm and does not bleed.	The hypertrophy caused by acute leukemia may be treated only by surgical removal; that caused by diphenylhydantoin therapy recedes with withdrawal of the drug.
Hereditary gingival fibromatosis	This is a rare disease inherited in an autosomal dominant fashion. The gingival tissue enlarges to cover the teeth. It is of normal color and does not bleed easily.	There is no treatment except surgical removal of gingival tissue. The hypertrophic tissue will recur following removal.
Acute necrotizing gingivitis (Vincent's infection; trench mouth)	Bacterial cause has been assumed but never proved. There is a sudden onset of punched-out, crater-like ulcerations of the marginal gingiva. The ulcerations have a whitish pseudomembrane, and they are surrounded by erythema. Any area of the gingiva may be affected. There is spontaneous bleeding of the gingiva. The breath has a fetid odor. There may be regional lymphadenopathy, fever, and malaise. Pain is severe, and mastication is often impossible.	Treatment consists of debridement and frequent mouth rinses with hot salt water or a hydrogen peroxide solution. Systemic antibiotics may be used but are usually not necessary.

Continued

DISEASE	CLINICAL FEATURES	TREATMENT
Acute herpetic gingivostomatitis	The herpes simplex virus is the cause of this illness. Fever, irritability, and regional lymphadenopathy usually precede intense inflammation of the gingiva. Pain accompanies the inflammation. Small vesicles erupt and then become shallow ulcers with red, elevated margins and gray craters. The gingiva, labial or buccal mucosa, soft palate, pharynx, sublingual mucosa, and tongue may be involved.	Ulcers heal spontaneously in 7 to 14 days. The erythema persists several days more. Viscous Xylocaine may be used to provide symptomatic relief while healing takes place.

Reference: Polson, A.M.: Pediatrics, *54*:190, 1974.

POPSICLE PANNICULITIS

Once the popsicle was invented, could popsicle panniculitis be far behind? This form of panniculitis is produced by the sucking on cold objects, such as popsicles and ice cubes. It is characterized by the presence of a reddish-purple discoloration of the cheeks. On occasion it may feel indurated. Tenderness and warmth are unusual.

The lesions are most obvious 24 to 48 hours after the cold injury. They are most commonly confused with a cellulitis. The patients with popsicle panniculitis are afebrile and feel well. The lesions subside without treatment, leaving no permanent injury.

The next time you see a red-faced child, inquire about prolonged sucking on popsicles or ice cubes. Misdiagnosis may leave you red-faced.

Reference: Epstein, E.H., Jr., and Oren, M.E.: N. Engl. J. Med., *282*:966, 1970.

"Happy the child that has for friend an old, sympathetic, encouraging mind, one eager to develop, slow to rebuke or discourage."

Arthur Brisbane

TACHE CÉRÉBRALE

Stroking the skin can often provide diagnostic information. Two major responses may be elicited when the skin over the abdomen, back, or chest is gently stroked with the fingernail. One response is tache cérébrale, and the other is dermatographia.

In tache cérébrale, the stroking produces a red streak that is flanked by thin, pale margins. This sign develops within 30 seconds of stroking and persists for several minutes. It has been noted to be present in patients with scarlet fever, hydrocephalus, a variety of febrile illnesses, and, most particularly, in meningitis. It can be used as an early clue to the presence of meningitis, particularly in the neonatal period.

In dermatographia, the stroking produces a white or pale line with red margins. This wheal is seen in patients with fair skin, in those with vasomotor instability, or in extreme form in patients with urticaria pigmentosa.

Reference: Martin, G.I.: J. Pediatr., *87*:322, 1976.

SPLENOMEGALY

Normally, the spleen's erythropoietic role ceases at birth. Its primary functions in postnatal life are the filtration of particulate matter and formed elements from the blood and the production of humoral factors required for the opsonization of infectious organisms. Splenomegaly may result from disease states in which these normal functions are required in excess. There are, however, other processes that result in splenomegaly. Reference to the following table should be of some help in making a diagnosis when the spleen is enlarged.

MECHANISM OF ENLARGEMENT	CLINICAL EXAMPLES	OTHER FINDINGS
Sequestration Loss of RBC deformability	Hemolytic anemias, i.e., sickle cell disease, thalassemia, RBC enzyme deficiencies	Jaundice, anemia No peripheral lymphadenopathy
Antibody coating of RBCs	Rh and ABO isoimmunization in the newborn. Autoimmune hemolytic anemia	Increased reticulocyte count, peripheral blood smear shows evidence of hemolysis
Proliferation Chronic immunologic stimulation	Viral infections, i.e., infectious mononucleosis, cytomegalovirus Severe bacterial pneumonia, bacterial endocarditis, typhoid fever, indolent septicemia	Generalized lymphadenopathy Atypical lymphocytes Other findings typical of the infectious process
Lipid Accumulation of lipid-laden macrophages in the spleen	Tay-Sach's disease Gaucher's disease Niemann-Pick disease Metachromatic leukodystrophy Gangliosidoses	Appropriate clinical and historical findings for these diseases

Continued

MECHANISM OF ENLARGEMENT	CLINICAL EXAMPLES	OTHER FINDINGS
Engorgement		

Portal hypertension	Chronic hepatitis
	Cystic fibrosis
	Wilson's disease
	Biliary atresia
	Ascending infection via
	   umbilical vein catheter
	   in the newborn
	Portal vein thrombosis
		Hepatomegaly
		Esophageal varices
		Internal hemorrhoids
		History of liver disease
		Leukopenia,
		   thrombocytopenia

Accumulation of blood in the splenic capsule	Splenic trauma	History of trauma

Acute splenic engorgement	"Sequestration crisis" of
	   sickle cell disease
		Child under 5 years
		Hypovolemia
		Anemia
		Findings of sickle cell
		   disease

Endowment		
Rare congenital causes of splenomegaly	Splenic hemangiomas Splenic cysts Splenic cystic hygroma	Positive spleen scan
iNvasion		
Malignancy	Leukemia Lymphoma Metastatic neuroblastoma Histiocytosis	Other findings consistent with these diseases
Granuloma	Sarcoidosis Tuberculosis Systemic fungal infection	

You may have noticed that the underlined letters in the headings above spell SPLEEN. Memorization of these general processes involved in splenic enlargement may help in understanding the disease state of your patient with an enlarged spleen. Remember, however, that approximately 30 per cent of normal term infants and 10 per cent of healthy infants at 1 year of age have a palpable spleen. By age 12, only 1 per cent of normal children have a spleen that may be felt as much as 1 cm below the costal margin.

Reference: Boles, E.T., Jr., Baxter, C.F., and Newton, W.A., Jr.: Clin. Pediatr., *2*:161, 1963.

"The child is surrounded by so much authority, so much school, so much dignity, so much law, that it would have to break down under the weight of all these restraints if it were not saved from such a fate by meeting with a friend."

Dr. Wilhelm Stekel

LIVER SIZE

The child admitted as a medical patient to a busy pediatric floor may be examined by many students and physicians. Palpation and percussion of the liver may be reflected in some write-ups as hepatic enlargement and in others as "within normal limits."

The liver size of 105 healthy children aged 5 to 12 years is depicted in Figure 1–5. Examination was by palpation and percussion in the right midclavicular line. Palpation of liver edge below the costal margin alone is an unreliable measurement, presumably because of diaphragmatic movement.

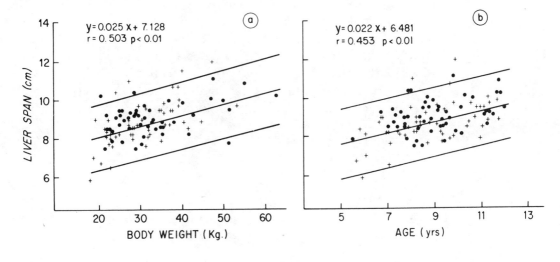

FIG. 1–5

Liver span (estimates of height in the right midclavicular line) in normal male and female children was obtained by palpating the lower border and percussing the upper border. The closed circles represent values for females, and the crosses represent values for males. Each mark is a *mean* of the measurements obtained by two investigators. The liver span is plotted against body weight in *A*, and against age in *B*. The middle lines are the regression lines, and the outer lines represent the 95 per cent confidence limits.

Reference: Younoszai, M.K., and Mueller, S.: Clin. Pediatr., *14*:378, 1975.

ABDOMINAL MASSES

The diagnostic considerations that accompany the finding of an abdominal mass are largely determined by the age of the patient, associated symptoms, and physical findings. Many abdominal masses detected on routine physical examination ultimately prove to be:

Fecal material
Distended urinary bladder
The abdominal aorta
A pregnant uterus

Fecal material in the colon is usually freely movable and easily compressible. If one suspects that the mass is fecal in origin and this cannot be confirmed by rectal examination, an enema should be given to the patient and the examination repeated.

A *distended bladder* may be palpated in the newborn who has not voided within the first 24 hours of life. This delay may signify the presence of abnormalities of the urethra, such as posterior urethral valves. Other causes of bladder distention include:

The use of anticholinergic drugs
Spinal cord tumors
Abnormalities of the spinal cord
Coma
The early postoperative period
Bladder irritation produced by an inflammatory lesion in the pelvis,
    such as an inflamed appendix or appendiceal abscess

If the mass is of bladder origin, it will appear to originate at a point below the symphysis pubis and may extend as high as the umbilicus. Rectal examination will usually confirm the presence of a distended bladder. If the child cannot be induced to void, catheterization may be required to confirm the diagnosis.

Abdominal Masses in Older Infants and Children

GASTROINTESTINAL MASSES

Ages 3 to 6 weeks

1. Most common mass is the "tumor" of *pyloric stenosis*.

2. *Duplications* of the gastrointestinal tract, usually of the small bowel, are generally accompanied by symptoms of intestinal obstruction. May be of neurenteric origin and associated with defects in the vertebral column.

Ages 6 months to 3 years

1. *Intussusception* is the most common mass. At this age it is usually secondary to:

> Enlarged mesenteric lymph nodes
> Polyps
> Meckel's diverticulum
> Henoch-Schönlein purpura

2. *Mesenteric cyst.* Associated with painless abdominal enlargement. May be of months to years in duration. Freely movable in the lateral direction and sometimes associated with a fluid wave or shifting dullness.

3. *Appendiceal abscess.*

4. Abscesses and fistulas secondary to *granulomatous colitis*.

NEOPLASMS

Most common tumors are neuroblastomas and Wilms' tumor.

Wilms' Tumor

Clinical features include:

1. Approximately 60 per cent occur before age 5 years.

2. May be associated with fever, pain, and hypertension.

3. Hematuria present in 20 per cent of patients at diagnosis.

4. Mass may extend to midline and into the iliac fossa.

5. Intestine displaced to the opposite side.

6. Calcifications uncommon.

7. Tumor spreads locally but also metastasizes to liver, lung, and brain.

8. Occurs with increased frequency in children with sporadic (in contrast to familial) aniridia.

9. Occurs with increased frequency in patients with congenital hemihypertrophy and congenital macrosomia (Beckwith's syndrome).

Neuroblastoma

Clinical features include:

1. About 50 per cent occur within first 2 years of life.
2. In about one-half of patients, tumor arises in the abdomen. In one-third of patients it is in the adrenal gland, and in an additional 18 to 20 per cent it arises from nonadrenal intra-abdominal sites.
3. Mass frequently crosses the midline.
4. Calcifications common on x-ray films of the abdomen.
5. Skeletal metastases common. Lung metastases uncommon.
6. Skin, hepatic, and nodal involvement may be present at time of diagnosis. Invasion of retrobulbar soft tissue frequently observed and produces proptosis of the eye as well as periorbital swelling and ecchymosis of the upper eyelid.
7. Initial signs and symptoms may reflect excessive catecholamine production by the tumor and include skin flushing, perspiration, tachycardia, hypertension, paroxysmal headaches, and intractable diarrhea.
8. Uncommon initial manifestations include signs of encephalopathy or opsoclonus.

A general list of the more common abdominal masses that may be encountered in infants and children is listed below.

Abdominal Masses in the Older Infant and Child

Renal malformations
Hydronephrosis
Duplication cysts of the intestine
Volvulus of the gut
Intussusception
Periappendiceal abscess
Mesenteric abscess
Mesenteric cyst
Hepatic cyst or abscess
Choledochal cyst
Pancreatic pseudocyst
Hepatoma
Hemangioma of the liver or spleen
Wilms' tumor
Neuroblastoma
Lymphoma
Ovarian cyst
Ovarian tumor

1

Initial evaluation should include a careful rectal examination, complete blood count, urinalysis, and flat plate of the abdomen. More precise studies will be dictated by the preliminary findings.

References: Arey, J.B.: Pediatr. Clin. North Am., *10*:665, 1963. Sutow, W., Vietti, T.J., and Fernbach, D.J.: Clinical Pediatric Oncology. St. Louis, C.V. Mosby Company, 1973.

"I remember seeing a picture of an old man addressing a small boy. 'How old are you?' 'Well if you go by what Mamma says, I'm 5. But if you go by the fun I've had, I'm 'most 100.' "

William Lyon Phelps

A DIAGNOSTIC APPROACH TO LYMPHADENOPATHY

Is the lymphadenopathy generalized or localized? Generalized lymphadenopathy is defined as enlargement of more than two noncontiguous node regions. Generalized lymphadenopathy is caused by generalized disease.

GENERALIZED LYMPHADENOPATHY

What are associated signs and symptoms?
Rash?
Hepatosplenomegaly?
Thyroid enlargement?
Joint involvement?
Heart and lung abnormalities?
Pallor?
Easy bruising?

Infections

Exanthems
Cytomegalovirus
Infectious mononucleosis
Infectious hepatitis
Typhoid fever
Malaria

Pyogenic
Tuberculosis
Syphilis
Toxoplasmosis
Brucellosis
Histoplasmosis

Collagen Vascular Disease

Lupus erythematosus
Rheumatoid arthritis

LOCALIZED LYMPHADENOPATHY

Signs of infection in the involved node?
Evidence of infection in the drainage area of node?
History of recent antigenic introduction in the node's drainage area?

Supraclavicular — Always consider mediastinal disease (tuberculosis, histoplasmosis, coccidioidomycosis, sarcoidosis). Always consider lymphoma. In absence of evidence of pulmonary infection, early biopsy indicated.

Axillary — Secondary to infections in the hand, arm, lateral chest wall, or lateral portion of the breast. May be result of recent immunization in the arm.

Epitrochlear — Secondary to infections on ulnar side of hand and forearm. Observed in tularemia when bite occurs on finger. Also seen in secondary syphilis.

Immunologic Reactions
Serum sickness, drug reactions
Granulomatous disease (sarcoid)

Storage Disease
Gaucher's disease
Niemann-Pick disease

Malignancies
Leukemia
Lymphoma
Histiocytosis
Neuroblastoma, metastatic

Hyperthyroidism

Inguinal — Infection in lower extremity, scrotum, penis, vulva, vagina, skin of lower abdomen, perineum, gluteal region, or anal canal. May be seen in lymphogranuloma venereum. May represent metastatic disease from testicular tumors or bony tumors of the leg. Immunization in leg.

Cervical — Generally the result of localized infection. See accompanying table for differential diagnosis.

Causes of Cervical Adenitis

CAUSE	COMMENT
Viral upper respiratory infections	Most common cause. Nodes soft, minimally tender, and not associated with evidence of redness and warmth of overlying skin.
Bacterial infection	Streptococcus and staphylococcus most common etiologic agents. Usually secondary to previous or associated infection in drainage area of node. More frequently unilateral. Signs of infection — tenderness, warmth, and redness generally present. Look for primary focus of infection in scalp, mouth, pharynx, and sinuses.
Tuberculosis	*Mycobacterium tuberculosis* infections generally bilateral, involve multiple nodes. Associated with evidence of chest disease and systemic signs. Atypical mycobacteria infections more commonly unilateral initially. Not associated, in general, with other foci of disease. With either agent, evidence of local warmth and redness uncommon.
Infectious mononucleosis	Fever, malaise, preceding upper respiratory infection often noted. Splenomegaly common. Atypical lymphocytes present. Epstein-Barr virus titers required for diagnosis in younger children.
Cytomegalovirus Toxoplasmosis	Indistinguishable clinically from Epstein-Barr virus infections. Requires serologic studies to make the diagnosis.
Cat-scratch disease	History of contact with young cat. May be preceded by history of fever and malaise. Adenopathy restricted to area drained by initial cat scratch.
Sarcoidosis	Disease bilateral. Chest x-ray almost always abnormal. May have keratitis, iritis and evidence of bone disease.
Hodgkin's disease	Common presenting symptom. Frequently unilateral at time of initial manifestation. Node is rubbery, nontender, and not associated with signs of inflammation. Make certain that supraclavicular involvement is not present. When present, strongly suspect lymphoma.
Non-Hodgkin's lymphoma	Bilateral at time of initial presentation in approximately 40 per cent of patients. Cervical and submaxillary nodes commonly involved together.

Algorithm

GENERALIZED LYMPHADENOPATHY

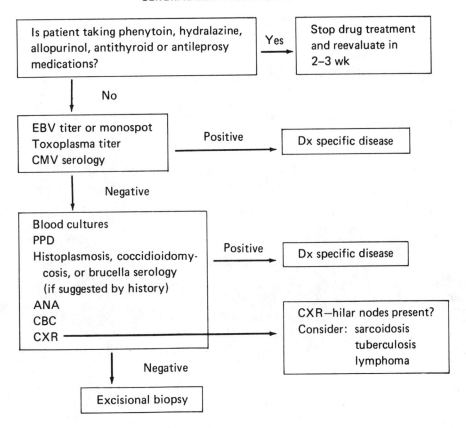

Algorithm

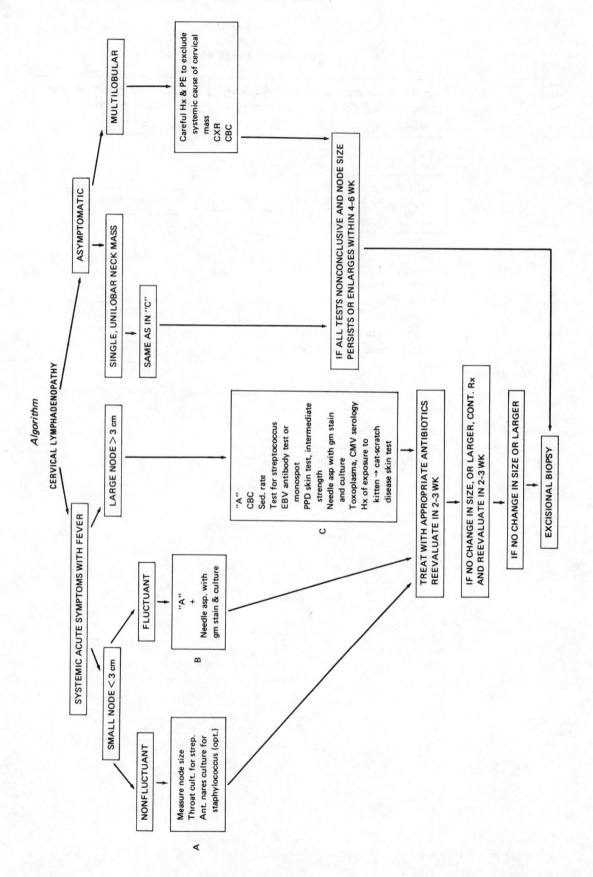

CERVICAL LYMPHADENOPATHY

ASYMPTOMATIC

MULTILOBULAR

Careful Hx & PE to exclude systemic cause of cervical mass
CXR
CBC

SINGLE, UNILOBAR NECK MASS

SAME AS IN "C"

IF ALL TESTS NONCONCLUSIVE AND NODE SIZE PERSISTS OR ENLARGES WITHIN 4–6 WK

SYSTEMIC ACUTE SYMPTOMS WITH FEVER

LARGE NODE > 3 cm

"A"
CBC
Sed. rate
Test for streptococcus
EBV antibody test or monospot
PPD skin test, intermediate strength
Needle asp with gm stain and culture
Toxoplasma, CMV serology
Hx of exposure to kitten → cat-scratch disease skin test

C

SMALL NODE < 3 cm

FLUCTUANT

"A"
+
Needle asp. with gm stain & culture

B

NONFLUCTUANT

Measure node size
Throat cult. for strep.
Ant. nares culture for staphylococcus (opt.)

A

TREAT WITH APPROPRIATE ANTIBIOTICS REEVALUATE IN 2–3 WK

IF NO CHANGE IN SIZE, OR LARGER, CONT. Rx AND REEVALUATE IN 2–3 WK

IF NO CHANGE IN SIZE OR LARGER

EXCISIONAL BIOPSY

Algorithm

LOCALIZED LYMPHADENOPATHY

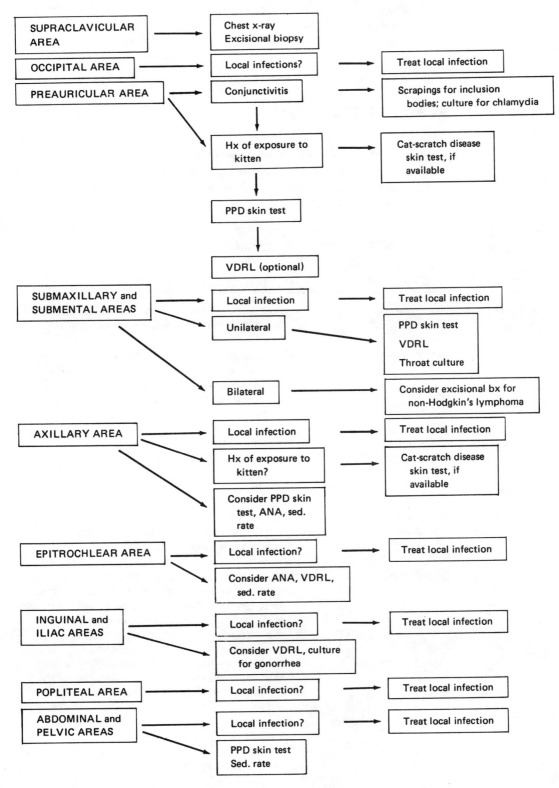

Reference: Bedros, A.A., and Mann, J.P.: Lymphadenopathy in children. Adv. Pediatr., *28:*341, 1981.

THE TESTES—SITUS INVERSUS

Usually the left testis hangs lower in the scrotum than does the right. When both testes are descended and the right testis is lower than the left, always suspect that the patient may have situs inversus.

SCROTAL SWELLING

Although most children with swelling of the scrotum have either a hernia or hydrocele, other conditions must be considered. A thorough history and physical examination can often point to a specific diagnosis prior to or obviating the need for surgical exploration.

Conditions Associated with Scrotal Swelling

CONDITION	CLINICAL CLUES
Hernia, direct	Uncommon, usually does not transilluminate; reducible unless incarcerated; usually tender.
Hernia, indirect	History of intermittent swelling in the inguinal region; fluid sometimes present (therefore, transillumination may be positive); usually tender; reducible unless incarcerated; peristalsis may be audible on auscultation.
Hydrocele	Frequent under 2 years of age; transillumination usually positive; nontender; not reducible; associated testicular enlargement is suggestive of tumor.
Torsion of testis or appendage	Acute onset of pain, followed shortly by swelling and discoloration; elevation of mass *increases* pain; surgical emergency.
Epididymo-orchitis	May be accompanied by signs of urethritis (e.g., dysuria); can be gonococcal in origin; associated fever common; painful; elevation of testis *decreases* pain; torsion can be ruled out only by surgical exploration.
Orchitis (true)	May be history of recent parotid swelling or other clues to mumps or enteroviral infection; painful; elevation of testis decreases pain.
Trauma	History usually positive; hematoma may be seen.
Edema, generalized	History and physical examination will often provide clues to primary process, as well as demonstrate edema of eyelids, sacrum, ankles, or other sites.

Edema, local	Examination may reveal source of local problem (e.g., insect bite or diaper dermatitis characteristic of detergent sensitivity); testis is nontender and normal in size.
Leukemia	Other systemic signs of illness usually present.
Anaphylactoid purpura	Characteristic rash usually present or beginning.
Filariasis	Peripheral eosinophilia.
Testicular tumor	Painless; may have associated hydrocele; sexual precocity or gynecomastia have been associated.
Cyst or angioma	May transilluminate; painless; not reducible; examination may disclose lesions elsewhere.

GYNECOLOGIC EXAMINATION OF THE YOUNG GIRL

The gynecologic examination is often avoided by the examiner and feared by the patient. Here is a method that allows a good view of the cervix and vagina without the use of a frightening instrument. The patient is asked to lie "on her tummy with her bottom in the air." As the buttocks are held apart by an assistant, the child is asked to take some deep breaths. The vaginal orifice falls open. Inspection may then be carried out with an ordinary otoscope head without the speculum. The otoscope provides light and magnification, allowing visualization of the cervix and vagina.

If a better view is required, the otoscope may be used along with a veterinary otoscope speculum. These specula are wider and longer than the human variety, but they fit the standard otoscope head.

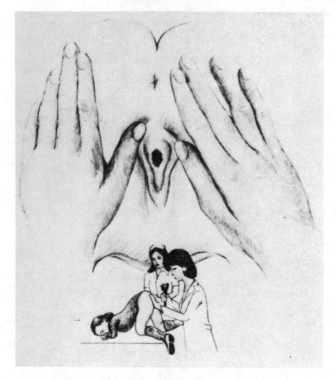

FIG. 1-6

References: Emans, S.J., and Goldstein, D.P.: Pediatrics, 65:758, 1980. Billmire, M.E., Farrell, M.K., and Dine, M.S.: Pediatrics, 65:823, 1980.

Speculum—The term speculum originally meant mirrors of polished metal. Later, when glass mirrors were used, the term was continued for what was called speculum metal of which the mirrors for reflecting telescopes were made.

LOCALIZED EDEMA—A SIGN OF SYSTEMIC DISEASE

Some generalized disorders may produce characteristic localized signs. One such sign is the presence of unusual edema. Listed below are some sites of localized edema and the disease process that should be considered.

Edema of the eyelids	Early finding of both roseola infantum and infectious mononucleosis
Edema of the forehead	Henoch-Schönlein purpura
Edema of the glottis	Angioneurotic edema
Edema of the neck	Diphtheria. Accompanied by lymphadenopathy
Edema over the sternum	Mumps
Edema of the hands and feet in the newborn period	Turner's syndrome Milroy's disease
Edema of the hands and feet in the older infant and child	Sickle cell disease ("hand-foot syndrome"). Edema usually accompanied by warmth and tenderness
Scrotal edema	Early manifestation of Henoch-Schönlein purpura
Pretibial edema	Hypothyroidism

THE BEST OF BARNESS

Despite the introduction of computerized axial tomography, the SMA–12, the bone scan, ultrasonography, and similar technologic advances, the detailed history and careful physical examination still remain the bedrock of the diagnostic process. The text entitled *Manual of Pediatric Physical Diagnosis* by Lewis A. Barness is a testimony to what can be learned by examination of the infant and child. On every page are multiple facts and helpful suggestions to guide you in performing a physical examination. Some of the pointers we like best are excerpted below.

Physical examinations are performed in children by taking full advantage of opportunities as they present themselves. . . . The order of an adequate examination, therefore, is more or less determined by the child rather than the physician.

A rectal examination is done whenever the patient has any symptom referable to the gastrointestinal tract.

Modesty should be respected in a child regardless of age.

The child with paradoxical hyperirritability may lie quietly on the examining table only to scream when picked up by the mother. This is a valuable sign since most children are calmed when picked up, and may indicate a serious disturbance in the central nervous system, particularly meningitis, or pain in motion such as occurs with scurvy, fracture, cortical hyperostosis, or acrodynia; or it may represent a serious disturbance in response to painful stimuli.

A musty or mousy odor is found in children with phenylketonuria or diphtheria.

Slight pulsations of the anterior fontanel occur in normal infants. Marked pulsations, however, may be a sign of increased intracranial pressure, venous sinus thrombosis, obstruction of the venous return from the head, or increased pressure due to an arteriovenous shunt, patent ductus arteriosus, or excitement.

Macewen's sign is one that many examiners like to elicit, but usually it has little significance in childhood. On percussing the skull with one finger, a resonant "cracked-pot" sound is heard. As long as the fontanel is open, this type of sound is physiological. After closure of the fontanel, the sound indicates increased intracranial pressure or a dilated ventricle.

Unilateral paralysis of the face, including the muscles of the forehead and eyelid, indicates a peripheral facial nerve lesion and may be due to trauma, otitis media, or other peripheral lesions. Recovery from the peripheral nerve palsy may occur in the upper portion of the face first, and at this time may resemble a supranuclear weakness.

Pediatrics—Derived from the Greek *pais* or *paido*, which means child, and *iatria*, which means medical treatment.

Children's pupils should react to light quickly. Reaction of the pupil on which the light shines is the direct reaction; of the opposite pupil, consensual reaction. The pupils of newborn infants are constricted until about the third week of age so that light reaction, while always sluggish in an infant with congenital glaucoma, is not a good test of glaucoma in the newborn.

Gray stippling around the optic disc is a sign of lead poisoning.

Unilateral papilledema with contralateral optic atrophy may be due to a frontal lobe tumor, Foster Kennedy syndrome.

A white disc may indicate optic atrophy, as occurs with osteopetrosis causing compression of the nerve, or with neurofibroma of the optic nerve. It also occurs following optic neuritis which affects the nerve far back of the eyeball, as with multiple sclerosis or methyl alcohol poisoning.

Patients with discharge and crusting below or on the edges of the alae nasi, particularly with redness of the surrounding skin, usually have infections with β-hemolytic streptococci.

With circumoral pallor the immediate area around the mouth appears white, while a strip just below the nose, the surface of the checks, and lower chin are red. This appearance may occur with any febrile disease, but is particularly noted in children who have just exercised or who have scarlet or rheumatic fever or hypoglycemia.

A palpatory thud (or audible slap) may be felt or heard over the trachea and may indicate the presence of a foreign body free in the trachea.

Children below the age of 3 years with upper airway obstruction rarely breathe faster than 50 per minute, while those with lower airway obstructive disease, such as bronchiolitis, frequently breathe at rates of 80 to 100.

It is occasionally difficult to distinguish the third heart sound from a gallop rhythm which indicates a failing heart. Occasionally, the three beats of the gallop can be felt on palpation; the third heart sound can never be felt as an impulse.

Free fluid may give one the impression of a non-tense abdomen even though peritonitis is present.

Intra-abdominal tenderness can be distinguished from muscle tenderness by asking the child to raise his head and then palpating. Intra-abdominal tenderness is lessened, while superficial tenderness is increased, by this maneuver.

A thrill over an enlarged liver is found with hydatid echinococcal cysts in the liver; a gurgling sound may be heard in the same area.

Auscultation over the femoral artery may reveal a booming sound or "pistol shot" characteristic of aortic insufficiency or other causes of increased pulse pressure. A double sound is indicative of the same.

Occasionally, a prostate will be palpated as a flat mass several centimeters up and on the midline anterior wall of the rectum. Any prostate felt larger than 1 cm before the age of 10 years may indicate precocious puberty or congenital adrenal hyperplasia.

Spina bifida occulta can occasionally be determined by pressing carefully over the area under suspicion when the trunk is flexed. The spinous processes above and below the spina bifida will feel thin and well formed, while that of the defective vertebra may feel split.

A painful limp, especially in the morning, is usually seen in children with tuberculosis of the hip.

Associated movements, or voluntary movement of one muscle accompanied by involuntary movement of another muscle, may sometimes be noted. These movements are regulated by the cerebellum. They occur as mirror movements in the Klippel-Feil syndrome, in diseases with increased intracranial pressure, and in patients whose handedness has been changed. Reciprocal movements occur normally in infants 2 to 4 months of age and usually decrease by 4 to 6 months; failure of these movements to appear or disappear at the proper times is an indication of brain damage.

A "reverse" Moro reflex consists of extending and externally rotating the arms, with rigidity following the usual stimulus. Such a reflex is seen in children over 5 days of age who have basal ganglia disease, including kernicterus of erythroblastosis fetalis.

Sweating is rare in the newborn, but may be present in babies with brain cortex irritation, anomalies or injuries of the sympathetic nervous system, or in babies whose mothers were morphine addicts.

Reference: Barness, L.A.: Manual of Pediatric Physical Diagnosis. 4th Ed. Chicago, Year Book Medical Publishers, 1972.

SYMPTOMS OF IMPORTANCE— ILLINGWORTH'S BAKER'S DOZEN

Failure to take note of these may have disastrous results.

1. Jaundice on the first day of life.
2. Vomitus containing bile in the newborn period, or vomiting with abdominal distention.
3. Vomitus containing streaks of blood in a baby, because it suggests hiatus hernia or reflux, and calls for investigation.
4. Diarrhea in any infant or young child, because of the rapidity with which dehydration may occur.
5. Stridor of acute onset.
6. Cough of really sudden onset, without an upper respiratory infection, because it suggests an inhaled foreign body.
7. Ear pain, because if it is due to otitis media, it requires immediate antibiotic treatment (and not drops in the ear).
8. Neck stiffness (in flexion), because it may signify meningitis.
9. Fits with fever, because although febrile convulsions are the most likely diagnosis, they may be due to pyogenic meningitis. Hence a lumbar puncture must be performed.
10. The onset of drowsiness with an infection, because it may represent pyogenic meningitis.

11. Loss of weight.

12. A severe attack of asthma, not responding to the usual treatment, because it may be fatal. A child with such an attack should be sent to the hospital.

13. Poisoning of any kind, because hospital investigation and treatment are needed. The dangerous latent period, between the time of ingestion of the poison and the onset of symptoms, is a particular hazard.

Reference: Illingworth, R.S.: Common Symptoms of Disease in Children. 3rd Ed. Oxford, Blackwell Scientific Publications, 1971, p. 309.

THE VULNERABLE CHILD SYNDROME

Parents of a child who was expected to die, or parents of an only child, or parents who have experienced the death of a child often react in a manner that produces a disturbance in the psychosexual development of their offspring. Learn to recognize the circumstances that produce "the vulnerable child" syndrome and its manifestations. The psychosexual disturbance manifests itself most commonly in the following ways:

1. *Difficulty with separation.* Child may be briefly entrusted to the care of grandparents, but baby sitters are rarely used. In extreme instances, mother and child never separate. Sleep problems are common. The child frequently sleeps with parents or in parents' room. Mother or father wakes frequently during the night to check on the status of the child.

2. *Infantilization.* Parents are unable to set disciplinary limits. Parent is overprotective, overindulgent, and oversolicitous. Child is overly dependent, disobedient, irritable, argumentative, and uncooperative. Children may be physically abusive to parents. Feeding problems are common.

3. *Bodily overconcerns.* Hypochondriacal complaints, recurrent abdominal pain, headaches, and infantile fears are prominent. School absence is common. Mothers express concern about minor respiratory infections, stool habits, "poor color," circles under the eyes, and blueness when crying.

4. *School underachievement.* Unspoken agreement that the child is only safe with mother may produce separation anxiety that results in poor school performance.

Predisposing Factors in the Production of the Vulnerable Child

1. Child is first-born to older parents who had resigned themselves to being childless.

2. Parents cannot have additional children as a result of a hysterectomy or other sterilization procedure.

3. The patient was born with a congenital anomaly.

4. The patient was born prematurely.

5. The patient has an acquired handicap, e.g., epilepsy.

6. The child has had a truly life-threatening illness, such as erythroblastosis, nephrosis, or severe asthma.

7. During pregnancy the mother was told that the fetus might die.

8. Mother had a postpartum depression.

9. Mother has ambivalent feelings about child, such as instances where child was born out of wedlock.

10. Parents have unresolved grief reaction as a result of loss of another child.

11. A hereditary disorder is present in the family, such as cystic fibrosis or muscular dystrophy.

12. There is a psychological need on the part of the parents to find something physically wrong with the child in order to displace unacceptable feelings about the patient. Child is frequently brought to physicians because of parents' suspicion of leukemia, brain tumor, rheumatic fever, or other serious illness.

Treatment

1. Recognize the circumstances that may produce a vulnerable child and try to reassure parents about the health of the infant or child before symptoms appear.

2. Make authoritative statements about the child's well-being based on a thoughtful, cumulative history, physical examination, and pertinent measurements and laboratory findings.

3. Point out to the parents and get them to accept the reasons for their unnecessary concern, the child's responsive behavior, and the mutual reinforcement that is present.

Do not produce the syndrome yourself with comments such as "I thought for sure he was going to die," or "If she hadn't gotten here when she did we wouldn't have been able to save her," or "You are very lucky parents that we saved your child."

Reference: Green, M., and Solnit, A.J.: Pediatrics, *34*:58, 1964.

"All the little ones of our time are collectively the children of us adults of the time, and entitled to our general care."

Thomas Hardy

THE CHRONIC OR RECURRENT HEADACHE

The chronic, or recurrent, headache always produces concern in parents, as well as in older children and adolescents. All fear that the headache signifies the presence of a brain tumor. Obviously, most recurrent headaches in older children and adolescents are not caused by brain tumors but are usually a result of stress and tension. Equally obvious is the fact that a serious disorder may be present; an orderly approach to the problem is required to allay the concerns of the patient and family, as well as your own.

As a general rule, most headaches in children under the age of 4 to 5 years have an organic basis, while headaches in children over 5 do not.

The location of the headache and its associated signs and symptoms provide important clues as to the cause.

LOCATION

Frontal

Frontal sinusitis; may be unilateral or bilateral. Pain on palpation of frontal sinuses may be present. Often exhibits a diurnal pattern.

Tumor of cerebral origin; may be unilateral or bilateral. Generally worse after a period of recumbency. May be associated with vomiting.

Ethmoid sinusitis; pain may be referred to area over the eyes.

Migraine; generally unilateral; may be seen during the first 4 years of life; cyclic vomiting prominent feature in young child; attacks more common in the morning or may awake patient from sleep; scotomas occur more commonly in older child; transient loss of vision may be reported; photophobia; unilateral neurologic deficit of transient nature. Family history of other affected individuals.

Hypertension; headache commonly reported as throbbing; may be associated with epistaxis.

Ocular disturbances.

Occipital and suboccipital

Cerebellar tumors; may be accompanied by frontal pain as well. Head tilting may be present; periodic vomiting.

Sphenoid sinusitis.

Tension. On examination, pain and tenderness may be present in muscles at base of skull and neck. Usually accompanied by a "feeling of pressure." Worse at end of day; does not cause arousal from sleep. May be a history of similar headaches in other family members. Patients may have a long history of nonspecific abdominal pain or other gastrointestinal complaints.

Many diseases have an increased incidence of intracerebral complications that may produce headaches. Some of these disorders include:

Cyanotic heart disease	Cerebral abscess; cerebral vessel occlusion.
Sickle cell anemia	Large vessel occlusion; small vessel hemorrhage.
Neurofibromatosis	Meningiomas and other intracranial tumors.
Hemophilia	Cerebral hemorrhage.
Leukemia	Meningeal or cerebral infiltrates.
Sturge-Weber syndrome	Cerebral hemorrhage

The diagnostic process should include:

A detailed history of nature of headaches; life stresses and history of other family members. Always ask about *pica* in younger children.

A blood pressure measurement.

An examination of the eye grounds.

A complete neurologic examination.

Palpation of the skull; auscultation of the skull for bruits.

Examination of the teeth as a source of infection.

Palpation and transillumination of the sinuses.

Urinalysis.

If history or neurologic examination suggests the presence of intracranial disease, then additional diagnostic procedures to consider would include skull films, electroencephalogram, brain scan, CT scan, and lumbar puncture.

CHILD ABUSE—CLUES TO DIAGNOSIS

When a child is thought to be abused, the index of suspicion may be increased or diminished by recalling a few pertinent facts concerning child abuse. A constellation of findings is often present which provides clues to the diagnosis. These findings refer to the abused child, the abusive parent, and the family dynamics.

A. The Abused Child
   1. Average age: under 4 years, most under 2.
   2. Average death rate: 5% to 25%. (Regional figures: highest reported rates from California, New York City; substantiated, 5.4%; unsubstantiated, 17%.)
   3. Average age at death: slightly under 3 years.
   4. Average duration of exposure to battering: 1 to 3 years.
   5. Sex differentiation: none.

B. The Abusive Parent
   1. Marital status: overwhelming majority of parents were married and living together at the time of the abuse.
   2. Average age of abusive mother: 26 years.
   3. Average age of abusive father: 30 years.
   4. Abusive parent: father slightly more often than mother.
   5. Most serious abuse: mother more often than father.
   6. Most common instrument for abuse: hairbrush.

C. Family Dynamics
   1. Thirty to 60 per cent of abusing parents claim to have been abused as children themselves.
   2. High proportion of premarital conception.
   3. Youthful marriages.
   4. Unwanted pregnancies.
   5. Illegitimacies.

6. Forced marriages.
7. Social and kinship isolation.
8. Emotional problems in marriage.
9. Financial difficulty.

The pertinent history, physical findings, and radiologic signs may be seen in the following table:

HISTORY
1. Parents often relate story that is at variance with clinical findings.
2. Multiple visits to various hospitals.
3. Familial discord or financial stress, alcoholism, psychosis, perversion, drug addiction, etc.
4. Reluctance of parents to give information.
5. Admittance to hospital during evening hours.
6. Child brought to hospital for complaint other than one associated with abuse and/or neglect, e.g., cold, headache, stomach ache, etc.
7. Date of injury prior to admission.
8. Parent's inappropriate reaction to severity of injury.
9. Inconsistent social histories.

PHYSICAL EXAMINATION
1. Signs of general neglect, poor skin hygiene, malnutrition, withdrawal, irritability, repressed personality.
2. Bruises, abrasions, burns, soft tissue swellings, hematomas, old healed lesions.
3. Evidence of dislocation and/or fractures of the extremities.
4. Coma, convulsions, death.
5. Symptoms of drug withdrawal.

DIFFERENTIAL DIAGNOSIS
1. Scurvy and rickets.
2. Infantile cortical hyperostosis.
3. Syphilis of infancy.
4. Accidental trauma.

RADIOLOGIC MANIFESTATIONS
1. Subperiosteal hemorrhages.
2. Epiphyseal separations.
3. Periosteal shearing.
4. Metaphyseal fragmentation.
5. Previously healed periosteal calcifications.
6. "Squaring" of the metaphysis.

Reference: Helfer, R.: Pediatrics Basics, *4*:11, 1975.

THE FAINTING CHILD

Causes of syncope are multiple. The etiology may frequently be suspected from an accurate history. Historical details of importance include:

1. The circumstances under which the syncope occurred.
2. Possible precipitating factors.
3. Prodromal symptoms and signs.
4. Suddenness of onset.
5. Duration.
6. Occurrence of convulsive movements.

If history alone is not sufficient to provide an etiology, laboratory tests may be helpful. The following is a list of causes of syncope along with the characteristics of each.

CAUSE	CHARACTERISTICS
Vasomotor	Due to a sudden drop in blood pressure. Frequently first noted during adolescence. Syncope may be precipitated by fear, sight of blood, pain, or other unpleasant stimulus. It is most likely to occur after fasting, in hot rooms, and after prolonged standing. Attacks are preceded by feelings of nausea, weakness, pallor, and sweating. No specific treatment is indicated, but the child should be instructed to sit or lie down to abort the attacks. It may also be helpful to explore with the child the cause for anxiety.
Hysterical	Such episodes are most common in adolescent girls and are thought to be an expression of unconscious, repressed, instinctive impulses. The episodes are not preceded by symptoms such as nausea, weakness, pallor, or sweating. The patient does not seem anxious. Moaning may be noted during the attack. Treatment consists of psychiatric exploration of the unconscious conflict.
Epilepsy	Seizures are unlikely to be mistaken for syncope; however, if epilepsy is considered, EEG and metabolic studies may be helpful.
Cardiac	Syncope may be the first manifestation of isolated pulmonic stenosis, primary hypertension, congenital or acquired heart block, or arrhythmia. Severe aortic stenosis and cyanotic heart disease (e.g., tetrology of Fallot) may also be associated with syncope. Syncope and sudden death have also been described in children with a prolonged Q-T interval on the EEG. Some of these children also have congenital deafness.

Respiratory	Syncope may occur in children with hypoxic episodes secondary to respiratory disease (e.g., asthma). Syncope may also follow severe episodes of coughing.
Anemia	Syncope due to anemia is often preceded by a light-headed feeling and giddiness.
Hyperventilation	Generalized weakness, tingling, and numbness of the hands, and possibly tetany may precede syncope due to hyperventilation. The patient may not refer to the over-breathing but may describe a sensation of smothering or choking. It may be helpful to duplicate the patient's symptoms by having him or her hyperventilate in the office and to abort the symptoms using a rebreathing bag. Treatment includes investigation with the patient of the stresses or anxieties that precipitate the episodes.
Hypoglycemia	The history should include occurrence of pallor and sweating prior to syncope. The relationship of syncopal episodes to meals is important.
Breath-holding	This occurs during the late first to early second year of life. It is triggered by injury, anger, or frustration. The child cries, gasps, holds his or her breath, turns blue or pale, and becomes unconscious or limp. Convulsions may occur. Differentiation from epilepsy may require an EEG and further observation. The only treatment required is parental reassurance.
Fused cervical vertebrae	The cause of syncope in these patients is unknown.

Reference: Green, M.: Fainting. *In* Green, M. and Haggerty, R. J. (Eds.): Ambulatory Pediatrics II. Philadelphia, W. B. Saunders Company, 1977.

2
NUTRITION

GUIDELINES FOR FEEDING NORMAL INFANTS

Although there are many ways to approach feeding in the infant who is not being breast fed, this approach suggested by the Committee on the Fetus and Newborn of the American Academy of Pediatrics is worth following.

BIRTH WEIGHT (gm)	AGE FOR FIRST GLUCOSE WATER OR WATER FEEDING (hr)	FIRST FORMULA FEEDING Age (hr)	Cal/oz	ml/kg	Frequency	SUBSEQUENT FEEDING Age When Given 20 Cal/oz (hr)	Incremental Increase in Volume per Feeding	ml/kg per Feeding	Age When Receiving 100–120 cal/kg/day
1500	6–14	8–16	10–14	1–4	every 2 hours	48	1 ml/kg every 3rd to 4th feeding	12–15	7 days
1501– 2000	3–9	6–12	10–14	5–7	every 3 hours	24– 36	1 ml/kg every 2nd feeding	18–22	5 days
2001– 2500	2–6	6–10	20	8	every 4 hours	from first feeding	2 ml/kg every feeding	25–30	2 days

Reference: Standards and Recommendations for Hospital Care of Newborn Infants, 6th edition. American Academy of Pediatrics, 1977.

"Whatsoever was the father of a disease, an ill diet was the mother."

FEEDING THE INFANT WITH FAILURE TO THRIVE

When writing diet orders for the infant who is underweight it is important to specify the minimum number of calories you wish the infant to receive and to specify their source.

Guidelines

1. Infants under 6 months of age can receive all their calories from a proprietary milk formula.
2. Infants 6 months to 1 year can receive 66 per cent of their calories from the formula and the remainder from solid foods.
3. Aim to feed 120 cal/kg of idealized weight. The idealized weight is the infant's weight for length or the 50th percentile for weight of an infant of the same age (select the larger of the two).
4. Approximately 80 cal/kg will be required for maintenance. Each 5 to 7 cal/kg above this level should produce a weight gain of 1 gm/kg/day.

Example. Infant weighs 5 kg (idealized weight is 6 kg). Child receives 720 cal/day. Infant should gain about 7 to 8 gm/kg/day or a total of 35 to 40 gm.

The Menu

Keep it simple; specify what he eats and when. Use the following facts to make up the diet.

Proprietary milks	67 cal/100 ml
Infant cereals	370 cal/100 gm dry weight
Mixed grains	(this is 2.5 cups of cereal)
Rice	
Barley	
Juices	
Apple juice	47 cal/100 ml
Orange juice	49 cal/100 ml
Vegetables	
Beets	40 cal/jar or about 7 to 8 tbsp
Carrots	30 cal/jar
Green beans	35 cal/jar
Peas	60 cal/jar
Sweet potatoes	90 cal/jar

2

Fruits
    Applesauce   60 cal/jar
    Peaches   110 cal/jar
    Banana with custard   100 cal/jar
    Pears   60 cal/jar

Meats
    Beef with vegetables   100 cal/jar
    Chicken with vegetables   100 cal/jar
    Turkey with vegetables   120 cal/jar
    Veal with vegetables   90 cal/jar

Desserts
    Chocolate custard   130 cal/jar
    Orange pudding   120 cal/jar

With this information you can compile your own calorie count each day if the nurses have been requested to record carefully the infant's intake. See how it matches up with the calories counted by the dietician.

Always prepare a flow sheet on the chart, with caloric intakes recorded along with weight gain and unusual stooling.

All these infants should receive vitamin supplements (A, C, D) if they are not receiving a full quart of a vitamin-enriched proprietary formula.

CLASSIFICATION OF NUTRITIONAL STATUS

> *Marasmus*—From the Greek word *marasmos*, which means wasting or withering.

Is your patient obese, or merely overweight? Conversely, is your patient mildly or severely malnourished? Figure 2–1 depicted below serves as a convenient and simple means of accurately classifying the nutritional status of patients under 5 years of age.

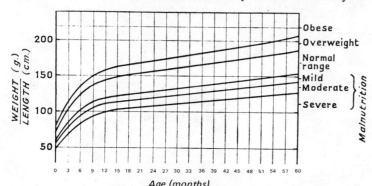

FIG. 2–1

To determine the nutritional status of a subject at a given age, the weight in grams is divided by the length in centimeters, and a mark is placed on the graph where the quotient coincides with the appropriate vertical age lines.

Reference: McLaren, D.S., and Read, W.C.: Lancet, *2*:219, 1975.

CALORIC EXPENDITURES IN INFANCY

How does the infant spend the energy that he derives from his caloric intake? As the infant grows, more is consumed by activity and less is required for growth.

Calorie Intake and Usage by Infant Boys

WEIGHT (kg)	INTAKE (kcal/kg)	USAGE (kcal/kg)			
		Basal Metabolism	Growth	Activity	Stool Losses
3	120	46	56	8	10
4	120	50	53	8	10
5	118	54	46	8	10
6	114	56	38	10	10
8	106	56	28	12	10
10	98	54	22	13	9

Reference: Holt, L.E., and Fales, H.L.: Am. J. Dis. Child., *21*:1, 1921.

INFANT FOODS—
CALORIES AND THEIR DISTRIBUTION

When you begin to add strained foods or junior foods to the infant's diet, you should be aware of the number of calories you are providing and where they are coming from. The table below provides estimates derived from analysis of a variety of products in each category.

Strained Foods

CATEGORY	KCAL/100 GM	PERCENTAGE OF CALORIES		
		Protein	Fat	Carbohydrates
Juices	65 (45–98)	2	2	96
Fruits	85 (79–125)	2	2	96
Vegetables				
Plain	45 (27–28)	14	6	80
Creamed	63 (42–94)	13	13	74
Meats	106 (86–194)	53	46	1
Egg yolks	192 (184–199)	21	76	3
High meat dinner	84 (63–106)	29	45	29
Desserts	96 (71–136)	4	7	89
Cereal	360 (349–393)	39	12	49
Cereal-fruit	85 (76–98)	18	6	76

Junior Foods

Fruits	85 (69–116)	2	2	96
Vegetables				
Plain	46 (27–71)	12	7	81
Creamed	64 (45–72)	13	17	70
Meats	103 (88–135)	56	43	1
Soup-dinner	61 (39–100)	15	27	58

Reference: Fomon, S.J.: Infant Nutrition. 2nd Ed. Philadelphia, W.B. Saunders Company, 1974, p. 410.

"It is through the idealism of youth that man catches sight of truth, and in that idealism he possesses a wealth which he must never exchange for anything else."

Albert Schweitzer

SIMPLIFIED PREDICTION OF RENAL SOLUTE LOAD

On occasion, it is important to know if the urine osmolality is appropriate for the infant on a particular diet.

A simple estimate of renal solute load may be based on dietary intake of nitrogen and of three minerals: sodium, potassium, and chloride. Each gram of dietary protein can be considered to yield 4 milliosmols of renal solute load (assumed to be all urea), and each milliequivalent of sodium, potassium, and chloride is assumed to contribute 1 milliosmol.

Estimated renal solute load from various feedings is listed in the table below.

Dietary Intake of Protein, Sodium, Chloride, and Potassium, and Estimated Renal Solute Load from Various Feedings

FEEDINGS (1000 ML)	DIETARY INTAKE				ESTIMATED RENAL SOLUTE LOAD		
	Protein (gm)	*Na (mEq)*	*Cl (mEq)*	*K (mEq)*	*Urea (mosm)*	*Na + K + Cl (mosm)*	*Total mosm*
Whole cow milk	33	25	29	35	132	89	221
Human milk	12	7	11	13	48	31	79
Boiled skim milk	46	35	40	49	184	124	308
Similac (20 kcal/oz)	15.5	11	17	19	62	47	109
Isomil (20 kcal/oz)	20	13	15	18	80	46	126

The estimated renal solute load and minimum urinary osmolality of a hypothetical 6 kg infant from various feedings are analyzed below.

Estimated Renal Solute Load and Minimum Urinary Osmolality of a Hypothetical 6 kG Infant from Various Feedings

FEEDING	ESTIMATED RENAL SOLUTE LOAD	OSMOLALITY OF 730 ML URINE
Whole cow milk	221 mosm	303 mosm/liter
Human milk	79 mosm	108 mosm/liter
Boiled skim milk	308 mosm	422 mosm/liter
Similac (20 kcal/oz)	109 mosm	149 mosm/liter
Isomil (20 kcal/oz)	126 mosm	172 mosm/liter

Reference: Ziegler, E.E., and Fomon, S.J.: J. Pediatr., *78*:561, 1971.

NONDAIRY FOODS RICH IN CALCIUM

Suppose you cared for a lactase-deficient child who required a high dietary calcium intake. What sorts of calcium-rich foods could you use rather than resorting to medicinal calcium supplements? A few examples of other-than-cow in origin calcium are as follows:

	CALCIUM: mg PER AVERAGE SERVING
Cereals	
Barley cereal, Gerbers, 1 cup	231
Oatmeal, ¾ cup	153
Pablum barley cereal, ¾ cup, cooked	2210
Pablum cereal, mixed, ¾ cup, cooked	2210
Cereal Flours	
Cornmeal, whole grain, 1 cup	354
Soy flour, low-fat, 1 cup	263
Wheat flour, self-rising, enriched, 1 cup	303
Fish	
Herring, canned, solids and liquids, 3½ oz	147
Mackerel, canned, 3½ oz	260
Sardines, Atlantic, canned in oil, 3½ oz	354
Smelt, Atlantic, canned, 3½ oz	358
Fruits	
Figs, dried, 3½ oz	126
Oranges, 1 large	96
Nuts	
Almonds, unblanched, 3½ oz	254
Brazil nuts, 3½ oz	186
Legumes and Seeds	
Soybean curd (Tofu), 4 oz	154
Beans, common, dried, ½ cup	144
Garbanzo beans, dried, ½ cup	150
Sunflower seed kernels, 3½ oz	120
Syrups and Sugars	
Molasses, cane, third extraction, blackstrap, 3½ oz	579
Maple sugar, 3½ oz	180
Vegetables	
Broccoli, cooked, 1 cup	132
Spoon cabbage, raw, 3½ oz	165
Collards, cooked, ½ cup	152
Dandelion greens, cooked, ½ cup	140
Lamb's-quarters, cooked, ½ cup	258

Reference: Hodges, R.E.: Nutrition in pregnancy and lactation. *In* Hodges, R.E. (ed.): Nutrition in Medical Practice. Philadelphia, W.B. Saunders Company, 1980, p. 55.

DIETARY SOURCES OF IRON FOR OLDER CHILDREN

Sometimes it is helpful to know which food sources are high in iron content when planning the diet of older children. Such food sources may be useful in the prevention of iron deficiency. On the other hand, it may be advisable for some patients to avoid these foods, such as those who are iron overloaded, e.g., subjects with thalassemia major. The four highest iron-containing foods per serving are: clams (4.2 mg Fe/2 oz), beef kidney (4.7 mg Fe/2 oz), raw oysters (3.4 mg/2 oz), and beef liver (4.7 mg Fe/2 oz.). The highest iron-containing foods expressed per 100 gm dry weight are cocoa powder (11.6 mg Fe), soybean flour (13 mg Fe), and brewer's yeast (18.2 mg Fe). If you mix the latter three together with water, then drink the mixture, you won't need a fuse to observe the detonation.

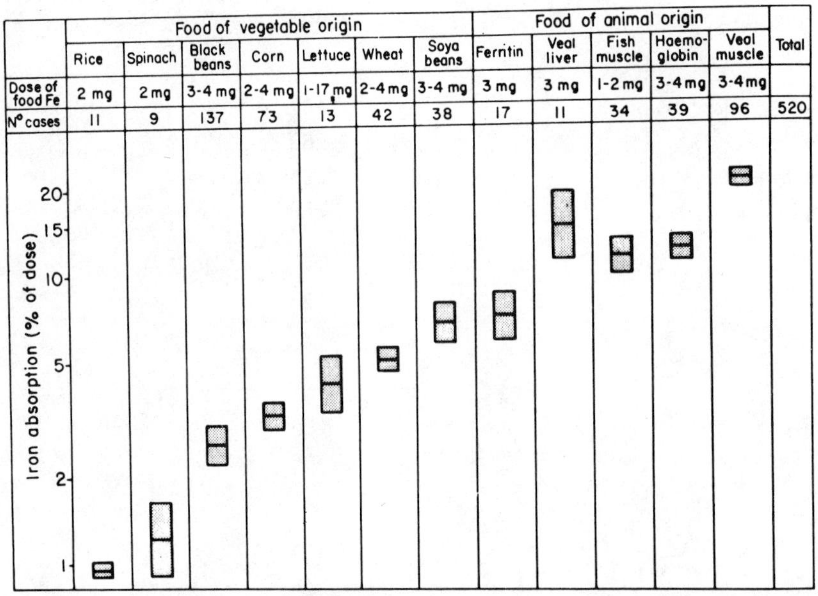

	Food of vegetable origin							Food of animal origin					Total
	Rice	Spinach	Black beans	Corn	Lettuce	Wheat	Soya beans	Ferritin	Veal liver	Fish muscle	Haemo-globin	Veal muscle	
Dose of food Fe	2 mg	2 mg	3-4 mg	2-4 mg	1-17 mg	2-4 mg	3-4 mg	3 mg	3 mg	1-2 mg	3-4 mg	3-4 mg	
N° cases	11	9	137	73	13	42	38	17	11	34	39	96	520

FIG. 2–2

Iron absorption from biosynthetically labeled food. Collaborative study of the Departments of Botany and Medicine, University of Washington at Seattle, U.S.A., and the Department of Pathophysiology, Instituto Venezolano de Investigaciones Cientificas, Caracas, Venezuela. The thick horizontal line represents the geometrical mean, and the cross-hatched area shows the limits of one standard error. (From WHO Tech. Rep. Ser., #503, 1972.)

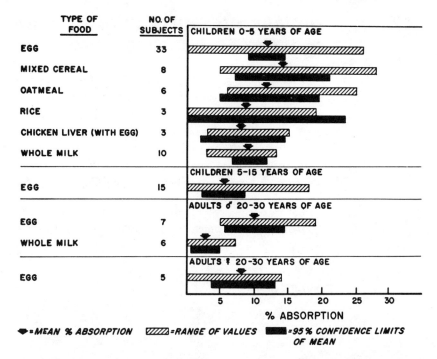

FIG. 2-3

Summary, to date, of studies of Fe^{59} absorption. The mean values in most groups of experiments are between 8 and 12 per cent absorption.

Excellent Dietary Sources of Iron

Liver
Oysters and other shellfish
Kidney
Heart
Lean meat
Dried peas and beans
Dried fruits
Dark molasses
Whole grain bread and cereals
Nuts
Certain fruits (apricots, prunes, peaches, raisins)

Tongue
Leafy green vegetables
Egg yolks
Meats in general

Reference: Mayo Clinic Diet Manual, 3rd ed. Philadelphia, W.B. Saunders Company, 1961, pp. 188–189.

POTASSIUM CONTENT OF COMMONLY INGESTED BEVERAGES AND VEGETABLES

We all know that patients on certain diuretics require a high potassium diet. But do you know whether prune juice or orange juice has more potassium per ounce? Can you state whether drip coffee, instant coffee, or cocoa has the most potassium? For the appropriate answers consult the following list.

FRUITS AND VEGETABLES WITH HIGH POTASSIUM CONTENT

Bananas, watermelons, cantaloupes, oranges, apricots, tomatoes, dried fruits (raisins, prunes, dates, figs), potatoes, broccoli, spinach

POTASSIUM CONTENT OF BEVERAGES

Per 8-oz Serving	K mEq
Prune juice	16.0
Tomato juice	14.2
Skim milk (fortified)	12.3
Cocoa	10.5
Orange juice	11.7
Grapefruit juice	9.2
Whole milk	8.6
Pineapple juice	8.6
Grape juice	7.4
Apple cider	6.1
Instant coffee	6.1
Drip coffee	4.9
Coca-Cola	3.2
Pepsi-Cola	0.2
Koolade	0

Reference: Adelman, R.D., and Hodges, R.E.: Nutrition and the kidney. *In* Hodges, R.E. (ed.): Nutrition in Medical Practice. Philadelphia, W.B. Saunders Company, 1980, p. 236.

DOCTOR, MY CHILD WON'T EAT

Everyone responsible for the care of children has heard this complaint from some anxious mother. Infants and children in this country will not voluntarily starve themselves. Most parents do not appreciate the fact that the child between 1 and 5 years of age is only gaining weight at the rate of about 2 kg per year and is not normally a large eater or an eater of three large meals per day. Meal time should be a pleasant time for both parents and children and not a test of wits or willpower.

Dr. Jay Arena, a pediatrician with both knowledge and experience, offers the following suggestions to pass on to parents when the complaint is, "Doctor, my child won't eat."

2

1. A quart of milk a day is great for the milk industry but not necessarily so for your child. One pint of milk (6 oz at each meal) is sufficient. Too much milk fills the stomach, dulls the appetite, and leaves little room for other important foods.

2. Serve small, attractive portions, emphasizing meat, eggs, and cheese. Don't expect him to eat all of each food served, even though you have strong feelings that it is "not enough to keep a bird alive."

3. Serve raw vegetables; many children prefer them to cooked vegetables.

4. Don't allow him to refuse what has been placed before him and then expect something different prepared for him alone, such as a bowl of fruit or cereal to sustain him through the night or until the next meal.

5. Thirty minutes is time enough; end the meal bravely and without emotion.

6. Don't use dessert as a bribe or reward for eating. If a dessert is part of his planned meal, don't insist that he clean up his plate or eat his other foods first.

7. Removing the tonsils is absolutely no guarantee that appetite will improve.

8. Vitamin supplements do not take the place of food; give no more than the recommended dose of polyvitamin supplement prescribed.

Reference: Arena, J.: Pediatric News, October, 1977, p. 18.

THE CREAMATOCRIT

Now that more mothers are breast-feeding their infants, every now and then a question arises about the caloric adequacy of a milk sample. A simple technique has been devised to provide a reasonable approximation of the caloric content of human milk. It takes advantage of the fact that fat is the major determinant of the energy value of the milk sample.

A sample of human milk is placed in a hematocrit tube and spun in a microcentrifuge at full speed for 15 minutes. The fat rises to the top of the column. The cream layer, easily visible, is read from the hematocrit capillary tube, and, like a hematocrit, is expressed as a percentage of the milk column in the tube. This is the "creamatocrit."

This number can then be employed in a formula which will provide you with the energy content of the milk expressed as kcal per liter. The formula is:

$$kcal/liter = 290 + 66.8 \times creamatocrit$$

For example: A human milk sample is found to have a creamatocrit of 5%. Its caloric value is:

$$290 + 66.8 \times 5$$

or

625 calories per liter.

Note: Creamatocrits should be read within one hour of centrifugation, because after that time the cream column begins to "unpack," and falsely elevated values are obtained.

Reference: Lucas, A., Gibbs, J.A.H., Lyster, R.L.J., et al.: Brit. Med. J., *1*:1018, 1978.

FEEDING THE LACTATING MOTHER

Breast-feeding increases the mother's nutritional requirements. You should be aware of these requirements so that you can assist her in planning her meals. Listed below are some guidelines designed to help all three of you — mother, baby, and doctor.

How Lactation Increases the Recommended Daily Dietary Allowances*
(Nursing mothers 18–50 years of age)

DIETARY INTAKE	DAILY INCREASE RECOMMENDED WHEN BREAST-FEEDING	SUGGESTED FOOD SOURCES FOR MEETING THESE INCREASED AMOUNTS
Energy (kcal)	500	All foods
Protein (gm)	20	Meats, fish, milk, cheese, eggs, beans
Calcium (mg)	400	Milk, egg yolk, tuna fish, salmon, cheese
Phosphorus (mg)	400	Milk, fish, beef, whole grains
Iodine (mcg)	50	Seafoods, oysters, shrimp, iodized salt
Magnesium (mg)	150	Beef, enriched bread, whole grains, deep green leafy vegetables
Zinc (mg)	10	Liver, oranges, strawberries, whole grains, deep green leafy vegetables
Vitamin A (I.U.)	2000	Milk, eggs, liver, butter, margarine, deep green leafy vegetables, yellow fruits and vegetables
Vitamin E (I.U.)	3.0	Vegetable oils, whole grains, cabbage
Vitamin C (mg)	35	Citrus fruits, deep green leafy vegetables, green peppers
Folacin (mg)	0.2	Liver, deep green leafy vegetables
Niacin (mg)	4.0	Beef, liver, whole grain, eggs, enriched bread
Vitamin B_1 (mg)	0.3	Pork, chicken, fish, liver, milk, enriched bread
Vitamin B_2 (mg)	0.5	Beef, milk, liver, deep green leafy vegetables, enriched bread
Vitamin B_6 (mg)	0.5	Beef, peas, whole grains, deep green leafy vegetables
Vitamin B_{12} (mcg)	1.0	Milk, beef, liver, salt-water fish, oysters

*National Research Council: Recommended Dietary Allowances, 8th ed. Washington, D.C., National Academy of Sciences, 1974.

EFFECT OF BREAST-FEEDING ON THE SIZE OF THE BREAST

A great deal of both mythology and misinformation concerns the cosmetic consequences of breast-feeding. Textbooks make categorical statements that suggest that breast-feeding has no ultimate effect on the size of the breast. If one asks women who have been pregnant, a different impression emerges. The following conclusions were obtained from a survey of 750 women.

GROUP	PERCENTAGE REPORTING CHANGE 6 MONTHS AFTER DELIVERY OR TERMINATION OF NURSING
Non–breast-feeding	27.9
Breast-feeding, 0–2 weeks	26.3
Breast-feeding, 2–6 weeks	27.0
Breast-feeding, 6 weeks–6 months	48.7
Breast-feeding, more than 6 months	48.4

Type of Changes

Non-breast-feeders or those breast-feeding for less than 2 weeks and noting a change:

Increase in breast size	60 per cent
Decrease in breast size	24 per cent
No change in size, less tone	16 per cent

Breast-feeding for more than 2 weeks and noting a change:

Increase in breast size	14 per cent
Decrease in breast size	50 per cent
No change in size, less tone	36 per cent

Only three women among the group noting a change in breast size following breast-feeding did not feed their subsequent children. All felt the cosmetic consequences were of little significance when contrasted with the psychological and nutritional benefits of nursing.

Reference: Oski, F.A.: Program, American Pediatric Society, 1968, p. 58.

HOW TO ENCOURAGE BREAST-FEEDING

Although most physicians, as well as many potential mothers, recognize the physiologic, immunologic, and psychologic virtues of human milk feeding, these alone appear to be insufficient to motivate the physician to encourage, and the mother to accept, breast-feeding.

There are several ways to remedy this situation. The physician should familiarize himself with the scientific facts about breast-feeding and then try to employ the following procedures.

Prenatally

1. Plan to meet and discuss the decision about breast-feeding with the expectant mother.

2. Do not say that it is "very easy and natural" or that it is "very hard and fraught with difficulties." The highly motivated, goal-oriented woman will be discouraged by the first approach, while the anxious mother will be dismayed by the second approach. State that it has a "reasonable probability of success."

3. Allow the expectant mother to meet and discuss breast-feeding with other women who have breast-fed their children, or provide her with an opportunity to witness mothers feeding their children. The incidence of successful breast-feeding is much higher among women who have had friends or relatives who have breast-fed their infants.

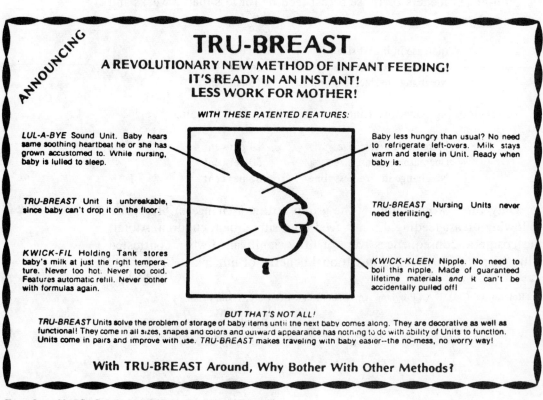

From Inter-NAPSAC, P.O. Box 267, Marble Hill, MO 63764.

FIG. 2-4

2

4. Explain prenatal breast care. Avoid soap on the nipples. The nipples may be prepared by briskly rubbing with a Turkish towel. Other excellent preparatory techniques include:

    a. Exposing the breasts to room air as much as possible.

    b. Allowing the nipples to rub against the clothing by going braless periodically.

    c. Exposing breasts to ultraviolet rays. Sun-bathing or a sun lamp are both suitable. Start slowly — avoid burns.

    d. Have breasts stimulated manually or orally. Employ nipple rolling several times per day. This is accomplished by taking nipple between thumb and forefinger and pulling it out firmly — just enough so that it can be felt but not enough so that it really hurts.

5. Explain that the criterion of adequate breast-feeding is weight gain by the infant. Excessive crying or frequent feeding does not indicate that her milk supply is inadequate or that the quality is poor.

Postnatally

1. Avoid sedation of the mother during labor. Oversedation of the mother will produce a sleepy infant with a decreased capacity for vigorous sucking during the first several days of life.

2. Place the baby to the mother's breast as soon after birth as possible. Optimally, this should be done within the first hour of life.

3. Encourage rooming-in. Try to pair the new mother with another woman who is breast-feeding.

4. If rooming-in is not possible, or desired, place the baby on a "demand" feeding schedule. If the baby is allowed to cry excessively before being brought to his mother, he will be exhausted. If he is brought while asleep, sucking may be unsatisfactory. Do not allow the infant to be fed in the nursery.

5. Have the mother suckle her infant for five minutes at each breast during each feed on the first day of life, ten minutes per breast on the second day, and 15 minutes per breast on the third day. Alternate the initial breast at each feeding.

6. Provide positive reinforcement in terms of weight gain. Explain that weight gain should not be anticipated during the first few days of life.

7. Plan to see or talk to the mother within three to seven days after discharge from the hospital.

8. Again remind the mother to clean her nipples with water — not soap. Avoid A and D ointment — it is irritating. If nipples are painful, suggest the application of anhydrous lanolin and not petrolatum. Try to keep nipples dry. Expose nipples as frequently as possible.

9. Remember that mastitis is not an indication to discontinue breast-feeding. The incidence of breast abscess is higher among women who discontinue breast-feeding than among women who do not.

Recommend that the expectant mother or the nursing mother read *The Complete Book of Breastfeeding* by Marvin S. Eiger and Sally W. Olds (Workman Publishing Company, New York). Read it yourself.

Reference: Weichert, C.: Personal communication.

3
GROWTH
AND
DEVELOPMENT

WATCHING FOR DEVELOPMENTAL LAGS
AND DISABILITIES

Most lists which indicate the normal stages of development do not really give a clue about when one should begin to be seriously concerned about developmental lags and disabilities. The following table includes many of the "red flags" often indicative of abnormal patterns of development. In many cases, the presence or absence of any one sign may mean nothing if the rest of development is normal. Certain signs, in and of themselves, are very important, however. For example, an infant who has no social smile at 6 months of age demands further investigation.

Indications For Further Evaluation For Developmental Delay

AT 3 MONTHS	Does not react to sudden noises
	Does not appear to listen to a speaker's voice
	Does not try to find the speaker's face with his eyes
	Has not begun to vocalize sounds
	Has been left to lie in a crib for hours without visual or auditory stimulation
	Does not raise the head when lying on the stomach
AT 6 MONTHS	Does not turn to the speaking person
	Does not respond to being played with
	Is not visually alert
	Never laughs or smiles
	Is not babbling
	Does not reach for or try to pick up a toy
	Is not learning to sit up
	Does not appear to be gaining weight
	Does not arch the back when lying on the stomach and raising the head
AT 1 YEAR	Has not been responding to "Pat-a-Cake," "Peek-A-Boo," or other baby games
	Is not imitating a variety of speech sounds
	Is not saying two or three words such as bye-bye, mama, dada
	Is not pulling up to a standing position
AT 18 MONTHS	Is not yet beginning to feed itself with a spoon
	Does not imitate speech or vocalize in jargon
	Is not moving about to explore
	Does not give eye contact
	Has not or does not spontaneously squat when picking up objects

AT 2 YEARS

Is not naming a few familiar objects and using a few two- or three-word phrases
Is not noticing animals, cars, trucks, trains
Is not beginning to play symbolically with housekeeping toys, little cars
Is not moving about vigorously, running, climbing, exploring
Avoids eye contact
Does not seem to focus eyes on a large picture
Engages in rocking or head banging for extensive periods of time
Is not walking up stairs

AT 3 YEARS

Does not seem aware of other children, of adults, of the weather, traffic, and so forth
Uses little or no speech
Does not engage in imitative play symbolic of adult activities
Avoids looking at pictures or pointing to pictures of familiar objects
Does not follow simple directions
Engages for long periods of time in repetitive behaviors like flipping pages of a magazine, or spinning a wheel on a little truck, head banging, and so forth
Cannot ride a tricycle if given plenty of opportunity to do so

AT 4 YEARS

Does not have at least partially understandable speech with sentences
Uses echolalic speech or frequent, bizarre, meaningless sounds
Does not focus visually on pictures
Does not seem interested in listening to a simple story about his or her experiences
Repeatedly tests all limits
Is so quiet and conforming that he or she never tests or tries anything new
Has pronounced fears and phobias
Frequently engages in flapping of the arms or flipping of the hands to express excitement
Runs about from one thing to another every minute or so without getting fully involved in an activity
Is still untrained in toileting (occasional slips do occur at this age)
Does not draw some sort of representation of human beings (at least a head and a few features), if crayons or pencils have been available to the child
Stays on the periphery of the playroom, paying no attention to other children for some weeks, after most children have overcome shyness and begun to play with or near other children
Avoids eye contact
Engages in head banging or rocking
Cannot tolerate change or frustration without frequent 2-year old tantrums

Reference: Young A., and Schliecker, I.: Preprimary Prevention Project. Mendota Mental Health Institute, 301 Troy Drive, Madison, Wisconsin.

RECOGNIZING SPEECH AND LANGUAGE PROBLEMS EARLY

Concern should be expressed when any one of the following conditions exist:

1. Child is not talking at all by the age of 2 years.
2. Speech is largely unintelligible after the age of 3.
3. Child is leaving off many beginning consonants after the age of 3.
4. Child is still not using two- to three-word sentences by the age of 3.
5. Child uses mostly vowel sounds in his speech.
6. Word endings are consistently missing after the age of 5.
7. Voice is a monotone, too loud, or too soft, or of a poor quality that may indicate a hearing loss.

COMPREHENSION

Comprehension follows an orderly sequence. Failures of comprehension may be the result of hearing difficulties or central nervous system defects. Listed below are sample questions and ages when appropriate response may be anticipated.

QUESTION	EXAMPLE	AGE MASTERED
1. Yes/no	Is this your coat?	2.0 years
2. What	What is that?	2.6 years
What-do	What are you doing?	2.6 years
Where	Where is your ball?	2.6 years
3. Whose	Whose book is that?	3.0 years
Who	Who painted this picture?	3.0 years
Why	Why is the boy running?	3.0 years
How many	How many blocks are here?	3.0 years
4. How	How do you open that box?	3.6 years
5. How much	How much candy is left?	4.0 years
How long	How long were you gone?	4.0 years
6. How far	How far did you walk?	4.6 years
7. How often	How often do you see her?	5.0 years
8. When	When is your grandma coming?	5.6 years

LANGUAGE DEVELOPMENT

The pediatrician should be familiar with the orderly progress of language development. Here are some guidelines that should prove helpful.

APPROXIMATE AGE	BABY SAYS
Birth to 4 weeks	Crying
4 to 16 weeks	Coos and makes "laughing" noises. Vocal play produces vowels and some consonant sounds involving tongue and lip activity. May engage in vocal dialogue with mother
20 to 24 weeks	Vocalizes when comfortable. Vowel-like cooing and considerable babbling, with consonants modifying the identifiable vowel. Makes some nasal sounds (m, n) and some lip sounds
6 to 7 months	Babbling now includes self-imitation (lalling). Many of the sound productions resemble one-syllable utterances that may include *ma, da, di, do*
8 to 9 months	Considerable self-imitative sound play. Is also likely to imitate (echo) syllables and words that others say
10 to 11 months	Repeats the words of others with increased proficiency. Responds appropriately to many word cues for familiar things and "happenings." Precocious child may have several words in his vocabulary
12 months	Still likely to imitate the speech of others, but so proficiently that he seems to have quite a lot to say. First labeling words for most children
By 18 months	Increased word inventory, possible from 3 to 50 words. Vocalizations reveal intonational (melody) pattern of adult speakers. May begin to use two-word utterances, 25 per cent intelligibility

APPROXIMATE AGE	BABY SAYS
24 months	Understands hundreds of words and sentences. Has a speaking vocabulary of 50 or more words. May begin to use two-word combinations, 50 to 70 per cent intelligibility
30 months	Vocabulary growth is proportionately greater than at any other period. Many, though not all, of the child's sentences are grammatically like those of the adults in his life. Understands most of what is said if it is within his experience. Almost total intelligibility
36 months	Speaking vocabulary may exceed 1000 words. Syntax almost completely "grown up." Can say what he or she thinks and make intentions clear
48 months	Productive vocabulary between 1500 and 2000 words; understands up to 20,000 words. Grammatically, has acquired much of what he or she is likely to acquire

3

EVALUATION OF ARTICULATION DISORDERS

The following test is designed to detect articulation disorders in the 2½ to 6 year old child.

The child's ability to articulate the underlined italicized sounds in the words below should be determined.

1. *t*able	9. *th*umb	17. gu*m*
2. shi*rt*	10. too*th*brush	18. *h*ouse
3. *d*oor	11. *s*ock	19. *p*encil
4. tr*un*k	12. vac*uu*m	20. *f*ish
5. *j*umping	13. *y*arn	21. *l*ea*f*
6. zip*per*	14. *m*o*th*er	22. ca*rr*ot
7. *gr*apes	15. *tw*inkle	
8. *fl*ag	16. wago*n*	

Evaluation should be made according to the following normal scores.

Age in Years	Normal Number of Sounds Articulated Correctly
2½–3	7 or more
3–3½	15 or more
4–4½	16 or more
4½–5	18 or more
5–5½	22 or more
5½–6	24 or more
6 and older	25 or more

The child should also be evaluated for intelligibility as words or phrases are put together. The child who is 2½ to 3 years old should be understood half the time or more. The child who is over 3 years of age should be readily understood.

An abnormal score on this simple test should provoke a complete neurologic assessment, an evaluation of the general development and intelligence, a physical examination of the oropharyngeal cavity, lateral head x-ray examination to determine degree of velopharyngeal closure, and a complete audiologic examination. Failure to determine the abnormality should lead to evaluation by a speech pathologist.

Reference: Silver, H.K.: *In* Kempe, C.H., Silver, H.K., and O'Brien, D. (Eds.): Current Pediatric Diagnosis and Treatment. Los Altos, California, Lange Medical Publications, 1976, p. 30.

THE LENGTH AND WIDTH OF THE PENIS

Occasionally the physician questions the appropriateness of the penile length or width of the infant or child being examined. Two studies have measured the size of the penis of normal premature and full-term infants and of children 2 months of age to adulthood. The penile length was determined by measuring from the pubic ramus to the tip of the glans penis by placing the end of a straight-edge ruler against the pubic ramus and applying traction along the length of the phallus to the point of increased resistance. The phallic diameter was determined by passing a hole gauge graduated in sixty-fourths of an inch over the phallus. The smallest diameter hole that could be passed over the glans easily was considered the penile width. The graphs derived from these measurements are below.

References: Schonfeld, W. A.: Am. J. Dis. Child., *65:*535, 1943. Feldman, K. W., and Smith, D. W.: J. Pediatr. *86:*395, 1975.

FIG. 3-1

Stretched phallic length of 63 normal premature and full-term male infants (●), showing lines of mean ± 2 SD. Correlation coefficient is 0.80. Superimposed are data for two small-for-gestational age infants (△), seven large-for-gestation age infants (▲), and four twins (■), all of which are in the normal range.

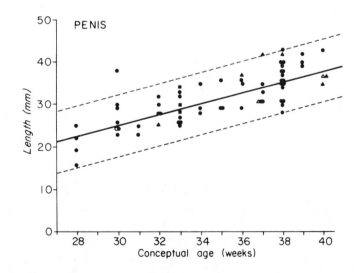

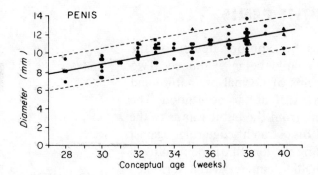

FIG. 3-2

Phallic diameter of 63 normal premature and full-term male infants (●), showing lines of mean ± 2 SD. Correlation coefficient is 0.82. Superimposed are data for two small-for-gestational age infants (△), seven large-for-gestational age infants (▲), and four twins (■), all of which are in the normal range.

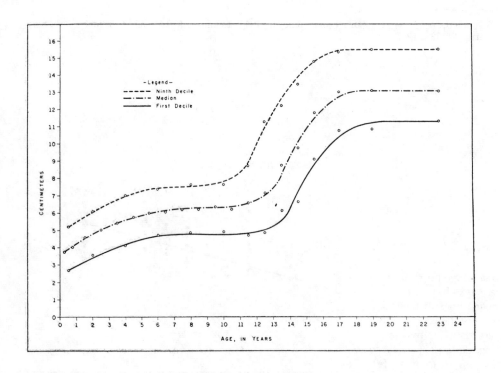

FIG. 3-3

Curve for growth of the penis in length from birth to maturity.

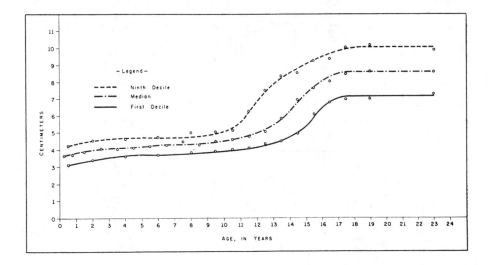

FIG. 3-4

Curve for growth of the penis in circumference from birth to maturity.

THE AGE OF APPEARANCE OF OSSIFICATION CENTERS

The hand is most frequently used to determine bone age. Radiologic examination of other bones may also reveal skeletal maturity. The following charts demonstrate the approximate age at which new centers of ossification should appear.

Reference: Wilkins, L.: The Diagnosis and Treatment of Endocrine Disorders in Childhood and Adolescence, 3rd ed. Springfield, Illinois, Charles C Thomas, Publisher, 1965, pp. 38, 39.

	BIRTH	I YR	2	3	4	5
Shoulder	0	Head of humerus (3 months)	Great tuberosity			
Elbow	0		Capitellum			Head of radius
Hand	0	Hamate (4 mos.) Capitate (6 mos.) Ep. radius		Triquetrum Ep. metacarpals Ep. phalanges	Lunatum	Trapezium Scaphoid
Hip	0	Head of femur (9 months)			Great trochanter	
Knee Ep. femur & tibia					Head of fibula	Patella
Foot Cuboid		Ext. cuneiform Ep. tibia	Ep. fibula	Int. cuneiform Ep. metatarsals	Mid cuneiform Navicular	

The new centers of ossification which appear at each year are shown in black.

6	7	8	9	10	11	12-13

6	7	8	9	10	11
Union head & tuberosity					
Int. epicondyle			Trochlea Olecranon		Ext. epicondyle
Trapezoid Ep. ulna				Pisiform	Styloid ulna
	Union ischium & pubis			Ep. lesser trochanter	
					Tibial tubercle
		Ep. os calcis			

The new centers of ossification which appear at each year are shown in black.

USE OF BONE AGE DETERMINATION IN THE DIAGNOSIS OF SHORT STATURE

The cause for short stature may often be determined by careful history and physical examination. Nutritional or emotional deprivation, chronic disease, or a history of short stature in other family members may provide an explanation for decreased height. Facial appearance may suggest a genetic or chromosomal abnormality. Organ enlargement may lead to a diagnosis of a storage disease.

Often, however, the diagnosis is not readily apparent. In these cases, it is helpful to begin with a comparison of skeletal maturation (bone age) to height age and chronologic age. The table lists the diagnoses that should be suggested by such a comparison, and the clinical features accompanying each diagnosis.

MEASUREMENT	DIAGNOSIS SUGGESTED	CLINICAL FEATURES
Bone age equal to or slightly behind chronologic age	Primordial short stature	Birth weight and length below normal for gestational age. Subsequent growth parallel to, but below, 3rd percentile Normal onset and progression of puberty. Minor skeletal abnormalities. Includes genetic and chromosomal aberrations, e.g., Down's syndrome and Turner's syndrome. Short stature as adult.
	Familial short stature	Normal length and weight for first 1 to 2 years of life. Height falls below 3rd percentile at 5 to 10 years of age. Puberty not delayed. "Normal" adult height not attained.
Bone age retarded in relation to chronologic age, but less retarded than height age	Constitutional short stature	Appropriate weight and length for gestational age at birth. Slow growth during childhood. Delayed onset of puberty. Other family members may remember similar growth pattern. Important to differentiate from hypothyroidism and growth hormone deficiency. Ultimately reach "normal" adult height.

MEASUREMENT	DIAGNOSIS SUGGESTED	CLINICAL FEATURES

	Metabolic disorders, e.g.:
	   Hypophosphatemic
	     rickets
	   Hypophosphatasia
	   Mucopolysaccharidoses
	   Glycogen storage
	     diseases
	   Renal tubular acidosis
	   Bartter's syndrome
	   Vasopressin-resistant
	     diabetes insipidus
		Clinical and laboratory findings consistent with these disorders

	Organic acidemias and
	   acidurias
	 Hemolytic anemias
	 Disorders of mineral
	   metabolism
	 Immunoglobulin or
	   white blood cell
	   abnormality
	 Others
		Clinical and laboratory findings consistent with these disorders.

	Chronic disease, e.g.:
	   Chronic infection
	   Hepatic disease
	   Pulmonary disease
	   Renal disease
	   Malabsorption
	   Malignancy
	   Collagen vascular
	     disease
	   Others
		Clinical and laboratory findings consistent with the disease; initial clue may be increased erythrocyte sedimentation rate.
		 May exhibit variable growth rate over several years.

Bone age equal to or advanced in comparison with height age	Familial short stature	See above
	Sexual precocity with androgen excess	Increased linear growth early in life with early closure of epiphyses. Clinical signs of androgen excess (facial, axillary, and pubic hair, penile or clitoral enlargement).
	Sexual precocity with estrogen excess	Early closure of epiphyses without prior augmentation of linear growth. Clinical signs of estrogen excess (breast enlargement, galactorrhea in females, and so on).

MEASUREMENT	DIAGNOSIS SUGGESTED	CLINICAL FEATURES
Bone age greatly decreased and less than or equal to height age	Hypothyroidism	Degree of growth retardation depends upon age of onset. Congenital hypothyroidism is associated with severe growth failure. In juvenile hypothyroidism, the growth retardation is more insidious. Delayed dental age.
	Cushing's syndrome (most often iatrogenic)	Truncal obesity, moon facies, violaceous striae, hirsutism, muscle weakness, hypertension.
	Hypopituitarism and growth hormone deficiency. Causes include: Congenital absence of pituitary Infection Reticuloendothelioses Vascular infarcts and anomalies Trauma Irradiation Surgical resection Malnutrition	Delayed dental age. Puberty often delayed. May have neurologic abnormalities.
	Maternal deprivation	May have impaired motor and intellectual development. May or may not be associated with malnutrition. May have growth hormone deficiency.

Reference: Gotlin, R.W., and Mace, J.W.: Curr. Probl. Pediatr. *2*:3, 1972.

CHILDHOOD
I used to think that grown-up people chose
To have stiff backs and wrinkles round their nose,
And veins like small fat snakes on either hand,
On purpose to be grand.
Till through the banisters I watched one day
My great-aunt Etty's friend who was going away,
And how her onyx beads had come unstrung.
I saw her grope to find them as they rolled;
And then I knew that she was helplessly old,
As I was helplessly young.

Frances Cornford

3

GROWTH VELOCITY

An increase in length is a direct result of growth of both the spine and lower extremities. While the growth in length or height of a typical child is nonlinear, it can be divided into time segments during which the increments are essentially linear. The tables below can be used to estimate whether a child's skeletal growth is normal.

Boys

GROWTH IN HEIGHT OR LENGTH (CM/YR), AGE 6 MO TO 10 YR

Percentile	6 mo	1 yr	2	3	4	5	6	7	8	9	10
97th	22.5	16.3	11.8	10.4	9.4	8.4	7.8	7.4	7.1	6.8	6.7
50th	18	12.6	8.9	7.9	7	6.4	6	5.8	5.5	5.3	5.2
3rd	13.5	9	5.8	5.4	4.8	4.5	4.3	4.2	4.1	3.7	3.6

Girls

GROWTH IN HEIGHT OR LENGTH (CM/YR), AGE 6 MO TO 8 YR

Percentile	6 mo	1 yr	2	3	4	5	6	7	8
97th	23.5	18.3	12.1	10.4	9.2	8.3	7.8	7.5	7.2
50th	19	13.8	9	7.8	7	6.5	6.1	5.7	5.5
3rd	14.5	10	6	5.3	4.7	4.5	4.3	4.2	4

Reference: Weaver, D.S., and Owen, G.M.: Postgrad. Med., *62:*93, 1977.

PREDICTED WEIGHT AND HEIGHT FROM AGE

If you know the age of a child and want a rough estimate of the weight and height:

Weight (lb) = age (mo) + 11

(for 3–12 mo)

Weight (lb) = age (yr) $\times$ 5 + 17

(for 1–6 yr)

Weight (lb) = age (yr) $\times$ 7 + 5

(for 7–12 yr)

Height (in) = (2½ x age) + 30

(for 2–14 yr)

Reference: Graef, J.W., and Cone, T.E.: *In* Manual of Pediatric Therapeutics. Boston, Little, Brown, and Company, 1980, p. 153.

MORE ON PREDICTED HEIGHTS

The formula of Tanner et al. demonstrates that height at age 3 years correlates better with height at maturity than it does at any other age:

Adult height = 1.27 x height + 54.9 cm (males)
(cm)   (at 3 yr)

Adult height = 1.29 x height + 42.3 cm (females)
(cm)   (at 3 yr)

If you cannot remember these formulas or your programmable calculator has been stolen, the commonly accepted statement that the child at age 2 has achieved one half his or her final height is quite satisfactory. For girls, however, 10 to 12 cm (2.54 to 4.00 in) must be subtracted from this predicted height. If the height at 3 years is known, an alternative to the Tanner equation to predict final adult height is to multiply the age 3 height by 1.87 for boys and 1.73 for girls.

Reference: Tanner et al.: Arch. Dis. Child., *31:*372, 1956.

ERUPTION OF DECIDUOUS TEETH

The eruption of the first tooth in an infant is accompanied by parental pride in the fact that yet another milestone is reached. Figure 3–5 indicates the age and the order in which deciduous teeth erupt. The dot represents the mean age, while the wavy line demonstrates normal variation. Exceptions to the sequence of eruption are uncommon. Late eruption is unlikely to be of significance; however, it has been associated with both hypothyroidism and rickets.

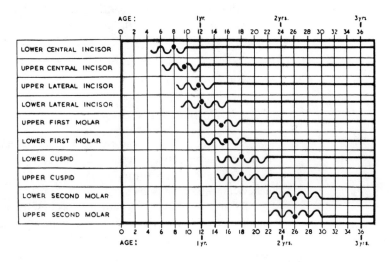

FIG. 3–5

Reference: MacKeith, R., and Wood, C.: Digestion and absorption. *In* Infant Feeding and Feeding Difficulties. London, J. & A. Churchill, 1971, p. 19.

"Adam and Eve had many advantages, but the principal one was that they escaped teething."

Mark Twain

TIPS ON TOILET TRAINING

Bowel control is not a simple physiologic reflex; it is a complicated behavior pattern profoundly influenced by maturity factors that are both neurologic and psychologic. For reasons that are difficult to understand, society has placed undue emphasis on early toilet training. This is often translated into a belief that "practice makes perfect." We ask our children to carry our cultural burden at a very early age; the child must do his "duty." We are prepared to extend liberties to our dogs that we will not extend to our children.

The facts of growth and maturity must be explained to parents. Most mistakenly believe that all infants should be toilet trained by 2 years of age, and that failure in this regard is a form of either perversity or, worse still, disobedience.

Steps in Normal Bowel Control

16 weeks: By this age the gastrocolic reflex has weakened somewhat, and there is a delay between feeding and defecation. A vigilant mother may note this delay and take the opportunity to place the child on the toilet. Success leads her to believe that the child is already trained.

28 weeks: Bowel movements become more irregular. They may occur unrelated to either waking or eating. Infants are generally indifferent to soiling.

40 weeks: The capacity to sit is usually well developed. Child may sit on toilet seat and look at mother and make imitative grunting movements. Occasionally a stool may be passed.

52 weeks: A higher order of neurologic maturation is taking place with the assumption of the upright posture. Child is usually not interested in sitting on toilet and making facial grimaces at this time.

15 months: If standing and walking have been achieved, the child may actually like to go to the toilet. Some children may instinctively assume a squatting position.

18 months: If the child has incorporated meaningful words like "toidy" into his growing vocabulary, and can relate it to bowel control and is ambulating without difficulty, he may be ready for toilet "training." The child must still understand the social significance of the act.

24 months: Most children by this age are "trainable." The child should be permitted to take over this responsibility. The child should have his own toilet seat. The seat should allow the child to place his feet squarely on the ground or on a bar so that he may develop the necessary intra-abdominal pressure. He may need help in removing his clothes.

30 months: Children of this age frequently display extremes and exaggerations of behavior. Bowel movements may become less regular.

36 months: Child has developed increased ability to withhold and postpone. Daily bowel movements may occur late in the day. The child is ready to accept the cultural burden.

48 months: The bowel movement has become a private affair. The child has a healthy "childlike" interest in the physical properties of the stool. He is frank, forthright, and independent.

The training process, therefore, requires a neurologically mature nervous system, a psychologically prepared child, and a healthy cultural setting. "Intestinal fortitude" is not a requirement.

The process may be facilitated but not expedited by:

1. An educated and relaxed attitude on the part of the parents.
2. The provision of a toilet seat or chair for the child.
3. Providing an opportunity for imitative behavior.
4. The avoidance of punishment or excessive rewards.
5. The avoidance of training during periods of stress in a child's life, such as a new sibling or a new home.
6. Providing training pants when appropriate.

References: Brazelton, T.: Pediatrics, *29*:121, 1962. Stehbens, J.A.: Pediatrics, *54*:493, 1974.

THE EVALUATION OF A CHILD WITH FAILURE TO THRIVE

Pediatricians are commonly required to evaluate infants and children who have "failed to thrive." This frequently encountered problem has many causes, although simple malnutrition is responsible for 75 to 90 per cent of all cases in the United States. Infants with genetic short stature and those with central nervous system deficits account for many of the remainder. An orderly approach to investigation coupled with careful history, physical examination, and simple observation can reduce both unnecessary laboratory investigation and the length of hospitalization.

A few useful general rules:

1. The malnourished infant or child will display a weight reduction out of proportion to his length reduction. His head circumference will be normal or near normal.

2. The infant of short stature will have a length reduction in proportion to or more than his weight reduction. His head circumference will be normal or even increased relative to his length.

3. In the child with a central nervous system deficit, both weight and length will be reduced proportionally, and the head circumference will generally be subnormal.

4. Chronic illness generally produces a proportional reduction in both length and weight, although the weight may be reduced more than the length.

5. Physical signs of neglect usually indicate malnutrition as the cause of the failure to thrive. These signs include: dirty nails, diaper rash, skin infections, flat occiput and "bald spot."

Initial laboratory tests should include:

Complete blood count

Macrocytic anemia (hypothyroidism, folic acid, or vitamin B_{12} deficiency, which may indicate disease of the small bowel)

Microcytic anemia (iron deficiency, gastrointestinal blood loss as a result of milk allergy, chronic infection)

Polycythemia (chronic lung disease, heart disease, dehydration)

Neutropenia (pancreatic insufficiency and bone marrow hypoplasia syndrome)

Leukocytosis (occult infection)

Thrombocytosis (neuroblastoma with metastases, granulomas of liver and bone marrow)

Urinalysis

Reducing substance (diabetes, renal tubular disease, disaccharide intolerance)

Urine pH (>6.5 — renal tubular acidosis?)

Sediment (WBCs — urinary tract infection; RBCs — nephritis)

Proteinuria (renal disease, renal tubular disease, aminoaciduria)

Ferric chloride

Specific gravity (<1.010 — diabetes insipidus)

Stool examination

Reducing substance (disaccharide intolerance)
Stool pH (below 6.0, disaccharide intolerance)
Occult blood (cow milk intolerance)
Ova and parasites

Tine test

Blood urea nitrogen, serum
sodium, potassium, chloride,
and carbon dioxide

If the initial history, physical examination, and simple laboratory tests are all normal, then the infant should be placed on a "therapeutic trial" of feeding. The infant's requirements for fluids, calories, and protein should be calculated, and intake and weight gain carefully recorded on a daily basis.

After several days of observation, the following conclusions may be drawn:

1. *Intake adequate* (120 cal/kg/day) and *weight gain* ensues.
   Conclusion: Inadequate feeding at home; maternal neglect or unsatisfactory parent-child relationship.

2. *Intake inadequate – no weight gain*
   Consider:

Poor swallowing	– neurologic or neuromuscular disorder
Eats small amounts	– cardiorespiratory disease, severe debilitation, chronic infection, hypothyroidism
Eats vigorously but spits, vomits, or ruminates	– psychological disorder, gastrointestinal anomalies, increased intracranial pressure, chronic subdural hematoma, metabolic abnormality

3. *Intake adequate – No weight gain.* Increase caloric intake to what would be optimal for patient's normal weight. If no weight gain after increase in diet, then malabsorption of some cause must be considered.

Abnormal physical findings or initial laboratory tests may provide you with clues to the diagnosis. Disorders that may produce failure to thrive may be broadly grouped into the classification listed below.

Inadequate Intake

Economic deprivation
Social deprivation
Psychic anorexia
Mechanical feeding problems
  Cleft palate
  Aerophagia
  Nasal obstruction
Avitaminosis C
Diabetes insipidus

Failure to Assimilate

Cystic fibrosis
Celiac disease
Milk allergy
Parasites
Postdiarrheal recovery phase
Portal hypertension
Aminoacidopathies
Hypoxemia
  Cardiac
  Pulmonary insufficiency

Increased Metabolism

Chronic infection
Malignancy
Collagen disease
Hyperthyroidism
Cerebral palsy–athetoid

Failure to Utilize (Sick Cells)

Renal acidosis
Renal alkalosis
Renal insufficiency
Hypercalcemia
Hepatic insufficiency – cirrhosis
Diabetes
Storage disease
  Glycogen storage disease
  Hurler's syndrome
Galactosemia

Bone Diseases

Chondrodystrophia
Ellis–van Creveld
Morquio's

Failure of Stimulation

> Cretinism
> > Pituitary
> > Primordial
> > Constitutional
>
> IUGR (intrauterine growth retardation)
> Gonadal dysgenesis
> Mental retardation
> > CNS anomalies and tumors
> > Subdural hematomas

AN APPROACH TO FAILURE TO THRIVE IN A BREAST-FED INFANT

Breast-fed infants who fail to thrive can do so for a variety of reasons. A flow chart listing the broad potential causes is as follows:

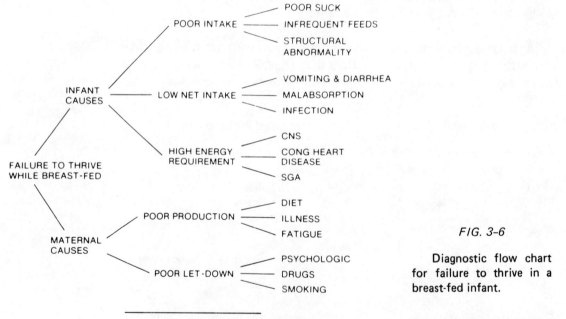

FIG. 3-6

Diagnostic flow chart for failure to thrive in a breast-fed infant.

Reference: Ballard, R.: Eleventh Ross Roundtable. Columbus, OH, Ross Laboratories, 1980, p. 68.

FAILURE TO THRIVE — A DIAGNOSTIC FLOW CHART

The diagnosis of "failure to thrive" can be encapsulated in the algorithm shown in Figure 3–7.

Reference: Fremont, MI, Gerber Medical Marketing Services, Gerber Products Company, 1979, pp. 6–7.

Failure to Thrive —
Diagnostic Flow Chart

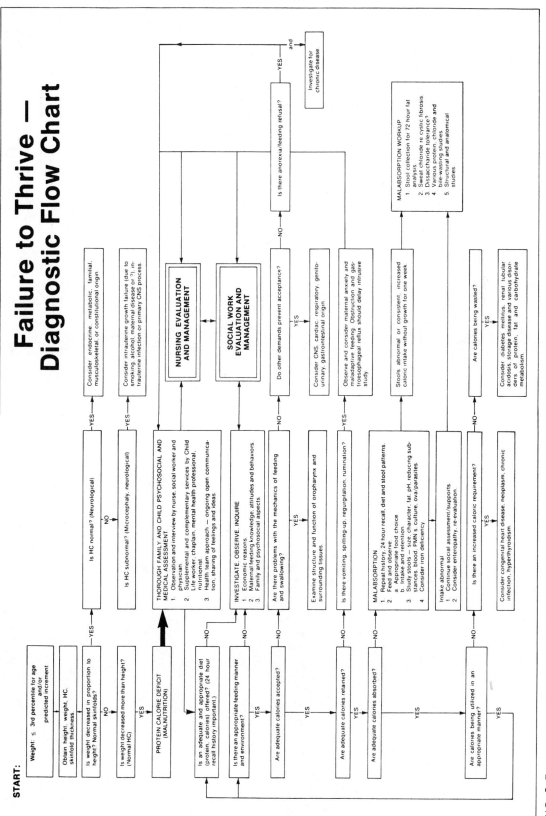

START:

Weight: ≤ 3rd percentile for age and/or predicted increment

Obtain height, weight, HC, skinfold thickness.

Is weight decreased in proportion to height? Normal skinfolds? — **NO** → Is HC normal? (Neurological) — **YES** → Consider endocrine, metabolic, familial, musculoskeletal, or constitutional origin.

— **NO** → Is HC subnormal? (Microcephaly, neurological) — **YES** → Consider intrauterine growth failure (due to smoking, alcohol, maternal disease or ?), intrauterine infection or primary CNS process.

Is weight decreased more than height? (Normal HC) — **YES** →

PROTEIN CALORIE DEFICIT (MALNUTRITION)

THOROUGH FAMILY AND CHILD PSYCHOSOCIAL AND MEDICAL ASSESSMENT
1. Observation and interview by nurse, social worker and physician.
2. Supplemental and complementary services by Child Life worker, chaplain, mental health professional, nutritionist.
3. Health team approach — ongoing open communication, sharing of feelings and ideas.

↔ **NURSING EVALUATION AND MANAGEMENT**

↔ **SOCIAL WORK EVALUATION AND MANAGEMENT**

Is an adequate and appropriate diet (protein, calories) offered? (24 hour recall history important) — **NO** →

Is there an appropriate feeding manner and environment? — **NO** → INVESTIGATE, OBSERVE, INQUIRE
1. Economic reasons
2. Maternal feeding knowledge, attitudes and behaviors.
3. Family and psychosocial aspects

Are adequate calories accepted? — **NO** → Are there problems with the mechanics of feeding and swallowing? — **YES** → Examine structure and function of oropharynx and surrounding tissues.

— **NO** → Do other demands prevent acceptance? — **YES** → Consider CNS, cardiac, respiratory, genitourinary, gastrointestinal origin.

— **NO** → Is there anorexia/feeding refusal? — **YES** → Investigate for chronic disease

Are adequate calories retained? — **NO** → Is there vomiting, spitting-up, regurgitation, rumination? — **YES** → Observe and consider maternal anxiety and maladaptive feeding. Obstruction and gastroesophageal reflux should delay intrusive study.

Are adequate calories absorbed? — **NO** → MALABSORPTION
1. Repeat history, 24 hour recall, diet and stool patterns.
2. Feed and observe
   a. Appropriate food choice
   b. Intake and retention
3. Study stools — size, character, fat, pH, reducing substances, blood, PMN's, culture, ova/parasites
4. Consider iron deficiency

Stools abnormal or consistent, increased caloric intake without growth for one week. →

MALABSORPTION WORKUP
1. Stool collection for 72 hour fat analysis.
2. Sweat chloride re cystic fibrosis
3. Dissaccharide tolerance?
4. Various protein, chloride and bile-wasting studies
5. Structural and anatomical studies

Intake abnormal
1. Continue social assessment/supports
2. Consider enteropathy, re-evaluation.

Are calories being utilized in an appropriate manner? — **NO** → Is there an increased caloric requirement? — **YES** → Consider congenital heart disease, neoplasm, chronic infection, hyperthyroidism

— **NO** → Are calories being wasted? — **YES** → Consider diabetes mellitus, renal tubular acidosis, storage disease and various disorders of protein, fat and carbohydrate metabolism.

FIG. 3–7

REFRACTIVE CAPACITY VERSUS AGE

A change in refractive capacity of the eyes occurs to some degree in just about all of us. A tendency toward hyperopia increases slowly for about the first eight years of life. This happens in spite of the fact that the eyeball grows rapidly during this period, because concurrent with eyeball growth is a relatively greater decrease in the curvature of the cornea and the lens. After 8 years of age hyperopia decreases gradually until adolescence, when vision is normally emmetropic. After the age of 20 there is a tendency toward myopia, which decreases after the midthirties. Presbyopia, the farsightedness associated with advancing age, is due to loss of elasticity in the lens. All this is of the following diopter magnitude as seen in Figure 3–8.

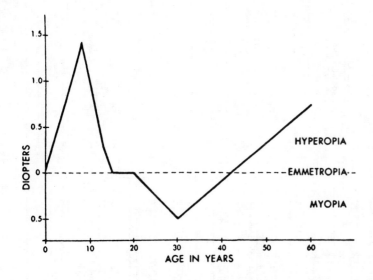

FIG. 3-8

Reference: Valadian, I., and Porter, D.: *In* Physical Growth and Development. Boston, Little, Brown & Company, 1977, p. 213.

THE GOODENOUGH DRAW-A-MAN TEST

The Goodenough draw-a-man test is one of the simplest developmental tests that may be done in the office. The rules and scoring criteria are given below.

3

Basal age = 3 years. For each four criteria, add 1 year to arrive at mental age, between ages 3 and 10 years. Instruct child to draw *a complete person;* no further instructions.

$$\frac{\text{Maturation age}}{\text{Chronological age}} \times \frac{100}{1} = \text{IQ}$$

Twenty-eight criteria for scoring:
1. Head present
2. Legs present
3. Arms present
4. Trunk present
5. Length of trunk greater than breadth
6. Shoulder indicated
7. Both arms and legs attached to trunk
8. Legs attached to trunk and arms to trunk at correct point
9. Neck present
10. Outline of neck continuous with that of head or trunk, or both
11. Eyes present
12. Nose present
13. Mouth present
14. Both nose and mouth in two dimensions, two lips shown
15. Nostrils indicated
16. Hair shown
17. Hair on more than circumference of head, nontransparent, better than scribble
18. Clothing present
19. Two articles of clothing, nontransparent
20. Entire drawing, with sleeves and trousers shown, free from transparency.
21. Four or more articles of clothing definitely indicated
22. Costume complete without incongruities
23. Fingers shown
24. Correct number of fingers shown
25. Fingers in two dimensions, length greater than breadth, angle subtended not greater than 180 degrees
26. Opposition of thumbs shown
27. Hand shown as distinct from fingers or arms
28. Arm joint shown; either elbow, shoulder, or both

Reference: Goodenough-Harris Drawing Test. New York, Harcourt Brace Jovanovich, 1963.

4
METABOLISM

PREDICTABLE FALL OF BUN
IN A DEHYDRATED CHILD

Children admitted to hospital with diarrhea and dehydration often have elevated blood urea nitrogen (BUN) levels. Usually this elevation is assumed to be prerenal and the abnormality is ignored, at least until just before discharge. Brill and coworkers found that the rate of fall of BUN in a dehydrated child with normal renal function was predictable. They plotted BUN levels against time on semilogarithmic graph paper. BUN had fallen to one-half the admission level in 24 hours or less in all children with uncomplicated dehydration and diarrhea.

Line A in Figure 4–1 represents the slope along which the BUN should fall in a child without renal disease or excess nitrogen load (e.g., gastrointestinal bleed). Lines B and C represent 2½ standard deviations on either side of that rate of fall.

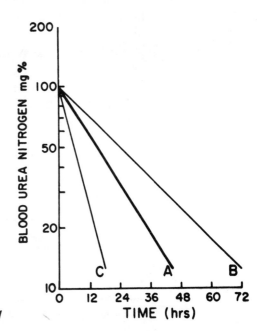

FIG. 4–1

Complicating disease should be sought in the dehydrated child whose BUN does not fall at a rate parallel to line A or within 2½ standard deviations from that rate.

Reference: Brill, C.B., Uretsky, S., and Gribetz, D.: J. Pediatr., *52*:197, 1973.

"In bringing up a child, think of its old age."

Joubert

SERUM OSMOLALITY

It is often important to estimate serum osmolality before the laboratory measurement becomes available. The following formula will make that estimation more accurate.

The short cut approach is

$$\text{Serum Osmolality} = \{Na(mEq/L) + K\ (mEq/L)\} \times 2 + \frac{Glucose}{18} + \frac{BUN}{3}$$

The normal value is 280.

CALCULATION OF PLASMA ONCOTIC PRESSURE

The plasma oncotic pressure is a major determinant of whether pulmonary edema will develop. Other variables, such as capillary and interstitial hydrostatic pressures, are difficult if not impossible to measure.

Equipment is available that will directly measure plasma oncotic pressure, but it is expensive and not yet widely in use. The albumin fraction of plasma is responsible for about 60 per cent of plasma oncotic pressure, with the globulin fraction constituting most of the remainder. A simple and fairly accurate formula (the Pappenheimer equation) can be used to calculate the plasma oncotic pressure. This formula is based on the total protein concentration of plasma where:

$$\text{Oncotic pressure (Torr)} = 2.1c + 0.16c^2 + 0.009c^3$$

where c = total plasma protein (gm/dl).

A Torr value greater than 18 to 20 is usually sufficient to prevent edema formation.

Reference: Weil, M.H., Morissette, M., Michaels, S. et al.: Critical Care Med., 2:229, 1974.

HYPOKALEMIA CAUSED BY DRUGS

Multiple diseases and clinical states cause hypokalemia. These include:

Persistent vomiting
Diarrhea
Unreplaced loss from nasogastric suction
Intestinal fistula
Congenital chloridorrhea (Darrow-Gamble syndrome)
Villous adenoma of the rectosigmoid
Renal tubular acidosis
Fanconi syndrome
Bartter syndrome
Chronic interstitial nephritis
Cushing syndrome
Hyperaldosteronism
Inadequate dietary intake
Leukemia in relapse

When these causes have been ruled out, drug-induced hypokalemia must be considered. The drugs that cause hypokalemia are listed below, according to the mechanism of potassium depletion.

Augmented Transport into Cells

Insulin and glucose
Poisoning with barium chloride or carbonate (not the insoluble radiologic suspension barium sulfate)

Gastrointestinal Losses

Laxative misuse causes direct losses in the stool as well as intravascular volume depletion, decreased renal blood flow, hyperreninemia, augmented aldosterone secretion, and finally increased urinary potassium loss.

Urinary Loss

By direct toxic effect on the kidney:

amphoterecin B
polymyxin B
outdated tetracyclines
gentamicin (possibly)

By enhanced distal nephron sodium-potassium exchange:

glucocorticoids
mineralocorticoids
licorice
carbenoxolone

By overwhelming the distal tubule with sodium ions:

> chlorothiazide
> diuretics that act on the loop of Henle
>   (furosamide and ethacrinic acid)
> massive sodium bicarbonate ingestion

By increasing the electrical negativity of the lumen of the distal tubule with a nonreabsorbable anion:

> carbenicillin
> other penicillins in very large doses

Potassium supplement may be given in anticipation of hypokalemia when these drugs are used. Other modes of treatment when hypokalemia occurs because of drugs include withdrawal of the offending drug and postfacto replacement of potassium losses.

Reference: Chesney, R. W.: Am. J. Dis. Child., *130:*1055, 1976.

THE ANION GAP

In these days of automated laboratory procedures, most sick patients will have their serum electrolytes measured. Obvious abnormalities are easily recognized. Hidden clues to diagnosis are also present in these numbers. Interpretation of the "anion gap" provides such a clue.

The principle of electroneutrality is always working and dictates that the sum of the positive charges, i.e., the mEq/L of cations, be exactly counterbalanced by the number of negative charges, i.e., the mEq/L of anions.

The principal cations in the plasma include sodium, potassium, calcium, and magnesium. The principal anions are chloride, bicarbonate, carbonic acid, dissolved carbon dioxide, albumin, globulin, sulfate, phosphate, and the organic acids, lactic and pyruvic acid.

Measurement of all the anions and cations is not required for interpretation of the patient's status. The serum sodium and potassium are representative of the extracellular fluid cations, and, in fact, account for 95 per cent of the cations present. Chloride and bicarbonate account for 85 per cent of the anions. Thus, the sum of the usually measured anions does not fully counterbalance the sum of the measured cations. Their difference is termed the anion gap. Because of potassium's relatively low and stable serum concentration, it has only a minor influence on the anion gap. Therefore the anion gap equation can be simplified to read as follows:

Anion gap = sodium − (chloride + bicarbonate)

The normal value for the anion gap is approximately 12.0 ± 2.0. The normal range for the anion gap is thus 8 to 16 mEq/L.

Causes of a high anion gap include:

Metabolic acidosis
Dehydration
Therapy with sodium salts of strong acids
Therapy with certain antibiotics
    Carbenicillin, large doses of sodium penicillin
Alkalosis

4

Specific causes of *high anion gap* metabolic *acidosis* include:

Uremia
Ketoacidosis
Lactic acidosis
Salicylate intoxication
Methanol intoxication
Paraldehyde toxicity

Specific causes of *normal anion gap* metabolic *acidosis* include:

Gastrointestinal bicarbonate loss
    Diarrhea or pancreatic fistula
Ureterenterostomy
Drugs
    Acetazolamide
    Sulfamylon
    Cholestyramine
    Acidifying agents (ammonium chloride, oral calcium chloride, arginine, hydrochloride, lysine hydrochloride)
    Rapid intravenous hydration
    Hyperalimentation
    Posthypocapnia
    Renal tubular acidosis

Causes of a *low anion gap* include:

Reduced concentration of unmeasured anions
    Dilution
    Hypoalbuminemia
Systematic underestimation of serum sodium
    Severe hypernatremia
    Hyperviscosity
Systematic overestimation of serum chloride
    Bromism
Retained nonsodium cations
    Paraproteinemia
    Hypercalcemia
    Hypermagnesemia

Reference: Emmett, M., and Narins, R. G.: Medicine, *56:* 38, 1977.

COMPOSITION OF BODY FLUIDS

The composition of intravenous fluids used to replace body fluid losses must be based on the source or site of these losses. Fluid losses from most body sites except the kidney vary from the equivalent of one-third to normal saline. The Na^+, K^+, Cl^-, HCO_3, and tonicity of the fluids from various body sources are as follows:

	Na^+ (mEq/L)	K^+ (mEq/L)	Cl^- (mEq/L)	HCO_3 (mEq/L)	pH	Osm (mOsm/L)
Gastric	50	10–15	150	0	1	300
Pancreas	140	5	50–100	100	9	300
Bile	130	5	100	40	8	300
Ileostomy	130	15–20	120	25–30	8	300
Diarrhea	50	35	40	50	Alk	
Sweat	50	5	55	0		
Blood	140	4–5	100	25	7.4	285–295
Urine	0–100*	20–100*	70–100*	0	4.5–8.5	50–1400

*Varies considerably with intake.

Reference: Graef, J.W., and Cone, T.E.: *In* Manual of Pediatric Therapeutics. Boston, Little, Brown & Company, 1980, p. 191.

SERUM AND URINE ELECTROLYTES

The usefulness of comparing serum and urine electrolytes is becoming increasingly apparent. The table illustrates this usefulness with respect to many of the more common causes of electrolyte imbalances.

Diagnostic Guide for Serum and Urine Electrolytes

Condition	SERUM VALUES					URINE VALUES			
	Na (mEq/L)	K (mEq/L)	Osm (mOsm/L)	BUN (mg/dl)	Creat.	Na (mEq/L)	K (mEq/L)	Osm (mOsm/L)	Urea (mg/dl)
Primary aldosteronism	140	↓	280	10	N	80	60-80	300-800	Low
Secondary aldosteronism	130	↓	275	15-25	↓	<20	40-60	300-400	800-1000
Na depletion	120-130	N or ↑	260	>30	N or ↑	10-20	40	600+	800-1000
Na overload	150+	N	290+	N or ↑	N	100+	60	500+	300
H$_2$O overload	120-130	↓	260	10-15	↓	50-80	60	50-200	300
Dehydration	150	↓	300	30 or N	N or ↑	40	20-40	800+	800-1000
Inappropriate ADH	<125	↓	<260	<10	↓	90	60-150	U$_{osm}$ > P$_{osm}$	300
Acute tubular necrosis									
Oliguric	135	↑	N or ↑	↑↑	↑	40+	20-40	300	300
Polyuric	135	N or ↑	275	↑	↑	20	30	300	100-300

Reference: Graef, J.W., and Cone, T.E.: *In* Manual of Pediatric Therapeutics. Boston, Little, Brown & Company, 1980, p. 187.

URINARY ELECTROLYTES

The cause of electrolyte abnormalities is usually self-evident, and urinary electrolyte evaluation is unnecessary. In cases where confusion arises, however, 24-hour urinary electrolyte measurement may be helpful. The following table correlates the clinical condition with urinary electrolyte values and the diagnostic possibilities.

DIAGNOSTIC PROBLEM	URINARY VALUE	PRIMARY DIAGNOSTIC POSSIBILITIES
Volume depletion	Na^+, 0–10 mEq/liter	Extrarenal sodium loss
	Na^+, >10 mEq/liter	"Renal salt wasting" or adrenal insufficiency
Acute oliguria	Na^+, 0–10 mEq/liter	Prerenal azotemia
	Na^+, >30 mEq/liter	Acute tubular necrosis
Hyponatremia	Na^+, 0–10 mEq/liter	Severe volume depletion; edematous states
	Na^+, ≥dietary intake	Inappropriate antidiuretic hormone (ADH) secretion; adrenal insufficiency
Hypokalemia	K^+, 0–10 mEq/liter	Extrarenal potassium loss
	K^+, >10 mEq/liter	Renal potassium loss
Metabolic alkalosis	Cl^-, 0–10 mEq/liter	Chloride-responsive alkalosis
	Cl^-, ≅dietary intake	Chloride-resistant alkalosis

For purposes of this table, it is assumed the patient is not receiving diuretics.

Reference: Harrington, J.T., and Cohen, J.J.: N. Engl. J. Med., *293*:1241, 1975.

UNUSUAL ODOR AS A CLUE TO DIAGNOSIS

It is 3:00 A.M. in the nursery, and a call from the nurse informs you that a 2 day old full-term infant, who had been perfectly fine until now, has turned sour. Not recognizing the pun, you sleepily arouse yourself to examine the patient. If you are fortunate, you note that the diaper of the seizing infant smells like sweaty feet. If you are doubly fortunate, you remember that odor long enough to order an amino acid analysis of serum and urine and discontinue all proteins in the patient's diet. That particular baby may have isovalericacidemia. It probably does not, since it is a very rare condition, but the sweaty feet syndrome is just one of several errors of metabolism that may be discovered in the nursery by an alert olfactory organ (see accompanying table).

Some of the above metabolic diseases may be quickly verified by adding 10 per cent ferric chloride drop by drop to 1 ml of the patient's urine.

Reference: Mace, J.W., Goodman, S.I., Centerwall, W.R., et al.: Clin. Pediatr., *15*:58, 1976.

Diseases Associated with Unusual Odors

DISEASE	ENZYME DEFECT	ODOR	CLINICAL FEATURES	TREATMENT
Diabetes mellitus	Lack of insulin or insulin activity	Acetone on breath	Polyuria, polyphagia, polydipsia, weight loss, acidosis, coma	Insulin administration
Phenylketonuria	Phenylalanine hydroxylase	Musty, "mousy," "horsey"	Progressive mental retardation, eczema, decreased pigmentation, seizures, spasticity	Diet low in phenylalanine
Maple syrup urine disease	Branched chain decarboxylase	Maple syrup	Marked acidosis, seizures, coma leading to death in first year or two of life or mental subnormality without acidosis or intermittent acidosis without mental retardation	Diet low in branched chain amino acids; protein restriction and/or thiamine in large doses
Oasthouse urine disease	Defective transport of methionine, branched chain amino acids, tyrosine, and phenylalanine	Yeast-like Dried-celery-like	Mental retardation, spasticity, hyperpnea, fever, edema	Restrict methionine in diet
Odor of sweaty feet, Syndrome I	Isovaleryl CoA dehydrogenase	Sweaty feet	Recurrent bouts of acidosis, vomiting, dehydration, coma, aversion to protein foods	Restrict leucine in diet
Odor of sweaty feet, Syndrome II	Green acyldehydrogenase	Sweaty feet	Onset of symptoms in first week of life with acidosis, dehydration, seizures, and death	High CHO diet(?) Low fat diet(?)

4

Syndrome	Enzyme defect	Odor	Clinical features	Treatment
Odor of cats syndrome	Beta-methyl-crotonyl-CoA carboxylase	Cat's urine	Neurologic disorder resembling Werdnig-Hoffmann disease, ketoacidosis, failure to thrive	Leucine restriction(?) Biotin administration
Fish odor syndrome	Unknown	Like dead fish	Stigmata of Turner's syndrome, neutropenia, recurrent infections, anemia, splenomegaly	Unknown
Fish odor syndrome	Trimethylamine oxidase	Like dead fish	Unusual odor of sweat, skin and urine. Normal development	Elimination of fish from the diet
Odor of rancid butter syndrome	Unknown	Rancid butter	Poor feeding, irritability, progressive neurologic deterioration with seizures and death; hepatic dysfunction; possibly same as acute tyrosinosis	Response to decreased phenylalanine and tyrosine intake(?)

"The childhood shows the man as morning shows the day."

Milton

CHANGES IN URINE COLOR

Parents as well as children may become alarmed when they note a change in the color of urine. Many drugs and natural substances can produce such alterations. A partial list of such agents and the colors they produce is given below.

URINE COLOR	DRUG OR CHEMICAL
Blue	Methylene blue Triamterene (Dyrenium)
Brown to black	Metronidazole (Flagyl) Nitrites Nitrofurans Phenacetin Rhubarb Senna
Green (blue plus yellow)	Amitriptyline (Elavil) Bile pigments Methocarbamol (Robaxin)
Purple	Phenolphthalein (urine pH $<$8.0)
Orange	Phenazopyridine (Pyridium)
Orange to red-brown	Rifampin Warfarin sodium
Pink to red to red-brown	Aminopyrine Cascara Deferoxamine (Desferal) Methyldopa (Aldomet) Phenazopyridine hydrochloride (Pyridium in acid urine) Phenolphthalein (urine pH $>$8.0) Phenothiazines Diphenylhydantoin (Dilantin) Senna (alkaline urine) Urates
Yellow or brownish	Aminosalicylic acid Bismuth Mercury Bilirubin Sulfonamides
Yellow or green	Methylene blue Carotene-containing foods

Pink	Beta-cyanine (beet pigment) in patients
	  with genetic defect or in children
	  with iron deficiency

Reference: Shirkey, H.C. (Ed.): Pediatric Therapy. 5th Ed. St. Louis, C.V. Mosby Company, 1975, p. 226.

THE THREE-STAGE CHEMICAL EVOLUTION OF RICKETS

Stage 1 (Intestinal Calcium Transport Decreased)

Serum calcium decreased
Serum phosphorus normal
Serum alkaline phosphatase normal
X-ray — normal
Tetany may occur

Stage 2 (Compensatory Hyperparathyroidism)

Serum calcium normal
Serum phosphorus decreased
Serum alkaline phosphatase increased
Serum bicarbonate decreased
Serum chloride increased
Aminoaciduria
X-ray — active rickets

Stage 3 (Parathyroid Response No Longer Sustains Normal Serum Calcium)

Serum calcium decreased
Serum phosphorus decreased
Serum alkaline phosphatase increased
Serum bicarbonate decreased
Serum chloride increased
Aminoaciduria
X-ray — florid rickets
Tetany may occur

References: Bergstrom, W.: Personal communication. Fraser, D., and Salter, R.B.: Pediatr. Clin. North Am., 5:417, 1958.

Rickets—or avitaminosis D, is named for its discoverer, Dr. Rickets, an "empiric" country practitioner in 17th century England. The term "rachitis," later applied to the same condition, was an apparent attempt by the medical profession to substitute a proper Latinized name for the more plebian rickets.

BLUE DIAPERS — A CLUE TO SYSTEMIC DISEASE

Blue diapers are seen in a variety of disorders. The "blue diaper syndrome" has been ascribed to the indican pigment seen in the urine of individuals with familial hypercalcemia and nephrocalcinosis. Actually, blue diapers can result from pigments in either the urine or stool. Stools with heavy growths of pseudomonas may stain the diapers blue. *Pseudomonas aeruginosa* produces two pigments — fluorescein (blue-green) and pyocyanine (dark blue). Urinary copper (such as in the copper-popper syndrome), amitryptyline, methylene blue, and tolonium may also cause blue discoloration of the urine, as do some dyes used as food coloring.

Reference: Baist, N. R., Bellinger, J. F., and Ramberg, D. A.: J. Pediatr., *81:*622, 1972.

CAROTENEMIA

Carotenemia is a benign condition caused by the ingestion of large amounts of food containing carotene. Carotene is a vitamin A precursor that is present in a variety of foods. Prepared infant foods often contain carotene-rich vegetables and fruits. Since gastrointestinal absorption of carotene is enhanced by cooking, puréeing, or mashing, infant foods provide an especially rich source of carotene.

Carotene deposition is usually detected first on the tip of the nose, the palms, the soles, the nasolabial folds, and the forehead. The yellow pigment may also be found on the chin, behind the ears, over the knuckles, and on the breasts, abdomen, and buttocks. Carotenemia may be distinguished from jaundice by the absence of scleral pigmentation in the former condition. If foods containing carotene are withdrawn from the diet, the skin reverts to normal color in two to six weeks.

The following is a list of foods containing carotene.

FOODS WITH HIGH CAROTENE CONTENT

Vegetables
Alfalfa
Asparagus
Beans, green and yellow
Beet greens
Broccoli
Carrots
Chard
Collard greens
Cucumbers
Endive
Escarole
Kale
Lettuce
Mustard
Parsley
Pumpkins
Rutabagas
Spinach
Squash
Sweet potatoes
Turnip tops
Watercress

Fruits
Apricots
Cantaloupes
Mangoes
Oranges
Papaya
Peaches
Prunes
Others
Butter
Eggs
Milk
Palm oil
Yellow corn

Deposition of carotene in the skin out of proportion to the amount of carotene in the diet has been associated with hypothyroidism and diabetes mellitus. Other diseases apparently predispose to carotenemia for reasons that are unknown. The following is a list of diseases that have been associated with carotenemia.

DISEASES ASSOCIATED WITH CAROTENEMIA
Hypothyroidism
Hypopituitarism
Diabetes mellitus
Liver disease
Nephrotic syndrome
Nephritis
Anorexia nervosa
Hypothalamic amenorrhea
Castration in males
Inborn error of metabolism

Reference: Lascari, A.D.: Clin. Pediatr. *20:*25, 1981.

GREEN HAIR

Green hair is as amazing to the physician as it is to the patient. It was noted as early as the 1800s, when there were scattered reports of it occurring in copper workers. In the early 1970s a small epidemic was reported at a state college in Framingham, Massachusetts. Most of the patients were women with "blond" hair whose "condition" occurred after the town had fluoridated its water supply. The fluorine acidified the water, which subsequently leached copper from piping. The copper was then deposited onto the hair during routine showering. The condition may be produced by chlorinated pool water in which copper-based algicides are used or by water that has a pH level so low that it leaches appreciable amounts of copper from the piping. Brass and mercury have also been associated with green hair.

You can suggest assaying the hair and water for copper content. Normal hair copper values range between 4 and 128 mg/kg hair. However, there is a simpler and less expensive alternative: tell your patient to stop swimming or showering in the offending water, and the green color will gradually fade from the hair with daily shampooing in copper-free water.

References: Lampe, R.M., Henderson, A.L., and Hansen, G.H.: J.A.M.A., *237:*2092, 1977. Parish, L.C.: N. Engl. J. Med., *292:*483, 1975. Cooper, R., and Goodman, J.: N. Engl. J. Med., *292:*483, 1975. Goldsmith, L.W., and Holmes, L.B.: N. Engl. J. Med., *292:*484, 1975.

5
THE
NEWBORN

THE JITTERY INFANT

It is frequently necessary to distinguish between the jittery infant and the infant with seizures. The movements of the jittery infant are characterized by tremulousness and, occasionally, by clonus. Keeping the following characteristics of jitteriness in mind can help in the distinction between these two conditions.

	JITTERINESS	SEIZURE
Abnormal gaze or eye movement	No	Usually
Stimulus-sensitive	Exquisitely	No
Predominant movements	Tremor	Clonic jerking
On passive flexion	Usually ceases	No change

The most commonly defined causes of jitteriness:

Hypoxic-ischemic encephalopathy
Hypocalcemia
Hypoglycemia
Drug withdrawal

Reference: Volpe, J.J.: Mead Johnson Symposium on Perinatal and Developmental Medicine, No. 6, 1974, p. 61.

RAPID ASSESSMENT OF GESTATIONAL AGE AT BIRTH

Determination of gestational age on the basis of time from the last menstrual period is fraught with many potential errors. Only in 85 per cent of cases is the date of the last menstrual period accurate. For this reason, assessment of gestational age on the basis of physical examination has become both popular and necessary. Some methods of scoring gestational age are time-consuming and potentially disturbing to a critically ill infant. Described below is a scoring system that is quite simple and sufficiently accurate. It is based upon a determination of the maturational characteristics of just four parameters: skin texture, skin color, breast size, and ear firmness. The total score in these areas permits an estimation of gestational age. The schema below is most accurate for infants of greater than 30 weeks gestation.

*Scoring of the Four Characteristics for Assessing
Gestational Age*

Skin texture. Tested by picking up a fold of abdominal skin between finger and thumb and by inspection.

0: very thin, with a gelantinous feel

1: thin and smooth

2: smooth and of medium thickness; irritation rash and superficial peeling may be present

3: slight thickening and stiff feeling with superficial cracking and peeling especially evident on hands and feet

4: thick and parchmentlike, with superficial or deep cracking

Skin color. Estimated by inspection when the baby is quiet.

0: dark red

1: uniformly pink

2: pale pink, although color may vary over different parts of body; some parts may be very pale

3: pale, nowhere really pink except on ears, lips, palms and soles

Breast size. Measured by picking up the breast tissue between finger and thumb.

0: no breast tissue palpable

1: breast tissue palpable on one or both sides, neither being more than 0.5 cm in diameter

2: breast tissue palpable on both sides, one or both being 0.5 to 1 cm in diameter

3: breast tissue palpable on both sides, one or both being more than 1 cm in diameter

Ear firmness. Tested by palpation and folding of the upper pinna.

0: pinna feels soft and is easily folded into bizarre positions without springing back into position spontaneously

1: pinna feels soft along the edge and is easily folded but returns slowly to correct position spontaneously

2: cartilage can be felt to the edge of the pinna, although it is thin in places and the pinna springs back readily after being folded

3: pinna firm, with definite cartilage extending to the periphery, and springs back immediately into position after being folded

*Mean Gestational Ages Derived from Total Scores of Skin
Color, Skin Texture, Ear Firmness and Breast Size*

SCORE	GESTATIONAL AGE	
	(d)	(w)
1	190	27
2	210	30
3	230	33
4	240	34½
5	250	36
6	260	37
7	270	38½
8	276	39½
9	281	40
10	285	41
11	290	41½
12	295	42

Reference: Parkin, J. M., Hey, E. N., and Clowes, E. S.: Arch. Dis. Child., *51:*259, 1976.

A DIAGNOSTIC APPROACH TO NEONATAL JAUNDICE

Determining the cause of jaundice in newborns is a recurrent diagnostic problem. In view of the fact that a variety of disorders may produce elevated bilirubin concentrations, an orderly and systematic evaluation is required in order to minimize unnecessary laboratory studies and most rapidly reach a correct diagnosis. The following guidelines may be employed.

Which Infants Require Diagnostic Evaluation

1. All patients with clinical evidence of jaundice during the first 24 hours of life.
2. All infants in whom the total serum bilirubin increases by more than 5 mg/dl per day.
3. All term infants in whom the serum bilirubin exceeds 12 mg/dl.
4. All premature infants in whom the serum bilirubin exceeds 15 mg/dl.
5. All infants in whom phototherapy is employed.
6. All infants in whom the conjugated bilirubin fraction exceeds 2 mg/dl.
7. All term infants in whom clinical jaundice persists beyond the first week of life, and all premature infants in whom clinical jaundice persists beyond the second week of life.

DATA COLLECTION SHEET FOR THE EVALUATION OF THE JAUNDICED INFANT

It is easy to forget an important item in the history, physical examination, and laboratory studies of the jaundiced infant. This checklist can help you from "leaving undone those things that ought to have been done."

Data Collection Sheet for the Jaundiced Infant

DATA

Mother
  Blood group and blood type
  Maternal serology
  History of previous pregnancies with respect to neonatal jaundice
  Race and/or ethnic origin
  Illness in pregnancy
  Drugs in pregnancy
  History of anemia or jaundice in family

Delivery
  Premature rupture of membranes
  Vacuum extraction
  Oxytocins
  Other drugs and anesthetics
  Apgar score

Infant Physical Examination
  General appearance (activity, cry, suck, hydration, plethora, pallor)
  Enclosed hemorrhage – cephalhematoma, ecchymoses
  Head size, length, weight
  Estimate of gestational age
  Fundi–chorioretinitis
  Liver and spleen size
  Umbilical stump
  Congenital anomalies

Infant History
  Age when jaundice first noted
  Vomiting
  Frequency, volume, and type of feeding
  Number of stools noted
  Drugs given to infant
  Was phototherapy employed prior to diagnostic procedures?
  Was hemoglobin followed sequentially?
  Was hemoglobin obtained at discharge?

Laboratory Studies

Blood type of infant, direct and indirect Coombs' test
Serology of cord blood
Bilirubin — Was conjugated fraction ever determined?
Hemoglobin
Reticulocyte count
Smear morphology
White cell count and differential
Comment regarding platelets
Urine-reducing substance
Any evaluation of sepsis (LP, cultures, IgM, serology)
G-6-PD screen
Hemoglobin electrophoresis
Consultations

A Schematic Approach to the Diagnosis of Neonatal Jaundice

Review maternal history, family history, facts of labor and delivery, infant's caloric intake, and stool history, and perform physical examination.

Initial laboratory studies: Hemoglobin, hematocrit, reticulocyte count, peripheral blood smear, white cell count and differential, urine for reducing substance, direct and indirect Coombs' test, maternal and infant blood groups.

Prolonged Jaundice

Consider: Hepatitis, biliary atresia, Down's syndrome, hypothyroidism, breast milk inhibitors, Crigler-Najjar syndrome, cyanotic heart disease, cystic fibrosis, alpha$_1$-antitrypsin deficiency.

Schematic Approach to the Diagnosis of Neonatal Jaundice

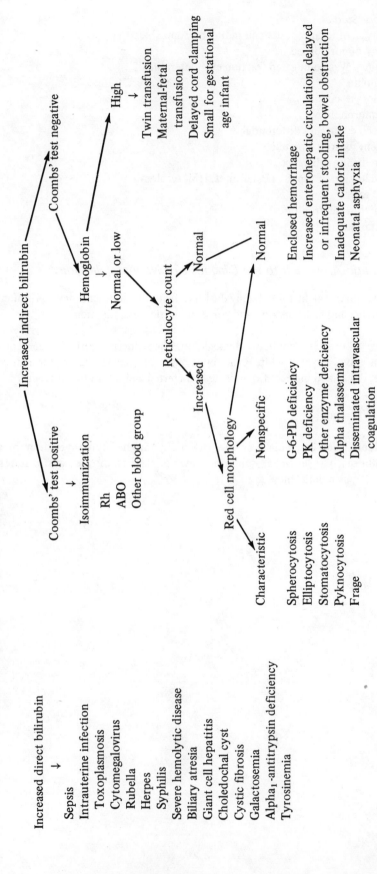

THE USE OF CLINICAL DATA IN DIAGNOSIS OF NEONATAL JAUNDICE

Once a methodical collection of data has taken place, the significance of the information must be appreciated. The tables below indicate what your findings should suggest.

Clinical Data

INFORMATION	SIGNIFICANCE
Family History	
Parent or sibling with history of jaundice or anemia	Suggests hereditary hemolytic anemia, such as hereditary spherocytosis
Previous sibling with neonatal jaundice	Suggests hemolytic disease due to ABO or Rh isoimmunization
History of liver disease in siblings or disorders such as cystic fibrosis, galactosemia, tyrosinemia, hyper-methioninemia, Crigler-Najjar syndrome, or alpha$_1$-antitrypsin deficiency	All associated with neonatal hyperbilirubinemia
Maternal History	
Unexplained illness during pregnancy	Consider congenital infections such as rubella, cytomegalovirus, toxoplasmosis, herpes, syphilis, or hepatitis
Diabetes mellitus	Increased incidence of jaundice among infants of diabetic mothers
Drug ingestion during pregnancy	Ingestion of sulfonamides, nitrofurantoins, or antimalarials may initiate hemolysis in G-6-PD deficient infant
History of Labor and Delivery	
Vacuum extraction	Increased incidence of cephalhematoma and jaundice
Oxytocin-induced labor	Increased incidence of hyperbilirubinemia
Delayed cord clamping	Increased incidence of hyperbilirubinemia among polycythemic infants
Apgar score	Increased incidence of jaundice in asphyxiated infants
Infant's History	
Delayed passage of meconium or infrequent stools	Increased enterohepatic circulation of bilirubin. Consider intestinal atresia, annular pancreas, Hirschsprung's disease, meconium plug, drug-induced ileus (hexamethonium)
Caloric intake	Inadequate caloric intake results in delay in bilirubin conjugation
Vomiting	Suspect sepsis, galactosemia, or pyloric stenosis; all associated with hyperbilirubinemia
Infant's Physical Examination	
Small for gestational age	Infants frequently polycythemic and jaundiced
Head size	Microcephaly seen with intrauterine infections associated with jaundice
Cephalhematoma	Entrapped hemorrhage associated with hyper-bilirubinemia
Pallor	Suspect hemolytic anemia

5

Petechiae	Suspect congenital infection, overwhelming sepsis, or severe hemolytic disease as cause of jaundice
Appearance of umbilical stump	Omphalitis and sepsis may produce jaundice
Hepatosplenomegaly	Suspect hemolytic anemia or congenital infection
Optic fundi	Chorioretinitis suggests congenital infection as cause of jaundice
Umbilical hernia	Consider hypothyroidism
Congenital anomalies	Jaundice occurs with increased frequency among infants with trisomic conditions

Laboratory Data

INFORMATION	SIGNIFICANCE
Maternal	
Blood group and indirect Coombs' test	Necessary for evaluation of possible ABO or Rh incompatibility
Serology	Rule out congenital syphilis
Infant	
Hemoglobin	Anemia suggests hemolytic disease or large entrapped hemorrhage. Hemoglobin above 22 gm/100 ml associated with increased incidence of jaundice
Reticulocyte count	Elevation suggests hemolytic disease
Red cell morphology	Spherocytes suggest ABO incompatibility or hereditary spherocytosis. Red cell fragmentation seen in disseminated intravascular coagulation
Platelet count	Thrombocytopenia suggests infection
White cell count	Total white cell count less than 5000/mm^3 or increase in band forms to greater than 2000/mm^3 suggests infection
Sedimentation rate	Values in excess of 5 during the first 48 hours indicate infection or ABO incompatibility
Direct bilirubin	Elevation suggests infection or severe Rh incompatibility
Immunoglobulin M	Elevation indicates infection
Blood group and direct and indirect Coombs' test	Required to rule out hemolytic disease as a result of isoimmunization
Carboxyhemoglobin	Elevated in infants with hemolytic disease or entrapped hemorrhage
Urinalysis	Presence of reducing substance suggests diagnosis of galactosemia

PROGRESSION OF DERMAL ICTERUS IN THE NEWBORN

The rate of rise of serum bilirubin in the newborn infant who is jaundiced should always be monitored by laboratory determinations. The pediatrician, however, through simple examination of the infant, may make some estimation as to the rate of rise of serum bilirubin.

Dermal icterus has been shown to progress in a cephalopedal fashion; that is, as the infant's bilirubin rises, more of the skin becomes icteric. The icterus begins at the head and neck and progresses caudally to the palms and soles. The following table correlates the level of indirect bilirubin with the area of skin that is icteric in full-term infants whose jaundice is not due to Rh incompatibility.

AREA OF THE BODY	RANGE OF INDIRECT BILIRUBIN (mg/100 ml)
Head and neck	4–8
Upper trunk	5–12
Lower trunk and thighs	8–16
Arms and lower legs	11–18
Palms and soles	>15

As icterus progresses, the area that had been jaundiced remains jaundiced, so that the entire body is icteric when the bilirubin rises above 15 mg/100 ml. The fading of the icterus as the bilirubin level falls affects all body areas at the same time, so that the intensity rather than the extent of the staining fades. The staining may progress more rapidly in the low birth weight infant, while the infant with Rh disease may demonstrate a relative lag in dermal staining.

Correct estimation of the extent of icterus involves the examination of the completely undressed infant under blue-white fluorescent light. Icterus may be detected by blanching the skin with pressure of the thumb and noting the color of the underlying skin. This is a more difficult determination to make in deeply pigmented black infants, but the palms and soles, at least, may be easily examined even in these patients.

Reference: Kramer, L.I.: Am. J. Dis. Child., *18*:454, 1969.

COMPARISON OF Rh AND ABO BLOOD GROUP INCOMPATIBILITY

If jaundice is noted in an infant at birth or shortly thereafter, blood group incompatibility between mother and infant may well be the cause. The following table compares the findings and recommended treatment in Rh and ABO incompatibility.

	Rh	ABO
Blood Group Setup		
Mother	Negative	O
Infant	Positive	A or B
Type of Antibody	Incomplete (7S)	Immune (7S)
Clinical Aspects		
Occurrence in first-born	5%	40–50%
Predictable severity in subsequent pregnancies	Usually	No
Stillbirth and/or hydrops	Frequent	Rare
Severe anemia	Frequent	Rare
Degree of jaundice	+++	+
Hepatosplenomegaly	+++	+
Laboratory Findings		
Direct Coombs' test (infant)	+	(+) or 0
Maternal antibodies	Always present	Not clear-cut
Spherocytes	0	+
Treatment		
Need for antenatal measures	Yes	No
Exchange transfusion		
Frequency	Approx. 2/3	Approx. 1/10
Donor blood type	Rh-negative	Rh — same as infant
	Group specific, when possible	Group O only
Incidence of late anemia	Common	Rare

THE MULTIPLE CAUSES OF HYDROPS FETALIS

As Rh isoimmunization becomes less common, the other causes of hydrops fetalis take on added diagnostic significance. The following are other recognized causes at birth of a grossly edematous newborn infant.

5

Severe Chronic Anemia In Utero

Isoimmunization due to ABO incompatibility or other blood groups
Homozygous alpha thalassemia
Fetal to maternal hemorrhage
G-6-PD deficiency with maternal drug ingestion

Cardiac Failure

Severe congenital heart disease
Premature closure of foramen ovale
Large arteriovenous malformation
Prolonged supraventricular tachycardia

Hypoproteinemia

Renal disease (congenital nephrosis, renal vein thrombosis)
Congenital hepatitis

Intrauterine Infections

Syphilis
Toxoplasmosis
Cytomegalovirus

Other

Maternal diabetes mellitus
Umbilical or chorionic vein thrombosis
Fetal neuroblastomatosis
Chagas' disease
Achondroplasia
Cystic adenomatoid malformation of the lung
Pulmonary lymphangiectasia
Choriocarcinoma in situ
Congenital Gaucher's disease
Urethral atresia
Placental chorioangioma

DETECTION OF ALPHA THALASSEMIA TRAIT IN THE NEWBORN

Heterozygotes for alpha thalassemia compose 2 to 7 per cent of the black population in America. Although this abnormality causes only minor hematologic changes, it may produce a mild microcytic anemia unresponsive to iron therapy.

Alpha thalassemia trait may be detected in the newborn by the identification of greater than 2 per cent hemoglobin Barts (tetramers of gamma chains) on hemoglobin electrophoresis. After the newborn period, the diagnosis is possible only on evaluation of globin chain synthesis.

Evaluation of red cell indices constitutes an efficient screening test for alpha thalassemia. *If the mean corpuscular volume of a black newborn is less than 94 μ^3, a hemoglobin electrophoresis should be performed.* Approximately 67 per cent of these infants will be heterozygotes for alpha thalassemia.

Reference: Schmaier, A.H., Maurer, H.M., Johnston, C.L., et al.: J. Pediatr., *83*:794, 1973.

NORMAL HEMOGLOBIN VALUES IN THE PREMATURE INFANT

How low does the hemoglobin level go in a healthy premature infant during the first 6 to 10 weeks of life? The experience at the Upstate Medical Center is depicted in Figure 5-1. All 50 infants studied had birth weights of less than 1500 grams. None had evidence of isoimmunization. All had hemoglobin values greater than 13.0 gm/dl on the eighth day of life. None were vitamin E deficient or had other nutritional causes for anemia. The solid line represents the mean value, while the shaded area represents all values recorded. It should be noted that the lowest mean hemoglobin value is reached at approximately 6 weeks of age. No infant had a hemoglobin value of less than 8.6 gm/dl at any time. The mean hemoglobin remained above 10.0 gm/dl. When hemoglobin values fall below 8.5 gm/dl during this period of life, something is wrong — a systematic search for an explanation will often be rewarded.

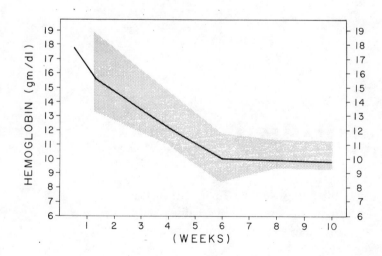

FIG. 5-1

THE NORMAL LEUKOCYTE COUNT IN THE NEWBORN

It is gradually being appreciated that the white blood cell count provides diagnostic information during the first week of life. Variations from normal, either increases or decreases in the total number of polymorphonuclear leukocytes or elevations in the band count, are usually a sign of infection. The following values can be used as a guide to normal values.

WEIGHT	AGE	ABSOLUTE NEUTROPHIL COUNT (mm³)	ABSOLUTE BAND COUNT (mm³)	B/N RATIO
Less than 2500 gm	0–96 hours	Up to 12,000	Up to 1,400	Up to 0.17
	>96 hours	2,000 – 4.700	<500	Up to 0.14
More than 2500 gm	0–96 hours	Up to 14,000	Up to 1,400	Up to 0.17
	>96 hours	2,400 – 4,500	<500	Up to 0.14

Elevations in counts were seen in noninfectious disorders, such as infants of diabetic mothers, meconium aspirations, hyaline membrane disease, hypoglycemia, neonatal seizures, and infants with 5-minute Apgar scores of 6 or less. In the absence of these complications, the presence of increased B/N ratios or increases or decreases in the absolute neutrophil count or increases in the absolute band count should be an indication for culturing of the infant and the initiation of antibiotic therapy. Low absolute neutrophil counts are currently most commonly associated with group B streptococcal sepsis.

Reference: Manroe, B., Browne, R., Weinberg, A.G., et al.: Pediatr. Res., *10*:428, 1976.

CONGENITAL INFECTION

The signs of congenital infection are varied. Diagnosis often depends upon history and physical examination. Use of the following table should facilitate your clinical evaluation.

DISEASE	TIME OF TRANSMISSION	TERATOGENIC EFFECTS	OTHER MANIFESTATIONS	LABORATORY DIAGNOSIS
Rubella	First trimester; early second trimester (problematical)	Cataracts, glaucoma, retinopathy, microphthalmia, microcephaly, congenital heart disease	Thrombocytopenia, hepatosplenomegaly, hepatitis, pneumonia, bone destruction, encephalitis, growth retardation	HI antibody, specific IgM antibody, viral isolation from body fluids
Toxoplasmosis	Throughout pregnancy	Microcephaly, hydrocephaly, cerebral calcifications, chorioretinitis	Encephalitis, myocarditis, hepatosplenomegaly, jaundice, diarrhea, vomiting, convulsions	CF, HI antibody, IgM-FTA specific antibody, placental culture
Cytomegalovirus	Throughout pregnancy	Microcephaly, cerebral calcifications, chorioretinitis	Same as toxoplasmosis	Isolation of virus from urine, specific IgM antibody
Herpes simplex	Intrapartum; ascending and direct contact	None	Cutaneous lesions (vesicles), visceral involvement, encephalitis, pneumonia, thrombocytopenia	Isolation of virus from throat, urine, vesicular lesions, CSF
Varicella	Intrapartum	Limb deformities?	Skin lesions, encephalomyocarditis, visceral involvement, pneumonia	Growth of virus on tissue culture, rise in maternal or infant's antibody

		Delayed effects on eyes, ears, teeth, joints, CNS	Osteochondritis, jaundice, hepatosplenomegaly, lymphadenopathy, rhagades, anemia	Darkfield examination for spirochetes, FTA-ABS, TPI immobilization
Syphilis	Second half of pregnancy	Delayed effects on eyes, ears, teeth, joints, CNS	Osteochondritis, jaundice, hepatosplenomegaly, lymphadenopathy, rhagades, anemia	Darkfield examination for spirochetes, FTA-ABS, TPI immobilization
Listeria	Intrapartum	Not known	Sepsis, meningitis, hepatitis, diffuse granulomatosis	Isolation of bacteria from blood, urine, or pus.
Gonococcus	Last trimester and at delivery	Not known	Sepsis, conjunctivitis, panophthalmitis	Gram stain and culture (Thayer-Martin medium)
Tuberculosis	Rarely transplacental; usually following delivery	Not known	Fever, anemia, pulmonary and systemic dissemination	Isolation of organism from gastric washing or maternal lesions, PPD unreliable during neonatal period

Reference: Revised from Evans, H.E., and Glass, L.: Mechanisms of infection. *In* Perinatal Medicine. New York, Harper & Row, 1976, p. 341.

THE DIAGNOSIS OF CONGENITAL SYPHILIS

The diagnosis of congenital syphilis can be made if:

1. Darkfield examination of the suspicious lesions is positive.
2. Infant's serologic titer is higher than the maternal titer.
3. Infant's titer is sustained during the first months of life.
4. Infant has a confirmed reactive serologic test after an initial negative test.
5. Infant has a confirmed serologic test at 3 months of age.

Remember, if the reagin antibody has been passively transferred, the serologic reaction will be negative in:

90 per cent of infants at 1 month of age
98 per cent of infants at 2 months of age
99 per cent of infants at 3 months of age

If the infant is infected, the serologic reaction will be positive in:

85 per cent of infants at 1 month of age
95 per cent of infants at 2 months of age
100 per cent of infants at 3 months of age

Reference: Solomon, L.M., and Esterly, N.B.: Neonatal Dermatology. Philadelphia, W.B. Saunders Company, 1973, p. 160.

PERSISTENT RHINITIS IN THE NEWBORN

Nasal congestion and rhinorrhea in the newborn may be a difficult problem, since neonates are often obligate nose breathers. The causes of persistent rhinitis in the newborn are listed below along with the treatment of each type.

ENTITY	CAUSE	TREATMENT
Transient idiopathic stuffy nose of the newborn	Unknown	Normal saline nosedrops may be instilled and then removed after a few minutes with cotton-tipped applicators or gentle suction on a rubber bulb syringe. If the congestion interferes with feeding, 2 drops of 0.125 per cent phenylephrine (Neo-Synephrine) may be instilled in the nose just before meals for several days.
Reserpine side-effects	Caused by mother's taking reserpine	Same as above.
Chemical rhinitis	Due to overtreatment of idiopathic stuffy nose with topical nasoconstrictors	Discontinue nosedrops. Use oral decongestants for 2 days.
Pyogenic rhinitis	These infants have bacterial infection despite absence of purulent discharge. Diagnose via cultures of discharge	Same as for idiopathic stuffy nose.
Congenital syphilis	Maternal syphilis	Penicillin.
Hypothyroidism	Congenital hypothyroidism	Thyroid hormone replacement.
Choanal atresia	Congenital defect	Place oral airway immediately. Definitive surgery by otolaryngologist.
Nasal fracture	Birth trauma	Diagnose by examination for subluxation of the nasal septum causing occlusion of the nasal passages. Refer to otolaryngologist.

Reference: Schmitt, B.D.: *In* Kempe, C.H., Silver, H.K., and O'Brien, D. (Eds.): Current Pediatric Diagnosis and Treatment. Los Altos, California, Lange Medical Publications, 1976, p. 251.

SCLEREMA NEONATORUM

Sclerema neonatorum is a condition that affects premature or debilitated newborn infants or older infants suffering from severe disease. Infants so affected have smooth, cool, tense, mottled purplish, hard skin that is apparently adherent to the subcutaneous tissues. The skin does not pit, nor can it be pinched into a fold. The process usually begins on the lower extremities and spreads peripherally through the fatty subcutaneous tissues. Sclerema neonatorum is a sign of life-threatening disease, and when it is noted, efforts should be made to identify the disease process.

1. The infant should be assumed to be infected until proved otherwise, and multiple cultures should be taken prior to the institution of antibiotic therapy.

2. Careful investigation should be made for congenital anomalies or signs of trauma so that appropriate treatment may be instituted.

3. Supportive measures, such as maintenance of optimum environmental temperatures, administration of intravenous fluids and blood when indicated, and digitalization if necessary, should be undertaken. Corticosteroids have not been shown to be of value, except when there is evidence of adrenal insufficiency.

Sclerema neonatorum should be distinguished from necrosis of fat that occurs in healthy infants during the first few months of life. Hardened areas attached to the skin but not to the deeper tissue develop over the bony prominences of the infant's body. These areas of fat necrosis disappear gradually, but may soften and become cystic before dissolving completely.

Sclerema neonatorum should also be differentiated from scleredema. Scleredema refers to a pitting edema that is usually generalized and occurs primarily in premature infants. The limbs affected by scleredema are swollen.

In the infant who is already moribund, sclerema neonatorum is a sign of impending death.

Reference: Warwick, W.J., Ruttenberg, H.D., and Quie, P.G.: J.A.M.A., *184*:680, 1963.

DISORDERS ASSOCIATED WITH BREECH PRESENTATION

5

The pediatrician summoned to be present for the breech delivery of an infant who is subsequently diagnosed as having the trisomy 18 syndrome may question the association of breech presentation and other disorders. A variety of anomalies and syndromes are more frequently present in infants presenting feet first:

Prader-Willi syndrome
Trisomy 13 syndrome
Trisomy 18 syndrome
Trisomy 21 syndrome
Smith-Lemli-Opitz syndrome
Fetal alcohol syndrome
Potter anomaly
Zellweger syndrome
Myotonic dystrophy
Werdnig-Hoffmann syndrome
de Lange syndrome
Familial dysautonomia
Hydrocephalus
Congenital dislocation of the hip
Anencephaly
Meningomyelocele

Breech presentation is also associated with:

Multiple births
Oligohydramnios
Polyhydramnios
Bicornuate or double uterus
Placenta previa

Normally, about 2.5 per cent of term infants are breech presentations. The frequency is two to three times higher in the smaller premature infants. The frequency of major malformations is three times as high as in those born in the vertex position. This difference is not the result of prematurity. The neonatal mortality rate for infants born by breech presentation is about 12 times the mortality rate in nonbreech deliveries. There is a 50 per cent incidence of major malformations in term infants who die after breech delivery. The frequency of neurologic abnormalities and motor retardation at age one year is 63 per cent higher in infants born by breech than by vertex presentation.

Reference: Braun, F.H.T., Jones, K.L., and Smith, D.W.: J. Pediatr., *86*:419, 1975.

NEONATAL CYANOTIC CONGENITAL HEART DISEASE

Cyanosis in the newborn may be a manifestation of a variety of disorders. Central nervous system disease, pulmonary disease, and anatomic lesions such as tracheoesophageal fistula and diaphragmatic hernia must be ruled out. If the cyanosis is considered to be of cardiac origin, the most likely anomaly may be deduced from the clinical findings, the chest roentgenogram, and the electrocardiogram.

Figure 5-2 lists the more common congenital defects to be expected with their typical physical and laboratory findings.

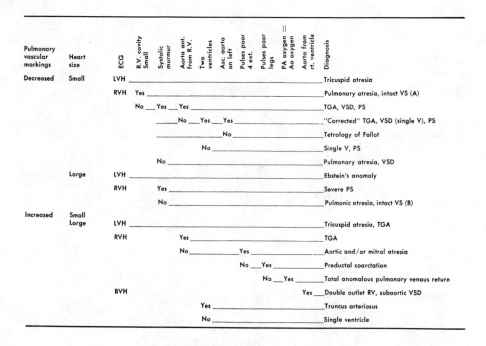

Reference: Rashkind, W.J.: Cardiovasc. Clin., *4*:275, 1972.

FIG. 5-2

TRACHEOESOPHAGEAL FISTULA

The diagnosis of tracheoesophageal fistula may be suggested by a variety of clinical observations. The five types of fistula are depicted in Figure 5-3 along with the symptoms and signs that typically accompany them.

5

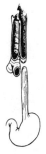

Type A
Symptoms and Signs:

Excessive mucus, aspiration
   of saliva.
Scaphoid abdomen.
No gas in bowel on x-ray.
Cannot pass catheter into
   stomach.
Gradually increasing respira-
   tory distress.
Polyhydramnios.

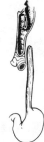

Type B
Symptoms and Signs:

Polyhydramnios.
Coughing, choking, and
   pneumonia from birth.
Scaphoid abdomen.
No gas in bowel on x-ray.

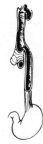

Type C
Symptoms and Signs:

Most common (80% of
   cases).
Excessive mucus.
Gradually increasing respira-
   tory distress.
Polyhydramnios frequent
   but not severe.
Gas in bowel on x-ray.

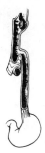

Type D
Symptoms and Signs:

Coughing, choking, and
   pneumonia from birth.
Gas in bowel on x-ray.

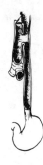
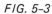

Type E
Symptoms and Signs:

Difficult to diagnose.
Coughing or cyanosis with
   feeding.
Chronic aspiration pneu-
   monia.

FIG. 5-3

The differential diagnosis includes pharyngeal muscle weakness, vascular rings, and esophageal diverticula.

Discovery of a tracheoesophageal fistula should alert the physician to the possibility that other congenital anomalies may be present. Anomalies that have been found to be associated include:

Vertebral
Anal
Cardiac
Renal
Limb

Reference: Brazie, J.V., and Lubchenco, L.O.: *In* Kempe, C.H., Silver, H.K., and O'Brien, D. (Eds.): Current Pediatric Diagnosis and Treatment. Los Altos, California, Lange Medical Publications, 1976, p. 81.

BULLOUS ERUPTIONS IN THE NEWBORN

Bullous eruptions in the neonatal period may be due to a variety of unrelated conditions, and prognosis and treatment vary with each. The following table lists the main points in the differential diagnosis of the major causes of bullous formation in the nursery setting.

Reference: Lewis, I.C., Steven, E.M., and Farquhar, J.W.: Arch. Dis. Child., *30*:277, 1955.

5

DISEASE OR CONDITION	CHARACTER OF LESIONS	DISTRIBUTION	MUCOSAL INVOLVEMENT	OTHER ECTODERMAL DEFECTS	SCARRING	COURSE
Epidermolysis bullosa	Clear blisters; sometimes hemorrhagic noninflammatory base	Sites of trauma or friction	Yes	Yes	Yes or no	Chronic or fatal
Bullous impetigo	Blisters, clear, opaque, purulent	General, particularly flexures	Possible	No	Yes	Short
Congenital syphilis	Bullae and maculo-papules	Palms, soles, trunk, and limbs	Yes	Yes	No (other than rhagades)	Short
Dermatitis herpetiformis	Vesicles and bullae in crops; also urticarial lesions	In infants face and limbs chiefly involved	Sometimes	No	Minimal in long-standing cases	One-third curable. Chronic or recurrent
Burns	Erythema, bullae, desquamation	Anywhere	No	No	Yes, if deep	Depends on type, depth, and therapy
Congenital porphyria	Red urine, photo-sensitivity of skin, erythema, bullae	Areas exposed to sunlight	No	Pigmented teeth	Pigmented scars	Chronic
Erythema multiforme bullosa	Dusky red circinate plaques, papules, bullae	Trunk, limbs, face	Yes	No	No	Short or recurrent
Dermatitis medicamentosa	May be vesicular	No particular site	No	No	No	Short
Papular urticaria	Papules, bullae, vesicles, pustules	Trunk only or limbs	No	No	No	Short or recurrent
Chickenpox	Vesicles, pustules	Trunk, face, limbs	Yes	No	Yes	Short
Smallpox	Vesicles, pustules	Limbs, trunk, face	Yes	No	Yes	Short

DISEASE OR CONDITION	CHARACTER OF LESIONS	DISTRIBUTION	MUCOSAL INVOLVEMENT	OTHER ECTODERMAL DEFECTS	SCARRING	COURSE
Kaposi's varicelliform eruption	Vesicles, pustules	Exposed parts	No	Pre-existing skin disease of infantile eczema or Besnier's prurigo	No	May be fatal
Herpes zoster	Vesicles	Classical girdle	No	No	Yes	Short
Bullous erysipelas	Raised tender erythema, bullae	Periumbilical, limbs, face, trunk	Rarely	Nil	Nil	Short with therapy
Benign familial pemphigus (Hailey's disease)	Vesicles and bullae	Anywhere	No	No	Nil	Benign chronic
Contact dermatitis	Often vesicles and bullae	Anywhere	No	No	No	Short
Phytophoto-dermatitis	Vesicles and bullae	Areas exposed to sunlight	No	No	No	Short
Acrodermatitis enteropathica	Crops scaling, vesiculo-bullous	Near orifices, around eyes, elbows, knees, hands, feet	Yes	Hair scanty	No	May be fatal

BOWEL GAS IN THE NEWBORN

The abdominal roentgenogram of the normal newborn infant reveals considerable bowel gas within three to six hours of birth. The infant swallows air, which is distributed throughout the intestine by peristalsis. Congenital anomalies such as duodenal atresia and tracheo-esophageal fistula may modify the normal gas pattern or even prevent air from entering the intestine at all.

The use of pancuronium bromide (Pavulon) in the intensive care nursery has introduced another cause of the gasless abdomen. Infants paralyzed with pancuronium for more efficient artificial ventilation cannot swallow. The autonomic innervation of the intestine is unaffected by this neuromuscular blocker, however, and the bowel gas that may have been present prior to its administration passes normally out of the gut.

Reference: Dillard, R.G., Crowe, J.E., and Sumner, T.E.: Am. J. Dis. Child., *134:*821, 1980.

DIAGNOSIS OF AMBIGUOUS GENITALIA AT BIRTH

The birth of a child is usually heralded by the welcome words "It's a girl," or "It's a boy." It is at that point that parents begin to define their relationship to their child. If sexual identification is impossible at birth, investigation should be undertaken immediately. The following chart will aid in such an investigation.

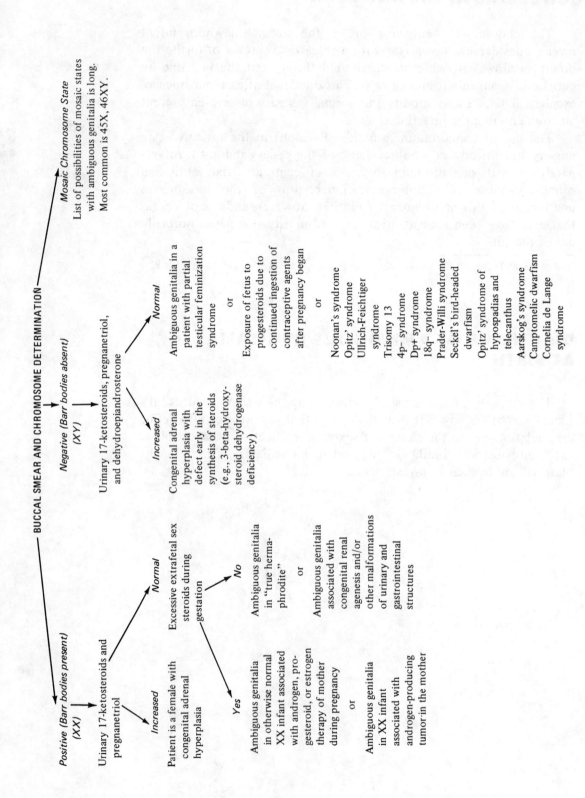

BUCCAL SMEAR AND CHROMOSOME DETERMINATION

Positive (Barr bodies present)
(XX)

Urinary 17-ketosteroids and pregnanetriol

Increased

Patient is a female with congenital adrenal hyperplasia

or

Ambiguous genitalia in otherwise normal XX infant associated with androgen, progesteroid, or estrogen therapy of mother during pregnancy

or

Ambiguous genitalia in XX infant associated with androgen-producing tumor in the mother

Normal

Excessive extrafetal sex steroids during gestation

Yes

No

Ambiguous genitalia in "true hermaphrodite"

or

Ambiguous genitalia associated with congenital renal agenesis and/or other malformations of urinary and gastrointestinal structures

Negative (Barr bodies absent)
(XY)

Urinary 17-ketosteroids, pregnanetriol, and dehydroepiandrosterone

Increased

Congenital adrenal hyperplasia with defect early in the synthesis of steroids (e.g., 3-beta-hydroxy-steroid dehydrogenase deficiency)

Normal

Ambiguous genitalia in a patient with partial testicular feminization syndrome

or

Exposure of fetus to progesteroids due to continued ingestion of contraceptive agents after pregnancy began

or

Noonan's syndrome
Opitz' syndrome
Ullrich-Feichtiger syndrome
Trisomy 13
4p− syndrome
Dp+ syndrome
18q− syndrome
Prader-Willi syndrome
Seckel's bird-headed dwarfism
Opitz' syndrome of hypospadias and telecanthus
Aarskog's syndrome
Camptomelic dwarfism
Cornelia de Lange syndrome

Mosaic Chromosome State

List of possibilities of mosaic states with ambiguous genitalia is long. Most common is 45X, 46XY.

Though the buccal smear evaluation is rapid, its interpretation may be difficult without accompanying karyotype analysis. The sex chromatin stains poorly in the newborn, and the diagnosis of certain mosaic states is difficult without chromosome identification. It is recommended that all newborns with ambiguous genitalia have both buccal smear and chromosome evaluation.

While awaiting the results of laboratory tests, daily serum sodium concentration should be ascertained for all newborns in whom genitalia are abnormal, since adrenal hyperplasia of the salt-losing form is a possible diagnosis. The sodium-losing crisis usually occurs at 8 to 10 days of life in these children.

Urinary 17-ketosteroids and pregnanetriol results are accurate in the second week of life. Rarely, the defect in congenital adrenal hyperplasia must be determined by urinary dehydroepiandrosterone or by chromatographic studies (in 3-beta-hydroxysteroid dehydrogenase defect) or by estimation or urinary or serum compound S (11-hydroxylase defect prior to clinically detectable hypertension).

Any male born with bilateral cryptorchidism, even if the genitalia appear otherwise normal, should have a karyotype analysis.

References: Zurbrügg, R.P.: Congenital adrenal hyperplasia; and Schlegel, R.J., and Gardner, L.I.: Ambiguous and abnormal genitalia. *In* Gardner, L.I. (Ed.): Endocrine and Genetic Diseases of Childhood and Adolescence. Philadelphia, W.B. Saunders Company, 1975.

THE ABDOMINAL MASS IN THE NEWBORN

Approximately one-half of the abdominal masses noted in the neonatal period reflect abnormalities of the genitourinary system. The major abnormalities presenting as an abdominal mass during this period of life are:

Kidney

Hypoplastic multicystic kidney, unilateral or bilateral
Hydronephrosis secondary to distal obstruction
Mesoblastic nephroma
Solitary cyst
Renal vein thrombosis

Liver and Biliary Tract

Hematoma of the liver
Hemangioma of the liver
Solitary cyst of the liver
Hepatoma
Choledochal cyst
Distended gallbladder secondary to cystic fibrosis

Gastrointestinal Tract

Duplication of the duodenum, jejunum, or ileum
Mesenteric cyst
Volvulus secondary to meconium ileus
Leiomyosarcoma of the intestine

Female Genital Tract

Ovarian cyst
Hydro- and hematocolpos

Retroperitoneal Teratomas

Adrenal Hemorrhage

Neuroblastoma

The finding of an abdominal mass in the newborn requires an immediate intravenous pyelogram and ultimate surgical exploration.

It should be noted that malignant tumors are uncommon at birth. Although Wilms' tumor was previously believed to occur with some frequency during this period of life, it is now realized that most of these tumors are mesoblastic nephromas. This tumor is histologically distinct in its fibroblastic appearance and shows only minimal nuclear polymorphism and mitotic activity. Even though these tumors may grow to large size and show evidence of local extension, they do not appear to metastasize, and cure may be achieved with surgery alone.

Reference: Arey, J.B.: Pediatr. Clin. North Am., *10*:665, 1963.

NEONATAL RENAL FAILURE: USEFULNESS OF DIAGNOSTIC INDICES

Separating prerenal from renal causes of oliguria may be difficult even under the best of circumstances. The table demonstrates the usefulness of determining the urinary sodium, urea, creatinine, and the ratios of these to serum, the renal function index (RFI), and fractional excretion of sodium (FENa) in the newborn.

5

SUMMARY OF VARIOUS DIAGNOSTIC INDICES IN NEONATES WITH OLIGURIA

Diagnostic Indices	Renal Failure	Prerenal Oliguria	P Value*
UNa† (mEq/liter)	63.41 ± 34.7	31.41 ± 19.5	<.01
U/S sodium	0.45 ± 0.22	0.23 ± 0.14	<.01
U/S urea	5.78 ± 2.89	29.64 ± 17.90	<.01
U/S creatinine	9.65 ± 3.57	29.24 ± 15.60	<.05
RFI	11.62 ± 9.61	1.29 ± 0.82	<.01
FENa urea	12.11 ± 11.50	1.01 ± 0.63	<.01
FENa creatinine	4.25 ± 2.18	0.95 ± 0.55	<.01

*Student's t-test.
†UNa = urine sodium.

where: RFI = (UNa)/(U/S Cr)
           FENa = (U/S Na)/(U/S Cr) or
                   (U/S Na)/(U/S Urea)
                   × 100 (expressed as percentage)
where: Na   = mEq/L while Cr = mg/dl

Reference: Mathew, O.P., et al.: Pediatrics, *65:*57, 1980.

THE STOMACH VOLUME OF THE INFANT

How big is the infant's stomach? How much can it hold? An infant's stomach is about the size of his fist. Unlike a fist, however, it has the capacity to expand. At birth, the stomach of a normal term infant has a 30 to 60 ml capacity. By the tenth day of life it will hold an amount equal to 3 per cent of the infant's weight, so that an infant

> *Gavage*—From the French word *gavage*, which means forced feeding; and originally derived from *gaver*, which means to gorge.

of 3.5 kg takes with pleasure a feed of 100 ml over a period of 15 minutes.

The 3 per cent rule holds, with some normal variation, during the first 6 months of life.

Reference: MacKeith, R., and Wood, C.: *In* Infant Feeding and Feeding Difficulties, 4th Ed. London, Churchill Livingstone, 1971, p. 20.

A TECHNIQUE FOR THE PALPATION OF THE KIDNEYS OF NEONATES

Congenital malformations of the urogenital tract occur in approximately 12 per cent of all newborns. In 0.5 per cent of all newborns, significant renal anomalies are present. These should be detected early in life in order to avoid subsequent complications. Almost all significant anomalies can be detected by careful abdominal palpation. A simple technique that will enable you to palpate the kidneys of 95 per cent of all neonates is as follows:

1. Support the infant in a semireclining position facing you by placing your left hand behind the infant's shoulders, neck, and occiput.
2. Place the fingers of your right hand in the infant's left costovertebral angle posteriorly.
3. Use the thumb of your right hand to search the infant's abdomen systematically, at first superficially and then deeply.
4. Deep palpation is performed by applying gentle, steadily increasing pressure subcostally in a posterior and cephalad direction. The thumb can then be slipped downward without reducing the posteriorly directed pressure. Usually, the upper pole of the kidney can be felt trapped between the descending thumb and the posteriorly placed fingers.
5. Next, change hands and examine the opposite side of the abdomen.

After practice on some two dozen infants, this technique can be mastered and subsequently performed in 30 seconds. Because of its high yield, it deserves your high skill and attention.

Reference: Perlman, M., and Williams, J.: Br. Med. J., 2:347, 1976.

DELAYED URINATION IN THE NEWBORN

One of the kindest acts a neonate can perform for his pediatrician is to urinate early in life. Ninety-nine to 100 per cent of all normal infants urinate at least once by 48 hours of age. Approximately 23 per cent will void first in the delivery room, and the act may not be reported to the nursery.

Failure to urinate by the first 1 to 2 days of life may be due to obstruction of urine flow or to inability to form urine. Causes of obstruction include

> Imperforate prepuce
> Urethral strictures
> Urethral diverticulum
> Hypertrophy of the verumontanum
> Neurogenic bladder
> "Megacystic syndrome"
> Ureterocele
> Renal tumors
> Cystic kidneys

Inability to form urine may result from

> Postnatal intravascular hypovolemia
> Restriction of oral fluids
> Bilateral renal agenesis
> Cortical necrosis
> Tubular necrosis
> Bilateral renal vein thrombosis
> Congenital nephrotic syndrome
> Congenital pyelonephritis
> Congenital nephritis

Nonspecific symptoms or signs such as excessive crying, irritability, poor feeding, pallor, emesis, mottled skin, or weak pulse may suggest the development of uremia.

The physical examination may be more useful in establishing a specific diagnosis.

Physical Examination

PALPATION OR PERCUSSION OF DISTENDED BLADDER	NO KIDNEYS PALPABLE	PALPABLE RENAL MASS
↓	↓	↓
Obstruction of urine flow	Bilateral renal agenesis	Renal vein thrombosis
↓	These infants are usually males and tend to have lowset ears, epicanthal folds, and a flattened nose	Infantile polycystic kidneys
Examine meatus for patency and look for epispadias or hypospadias		Hydronephoris
		Cystic dysplasia
A urethral diverticulum may give rise to a bulge along the dorsum of the penis		Neoplasm

Reference: Moore, E.S., and Galvez, M.D.: J. Pediatr., *80*:867, 1972.

NEONATAL HEMATURIA

Gross hematuria is a rare presentation during the first month of life. The findings in one series of 35 patients are demonstrated below.

CAUSE	NO. OF PATIENTS	AGE AT ONSET				DURATION (DAYS)	REMARKS
		1st WEEK	2nd WEEK	3rd WEEK	4th WEEK		
Unknown	11	8	2	1	...	1–3	1 died of hyaline membrane disease and pneumothorax; normal BUN level in 9, elevated in 2
Renal vein thrombosis	7	3	1	3	...	2–5	3 had diabetic mothers; Bun level >40 mg/100 ml in all; 4 had thrombocytopenia
Polycystic disease of kidney	6	6	...	...	...	2–4	5 died in neonatal period, one at 4 months; all had increased BUN, 40 to 80 mg/100 ml
Obstructive uropathy							
Hydronephrosis	3	1	...	2	...	1–5	BUN level 25 to 30 mg/100 ml; 2 with hydronephrosis underwent difficult delivery; 3 had pyuria and bacteriuria; palpable mass present in 2
Ureteral valve	3	2	...	...	...	2–4	
Bladder neck	1	1	...	...	1	4	
Sponge kidney	3	...	...	2	1	1	Death within 4 to 6 months of age
Wilms' tumor	1	...	...	...	1	2	Survived, patient doing well 4 years later

Abdominal masses were palpated in all patients later found to have renal vein thrombosis or polycystic kidneys. Intravenous pyelograms were normal in all patients in whom no cause was found for the hematuria, in the patients with posterior urethral valves, and in the one with bladder neck obstruction. IVP was abnormal in all other patients. Voiding cystourethrogram demonstrated the abnormality in the patients with obstruction.

Conclusion: Abdominal palpation, IVP, and blood urea nitrogen levels are warranted in all newborns presenting with gross hematuria. If the diagnosis is still unavailable, voiding cystourethrogram is in order. A significant number of these patients, however, will have no evident cause for their hematuria, and will recover spontaneously.

5

Reference: Emanuel, B., and Aronson, N.: Am. J. Dis. Child., 128: *204*, 1974.

NEONATAL PHRENIC NERVE PALSY— THE "BELLY DANCER'S SIGN"

Unilateral diaphragmatic paralysis with or without brachial plexus injury may present in neonates as "respiratory distress." The chest roentgenogram may be misleading unless obtained in deep inspiration. Fluoroscopy is required to demonstrate paradoxical motion of the diaphragm on the involved side.

It should be remembered that the existence of diaphragmatic paralysis can be recognized by merely observing the movement of the umbilicus during the respiratory cycle. To perform this maneuver, note the position of the umbilicus at full expiration. Mark this position by placing your pen at the spot. During inspiration, the umbilicus can be seen to shift upward and toward the side of the paralyzed diaphragm. Other suggestive physical findings include unexplained tachypnea without dyspnea, slightly decreased breath sounds on the paralyzed side, fine inspiratory rales on the paralyzed side if atelectasis is present, widening of the subcostal angle on the affected side during inspiration, and flattening of the epigastrium on the side of the paralyzed diaphragm during inspiration. The movement of the umbilicus is the sign most easily identified.

References: Nichols, M.M.: Clin. Pediatr., *15*:342, 1976. Light, J.S.: J. Pediatr., *24*:627, 1944.

FETAL-MATERNAL HEMORRHAGE—AN ESTIMATE OF VOLUME

Fetal red blood cells resist the elution of hemoglobin by acidic solutions. This characteristic allows quantitation of the amount of blood that may have been transfused from the fetus to the mother. The method for doing this is as follows:

1.   Obtain a small quantity of blood from the mother and prepare thin red cell films on microscopic slides within 2 hours.
2.   Fix in 80 per cent ethanol for 5 to 10 minutes, rinse with tap water, and dry
3.   Place a Coplin stain jar in a water bath at 37°C.
4.   Mix 37.7 ml of 0.1 M citric acid with 12.3 ml of 0.2 M Na_2HPO_4. Check pH and adjust to 3.3, if necessary, by adding additional citric acid or Na_2HPO_4. Pour into the Coplin jar.
5.   When the solution has reached 37°C, place the fixed slides in the jar. Incubate for 5 minutes.
6.   Remove slides; rinse with tap water; dry.
7.   Stain with hematoxylin 1 minute. Rinse with tap water. Stain with eosin 1 minute; rinse with tap water and dry.
8.   Examine under low power first to scan for occasional eosin-staining cells. These are the fetal cells. Maternal cells are seen under oil and appear as ghosts (colorless).
9.   The formula for estimating the volume of red cells transfused from fetus to mother is calculated by multiplying an adjusted maternal red cell mass (2400 ml) by the ratio of fetal to maternal cells from the maternal blood film where:

$$\text{Fetal-Maternal Hemorrhage} = 2400 \times \frac{\text{dark-stained cells}}{\text{unstained cells}}$$

A commercial kit called "Foetal Hemoglobin Rapid Method" is available through Boehringen-Mannheim, 219 E. 44th St., New York, New York.

Reference: Queenan, J.T.: Modern Management of the Rh Problem, 2nd ed. New York, Harper & Row, 1977, p. 244.

THE INFANT WITH A METABOLIC ERROR

Inborn errors of metabolism are suspected much more often than they are proven. The practicing physician has difficulty recognizing the clinical presentation of a host of metabolic disorders that are rarely seen in practice. The list below includes only those inborn errors of metabolism that present in the neonatal period.

Inborn Errors of Metabolism in the Neonatal Period

DISORDERS OF CARBOHYDRATE METABOLISM

(1) Galactosemia (galactose-1-phosphate uridyl transferase deficiency)
(2) Hereditary fructose intolerance (fructose-1-phosphate aldolase deficiency)
(3) Fructose-1, 6-diphosphatase deficiency
(4) Glycogen storage disease, type I (von Gierke's disease, glucose-6-phosphatase deficiency)
(5) Glycogen storage disease, type II (Pompe's disease, α-1,4-glucosidase deficiency)
(6) Glycogen storage disease, type III (limit dextrinosis, debrancher deficiency)
(7) Glycogen storage disease, type IV (amylopectinosis, brancher deficiency)
(8) GM_1 gangliosidosis, type I (generalized gangliosidosis, β-galactosidase deficiency)
(9) GM_3 gangliosidosis
(10) Wolman's disease (acid lipase deficiency)
(11) Niemann-Pick disease, types A and B (sphingomyelinase deficiency)

DISORDERS OF MUCOPOLYSACCHARIDE METABOLISM

(12) Hurler's syndrome (mucopolysaccharidosis I, α-L-iduronidase deficiency)
(13) Hunter's syndrome (mucopolysaccharidosis II, iduronosulfate sulfatase deficiency)
(14) β-Glucuronidase deficiency

UREA CYCLE DEFECTS

(15) Carbamoylphosphate synthetase deficiency (hyperammonemia type II)
(16) Ornithine transcarbamoylase deficiency (hyperammonemia type II)
(17) Citrullinemia
(18) Argininosuccinic aciduria
(19) Arginase deficiency

DISORDERS OF AMINO ACID METABOLISM OR TRANSPORT

(20) Maple syrup urine disease
(21) Hypervalinemia
(22) Hyperlysinemia
(23) Hyper-β-alaninemia
(24) Nonketotic hyperglycinemia
(25) Phenylketonuria
(26) Oasthouse urine disease (methionine malabsorption)

DISORDERS OF AMINO ACID METABOLISM OR TRANSPORT

(27) Tyrosinemia
(28) Hypermethioninemia
(29) Homocystinuria
(30) Hartnup disease
(31) Hypersarcosinemia
(32) Pyroglutamic acidemia

DISORDERS OF ORGANIC ACID METABOLISM

(33) Methylmalonic acidemia
(34) Propionic acidemia (ketotic hyperglycinemia)
(35) Isovaleric acidemia
(36) Butyric and hexanoic acidemia (green acyl dehydrogenase deficiency)
(37) β-Methylcrotonyl-CoA carboxylase deficiency

MISCELLANEOUS DISORDERS

(38) Adrenogenital syndrome
(39) Lysosomal acid phosphatase deficiency
(40) Renal tubular acidosis
(41) Nephrogenic diabetes insipidus
(42) Menke's kinky hair syndrome
(43) Orotic aciduria
(44) Congenital lactic acidosis
(45) Cystic fibrosis
(46) Hypophosphatasia
(47) Fucosidosis
(48) Crigler-Najjar syndrome
(49) Alpha$_1$-antitrypsin deficiency
(50) I-cell disease (mucolipidosis II)
(51) Albinism
(52) Lesch-Nyhan syndrome

The following tables list the above disorders according to their clinical presentation and laboratory tests that may confirm a suspected diagnosis.

Major Clinical Manifestations of Inborn Errors of Metabolism in the Neonatal Period

CLINICAL FINDING	ASSOCIATED DISORDERS*
Failure to thrive, poor feeding	Essentially all
Lethargy	8, 9, 15-24, 28, 32-35, 42, 44
Vomiting	1-4, 10, 15-22, 25, 27, 31-35, 38-42, 52
Diarrhea	1, 10, 27, 30, 45
Jaundice	1, 2, 7, 10, 11, 15, 48, 49
Hypotonicity or hypertonicity	1, 3-5, 8, 9, 15-20, 24, 26, 31-34, 37, 42, 44, 47, 52
Seizures	1, 2, 4, 6, 9, 15-20, 22-24, 26, 33, 34, 38-42, 44, 46
Hepatomegaly	1-14, 16, 18, 27, 28, 31, 33, 38, 47, 49, 50
Dehydration	15-19, 34, 38, 41
Coarse facial features	8, 9, 12-14, 50
Abnormal urinary odor	20, 25-28, 35-37
Respiratory distress	5, 9, 16, 18, 44
Gingival hyperplasia	8, 9, 50
Macroglossia	5, 8, 9

*Numbers refer to those listed in previous table.

Laboratory Findings Associated with Inborn Errors of Metabolism in the Neonatal Period

LABORATORY FINDING	ASSOCIATED DISORDERS*
Metabolic acidosis	2-4, 6, 15, 32-36, 40, 44
Hypoglycemia	2-4, 6, 20, 27, 28, 33, 39, 44, 49
Reducing substances in urine	1, 2, 27
Ferric chloride test (Phenistix) positive on urine	20, 25-27
Hyperammonemia	15-19, 22
Neutropenia	15, 27, 33-36, 43
Thrombocytopenia	27, 33-37
Vacuolated lymphocytes on peripheral smear	4, 8, 10-13, 47

*Numbers refer to those listed in previous table.

Disorders Associated with Abnormal Urinary Odor

DISORDER	ODOR
Phenylketonuria	Musty
Tyrosinemia	Musty
Maple syrup urine disease	Maple syrup or burnt sugar
Oasthouse urine disease (methionine malabsorption)	Dried malt or hops
Hypermethioninemia	Boiled cabbage or rancid butter
Isovaleric acidemia	Cheesy or sweaty feet
β-Methylcrotonyl-CoA carboxylase deficiency	Cat urine

Disorders Associated with Positive Ferric Chloride Reaction

DISORDER	MAJOR COMPOUND IN URINE	COLOR
Phenylketonuria	Phenylpyruvic acid	Green
Tyrosinemia	p-Hydroxyphenylpyruvic acid	Green, fading rapidly
Maple syrup urine disease	Branched-chain ketoacids	Gray-green
Oasthouse urine disease	α-Hydroxybutyric acid	Purple
Histidinemia	Imidazolpyruvic acid	Blue-green
Alkaptonuria	Homogentisic acid	Dark brown
Diabetic ketoacidosis	Acetoacetic acid	Cherry red
Melanoma	Melanin	Black
Pheochromocytoma	Catecholamines	Blue-green
Formiminotransferase deficiency	Imidazolcarboxamide	Gray-green
Drug intoxication	Salicylates	Purple
	Phenothiazines	Purple
	p-Aminosalicylic acid	Red-brown
	Lysol	Green
Conjugated hyperbilirubinemia	Bilirubin	Green

*Disorders That May Be Associated With Reducing
Substances in Urine*

DISORDER	COMPOUND
Galactosemia	Galactose
Hereditary fructose intolerance	Fructose
Tyrosinemia	p-Hydroxyphenylpyruvic acid
Galactokinase deficiency	Galactose
Essential fructosuria	Fructose
Diabetes mellitus	Glucose
Renal glycosuria	Glucose
Fanconi's syndrome	Glucose
Pentosuria	Xylulose
Severe liver disease with secondary galactose intolerance	Galactose

Reference: Burton, B.K., and Nadler, H.L.: Pediatrics, *61*:398, 1978.

TECHNIQUE FOR PALPATION OF THE FEMORAL ARTERY

It's your tenth examination of a newborn in one morning. You know it's important to be sure the femoral artery pulsation is good, but you can't be sure you feel it. There is no technique that will always be successful, but if you've always used your index finger, why not try your thumb for a change and see if that works.

Simply grasp the baby's right thigh and knee with your left hand (or the baby's left thigh and knee with your right hand). Your thumb will naturally fall into the infant's groin over the long axis of the femoral artery.

The thumb is traditionally not supposed to be used for palpation, but if it works, use it.

Reference: Bjarke, B.: Acta Paediatr. Scand., *66*:265, 1977.

FOOT LENGTH — A POTENTIALLY USEFUL MEASUREMENT IN NEONATES

Sometimes it is not possible to get all the anthropometric measurements you would like in critically ill newborns. One often overlooked, but very readily determined and useful, measurement is that of foot length. In preterm, appropriate for gestational age, infants, the correlation between foot length and birth weight is excellent (r = 0.95), as is the relationship between foot length and crown-heel length (r = 0.96). These data indicate that, if necessary, birth weight and crown-heel length of premature babies can be estimated from a measurement of foot length. When encumbrance of the incubator and intensive care apparatus preclude a weight or body length measurement, drug doses and intravenous fluid replacements normally based on these measurements can be indirectly calculated from the foot length. Figures 5–4 and 5–5 show these relationships.

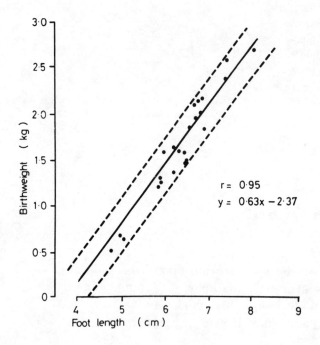

r = 0.95
y = 0.63x − 2.37

FIG. 5-4

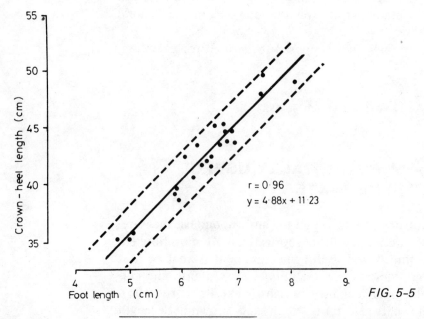

r = 0.96
y = 4.88x + 11.23

FIG. 5-5

Reference: James, D.K., Dryburgh, E.H., and Chiswick, M.L.: Arch. Dis. Child., *54:*226, 1979.

BIRTHMARKS

After sex, fingers, toes, and hair color have been identified, parents of newborns may begin asking questions about "birthmarks." We know that mongolian spots, salmon patches, pigmented lesions, and straw-berry marks are common, but how common are they? The following chart lists the frequency with which the various birthmarks were seen in 1058 infants under 72 hours of age.

BIRTHMARK	PER CENT OF INFANTS
Strawberry marks	2.6
Port-wine marks	0.3
Salmon patches	40.3
Pigmented lesions in whites	2.4
Pigmented lesions in blacks	19.7
Mongolian spots in whites	9.6
Mongolian spots in blacks	95.5
Mongolian spots in Asiatics	81.0
Mongolian spots in Latins	70.1

It should be remembered that strawberry marks are often not visible at birth.

Salmon patches are most frequently seen on the nape of the neck ("stork bite"), eyelids, glabella, or mid-forehead ("angel's kiss") of neonates.

Pigmented lesions include nevi, *café au lait spots,* and all sharply demarcated macules.

Erythema toxicum neonatorum, although not a birthmark, was found in 30.3 per cent of the infants examined.

Reference: Jacobs, A.H., and Walton, R.G.: Pediatrics, *58*:218, 1976.

SITE AND DEPTH OF HEEL SKIN PUNCTURES IN THE NEWBORN

Every day, including Sundays, literally thousands of newborn infants have heel punctures performed in order to obtain blood samples.

Many of these punctures are badly performed. Little attention is paid to normal anatomy. Serious complications of heel punctures in newborns include calcaneal osteomyelitis and necrotizing chondritis.

The skin's primary arterial blood supply comes from an arterial network at the junction of the lower dermis and upper subcutaneous tissue. Branches from one side of this network supply blood to the subcutaneous tissue, and those from the other side supply the dermis. A large network of veins is also present at the dermal subcutaneous junction. Because of the anatomy, most of the blood obtained from a skin puncture flows from vessels at the dermal subcutaneous junction, and for this reason it is not necessary to extend the puncture any deeper to obtain adequate blood flow.

How deep is this junction? Figure 5–6 illustrates the distance from the skin to the subcutaneous junction (S–S) and the distance from the skin to the periosteum of the calcaneus (S–P) as a function of body weight. A lancet puncture of 2.4 mm will extend below the dermal subcutaneous junction, but will not penetrate the perichondrium in even the smallest infants. Do not go deeper than 2.4 mm.

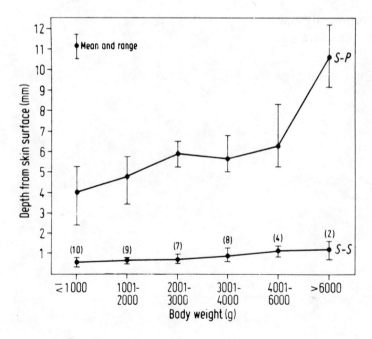

FIG. 5-6

The side-to-side limits of the calcaneus are illustrated in Figure 5-7. A line extending posteriorly from a point between the fourth and fifth toes and running parallel to the lateral aspect of the heel, and another line extending posteriorly from the middle of the big toe and running parallel to the medial aspect of the heel, serve as useful guidelines. Heel punctures should be performed on the plantar surface of the heel and beyond the lateral and medial limits of the calcaneus. These safe areas are marked by the hatched lines in the illustration. Don't be responsible for bone spurs.

5

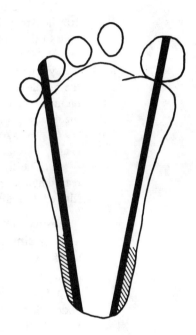

FIG. 5-7

Reference: Blumenfeld, T.A., Turi, G.K., and Blanc, W.A.: Lancet, *1:*230, 1979.

THORACIC TRANSILLUMINATION — AN AID TO THE DIAGNOSIS OF PNEUMOPERICARDIUM

Pneumopericardium is now seen with ever-increasing frequency because of the use of mechanical ventilation and continuous positive airway pressure. The diagnosis of pneumopericardium should be confirmed by x-ray examination of the chest, but in the case of acute tamponade it may not be possible to wait for these studies. In that situation you can employ a high-intensity fiberoptic light to illuminate the air in the thorax in order to diagnose and treat pneumopericardium.

The procedure, which can be performed with the patient in an incubator or under a radiant warmer, is as follows:

1. An area of abdominal skin to the right and caudal to the xiphoid is cleaned with an antiseptic and infiltrated with a local anesthetic agent.

2. The overhead light intensity where the infant is located should be reduced, but a dark room is not necessary.

3. The fiberoptic light source is placed initially on the left chest in the third or fourth intercostal space near the midclavicular line. Final placement of the light is determined by moving it over the thorax until the orange glow of light reflected from the pericardial air and transmitted through the chest wall is brightest; the silhouette of the beating heart will also be evident.

4. A 1.5-in, 20- or 22-gauge, short-bevel spinal needle with the stylet removed, attached to a 30-ml syringe, is inserted through the skin of the abdomen to the right of the xiphoid.

5. With the syringe and needle held 30 degrees above the plane of the trunk, the syringe plunger is gently pulled back to develop a small negative pressure, and the needle is advanced inferior to the xiphoid toward the heart, silhouetted by the illuminated, air-filled pericardial sac. When the pericardial air flows into the syringe, the orange glow of light quickly disappears.

6. The syringe and needle are then quickly withdrawn to prevent lacerating the heart.

7. The light source is removed, but can be used periodically to observe for reaccumulation of air. The light should not be used for extended periods unless it is filtered, to reduce the chance of thermal injury to the skin.

Since reaccumulation of air is expected in one third of the patients after a single needle aspiration, a modification of the method can be used whereby a 16-gauge Portex epidural catheter (Smiths Industries, Inc., Wilmington, MA) is inserted through an 18-gauge Touhy needle into the pericardial sac. The catheter should move easily through the needle lumen, but it is important that it should fit snugly. The narrowed tip of the plastic catheter is cut off to reduce the possibility of occlusion. The catheter, attached to a 30-ml syringe, is passed through the Touhy needle until it is visualized in the opening of the beveled tip; it is then retracted a few millimeters. The needle with the catheter is inserted through the skin of the abdomen to the right of the xiphoid. With the needle held 30 degrees above the plane of the trunk, the syringe plunger is gently pulled back by an assistant, and the needle is advanced inferior to the xiphoid into the illuminated, air-filled pericardial sac. Pericardial air is allowed to flow into the syringe until the orange glow of light diminishes in size but does not disappear. The catheter is carefully advanced 2 to 3 cm into the pericardial sac. The needle is withdrawn over the catheter and the remaining pericardial air is withdrawn by the syringe. The catheter is anchored to the skin by means of a suture, and continuous 10 cm H_2O suction is applied. The catheter should remain in place until there is no further need for respiratory assistance.

Reference: Cabatu, E.E., and Brown, E.G.: Pediatrics, *64:*958, 1979.

6
INFECTIOUS DISEASES

DIAGNOSIS OF STREPTOCOCCAL PHARYNGITIS

The diagnosis of streptococcal pharyngitis cannot reliably be made in the absence of a positive throat culture. The following table gives criteria for grouping patients according to high, medium, and low clinical index of suspicion of streptococcal sore throat.

HIGH	MEDIUM	LOW
Symptoms (or history)		
Close exposure to known streptococcal sore throat	Fever	Minimal fever
Fever greater than 101.5° F	Moderately sore throat	Slightly sore or scratchy throat
Severely sore throat	Abdominal pain	
Signs		
Scarlatiniform rash	Slightly tender, slightly enlarged peritonsillar lymph nodes	Palpebral conjunctivitis
Tender, enlarged peritonsillar lymph nodes	Moderately red pharynx	Slightly red or injected pharynx
Beefy red pharynx	Medium exudate	Thin, wispy exudate in crypts
Moderate exudate		Hoarseness, cough
Petechiae on soft palate or uvula		

Reference: Peebles, T.C.: Pediatr. Clin. North Am., *18*:145, 1971.

6

THE RESPONSE TO PENICILLIN IN STREPTOCOCCAL PHARYNGITIS

If your patient has a streptococcal pharyngitis and you initiate treatment with appropriate doses of penicillin, how soon should you expect to observe a disappearance of the signs and symptoms of the disease?

The following facts should help you in deciding if your diagnosis and treatment were correct.

SYMPTOM	MEAN DURATION (HOURS)
Sore throat	28.8
Headache	41.1
Abdominal pain	48.0
Vomiting	56.0

SIGN	MEAN DURATION (HOURS)
Fever	44.0
Pharyngeal injection	42.0
Pharyngeal petechiae	40.0
Pharyngeal exudate	40.0

As a general rule, your patient should manifest some evidence of improvement within 48 hours of the start of treatment. The duration of signs and symptoms is somewhat shorter in patients who are treated within 24 hours of the onset of fever.

Reference: Bass, J.W., Crast, F.W., Knowles, C.R., et al.: J.A.M.A., *235*:1112, 1975.

THE ETIOLOGY OF VIRAL DISEASE

Certain constellations of findings in children should suggest the possibility of viral infections. The table lists the viruses that may be responsible for these findings.

Roseola—Latin diminutive of *roseus*, meaning rosy.

Viral Agents Often Associated with Various Pediatric Syndromes

CLINICAL SYNDROME	VIRUSES
Neonatal viral disease	CMV, rubella, HSV, coxsackie
Lymphadenopathy	EBV, CMV, cat-scratch disease
Pharyngitis	Adenovirus, EBV, HSV, enteroviruses, influenza, parainfluenza
Other acute respiratory disease	Adrenovirus, respiratory syncytial virus, influenza, parainfluenza, enteroviruses, rhinovirus, measles (after killed vaccine), EBV
Parotitis	Mumps, parainfluenza, LCM, coxsackie B
Encephalitis and aseptic meningitis	Mumps, measles, polio, ECHO, coxsackie, HSV, LCM, arboviruses
Myocarditis	Measles, mumps, coxsackie B, ECHO, EBV
Pericarditis	Coxsackie B, influenza, EBV
Hepatitis	Hepatitis A, hepatitis B, EBV, CMV
Fever without localizing signs	ECHO, coxsackie, parainfluenza, adenovirus, influenza
Rash — petechial	Adenovirus, EBV, measles (after killed vaccine)
Rash — maculopapular	Measles, rubella, coxsackie, ECHO
Rash — poxlike	Varicella-zoster, HSV, vaccinia, variola
Rash — palms/soles	Coxsackie, ECHO, EBV, measles (after killed vaccine)

CMV = Cytomegalovirus; EBV = Epstein-Barr virus; HSV = herpes simplex virus; LCM = lymphocytic choriomeningitis.

Although viral diagnostic techniques are relatively slow and expensive, their use is called for in many situations:

For exclusion of malignancy or treatable nonviral infection (e.g., massive cervical adenopathy)

To allow discontinuation of antibiotic therapy (e.g., neonatal viral versus bacterial sepsis)

To justify use of antiviral drug or globulin (e.g., neonatal herpes)

Fatal undiagnosed illness

For early recognition and/or confirmation of outbreak

For increased knowledge of epidemiology and transmission of viral agents

To demonstrate susceptibility or immunity of an individual to specific viral disease (serologic study only)

Serologic studies are almost always indicated as part of viral diagnostic studies. The outstanding major exception is in attempts to document infections caused by the enteroviruses, ECHO and coxsackie, since there are more than three dozen non–cross-reacting serotypes. For these agents, most state or other reference laboratories will perform serologic studies only if a specific enterovirus has been isolated.

An acute (within seven days of onset of illness) serum specimen should be obtained (and saved) from any child with undiagnosed illness for later use in viral or other studies. Convalescent serum, if indicated, can be obtained 14 to 28 days later.

The table on the next page suggests the timing and sites of additional specimens useful in viral diagnosis.

Viral cultures differ from routine bacteriologic cultures in several important respects. Attention to the following points will improve the possibility of viral isolation.

1. Specimens to be cultured should be bacteriologically sterile whenever possible.

2. Most viruses are destroyed by drying; swabs should be sent to the laboratory in some type of viral "transport medium" (e.g., Hanks solution).

3. Specimens should be obtained as early in the disease course as possible and should be inoculated immediately.

4. If the specimen cannot be inoculated into tissue culture immediately, the sample should be stored at 4°C and inoculated as soon as possible.

5. A brief clinical history should accompany all specimens in order to help the virology laboratory decide which tissue cultures, and thus which viruses, are most appropriate to the situation.

References: Moffet, H.L.: Pediatric Infectious Diseases. Philadelphia, J.B. Lippincott Company, 1975. Gershon, A.A.: Pediatr. Clin. North Am., *18*:73, 1971.

Specimens in Viral Diagnosis of Specific Clinical Findings

	THROAT SWAB	STOOL	URINE*	CEREBROSPINAL FLUID	VESICLE FLUID†	OTHER
Optimal time (days) after onset to collect	≤3	≤14	≤3	≤7	As soon as possible	
Clinical Findings						
Neonatal disease	X	X	X	X	If present	Neonatal and maternal sera, repeat in 3 months
Lymphadenopathy	X		X			Urine cytology, rapid mononucleosis slide test
Pharyngitis	X		X			Rapid mononucleosis slide test
Other acute respiratory disease	X	X	X			
Parotitis/orchitis	X		X	If symptomatic		
Encephalitis/meningitis	X	X	X	X	If present	
Myocarditis	X	X	X			Rapid mononucleosis slide test
Hepatitis	X		X			Urine cytology
Rash	X	X	X			
Fever without localization	X		X			
Autopsy	X	X				Cultures of brain, liver, lung, kidney

*Urine for cytomegalovirus may be submitted at any time during the illness.
†Examination of vesicle base scraping stained with Wright or Wright-Giemsa stain (Tzanck prep) may be helpful.

Coryza—A combination of the Greek for "head" and "I boil." Coryza meant a cold in the head or a running at the nose.

DIFFERENTIATING AMONG THE COMMON RESPIRATORY TRACT DISEASES IN CHILDREN

The ability to differentiate among respiratory tract disorders is important not only because of treatment, management, and clinical course but also in view of potential complications. The use of pertinent clinical history, and careful attention to inspection of the child, can render a definitive diagnosis in 80 per cent of cases without further examination or laboratory tests.

6

AGES	CROUP 3 Mo–3 Yr	EPIGLOTTITIS 3–6 Yr	BRONCHITIS 3 Yr and Older	BRONCHIOLITIS 1 Mo–2 Yr	PNEUMONIA All Ages	ASTHMA 3 Yr and Older
Etiology	*Parainf. 1,2,3 Influenza A Adenovirus Rhinovirus Resp. syncytial virus	*H. influenzae, type B Occ. diphtheria	*Viruses Myxovirus Resp. syncytial virus Adenovirus Bacteria	*Resp. syncytial virus	*Viruses S. pneumoniae Mycoplasma	Resp. Tract
Pathogenesis	Subglottic	Supraglottic	Major bronchi	Bronchioles	Alveoli	
Rapid onset	No (O), except Spasmodic	Yes (+++)	No (O)	No (O)	No (O)	Yes—No (+-++)
Stridor	++	+++	0	+	0	0
Dysphonia	+++	+++	0	0	0	0
Fever	0-+	+++	0-+	+-0	+-+++	0-+
Prostration	0-+++	0	0-+++	0	0	0
Family Hx	0	0	0	0	0	+++
Response to adrenalin	0	0	0	0	0	+++
Wheezing	0	0	0	+++	0	+++
Rhonchi	0	0	++	+	++	++
Influenced by weather	++(?)	0	0	0	0	0-++
Stridor	+-+++	+++	0	0	0	0
Expiratory effort	0	0	0	+-+++	0	+-+++
Productive cough	0	0	0-++	0	+-+++	0
Cyanosis	0	0	0	0-+++	0-+++	0-++
Retractions	+-+++	++	0	+-+++	0-++	0-+++
Rales	0	0	0	+++ (I & E)	+++ (I)	0
Hyperinflated lungs	0	0	0	+++	0	+++
Elevated WBC	0	++	0	0	0-+++	0-+

Continued

AGES	CROUP 3 Mo–3 Yr	EPIGLOTTITIS 3–6 Yr	BRONCHITIS 3 Yr and Older	BRONCHIOLITIS 1 Mo–2 Yr	PNEUMONIA All Ages	ASTHMA 3 Yr and Older
Complications	Pneumothorax Mediastinal emphysema	Pneumothorax Mediastinal emphysema Pyarthrosis Meningitis	Pneumonia	Bacterial infection Pneumothorax Mediastinal atelectasis	Otitis media Sinusitis Empyema Atelectasis	Atelectasis Pneumothorax Pneumomediastinum Pneumonia

0 = Absent.
+ = Slightly present.
++ = Moderately present.
+++ = Always present, marked.
*Organism most commonly found.

Reference: Helfinger, D.C.: Continuing Education, *11*:75, 1979.

CROUP SYNDROMES

Differentiation between epiglottitis, laryngotracheobronchitis (LTB), and spasmodic laryngitis is a common task for the pediatrician. The accompanying table may simplify your efforts. Remember that a foreign body and retropharyngeal abscess may give similar clinical pictures.

	EPIGLOTTITIS	LTB	SPASMODIC LARYNGITIS
Primary age	3–8 years	<3 years	1–3 years
Etiology	Usually *Hemophilus influenzae*, occasionally pneumococcus or viral	Viral	Uncertain; viral (?)
Onset	Rapid	Gradual	Sudden, usually at night
Mean duration of illness before hospitalization	8.6 hours	1.9 days	—
Presenting complaints	High fever, respiratory distress in younger child, drooling and dysphagia in older child	Cough, hoarseness, fever, inspiratory stridor	No fever
Mean temperature	102.2 F	102.2 F	Normal
Physical examination	Diminished breath sounds, pallor, inspiratory rhonchi	Diminished breath sounds, inspiratory rales	Diminished breath sounds, labored respirations
Laryngeal findings	Inflammation of periglottic structures, especially edematous red epiglottis	Edema of vocal cords and subglottic area	Laryngeal spasm
Mean white blood count	24,300	13,200	—
Percentage neutrophils	85%	63%	—
Clinical course	Rapidly progressive, *medical emergency*	Self-limited, may last ≤ 1 week	Self-limited but may be recurrent
Bacterial complications	Other organs may be seeded	Rare	None

Continued

Croup—From the Scottish word *croak*, which describes the sound these children make.

	EPIGLOTTITIS	LTB	SPASMODIC LARYNGITIS
Treatment	Antibiotics and airway maintenance. *Hospitalization is mandatory*	Humidification and support	Humidification, relief of laryngospasm, reassurance

Reference: Eichenwald, H.P.: Hospital Practice, *11*:81, 1976. Rabe, E.F.: Pediatrics, 2:255; 415; 559, 1948.

"The family is a unit composed not only of children, but of men, women, the occasional animal, and the common cold."

Ogden Nash
Family Reunion

IS IT A VIRAL OR A BACTERIAL UPPER RESPIRATORY TRACT INFECTION?

It seems that never a day goes by when you don't have to make a decision regarding the etiology of an upper respiratory tract infection. On clinical grounds alone, how do you reach a conclusion to treat a viral infection expectantly or a bacterial one energetically?

Dr. Reginald Lightwood, one of England's premier pediatricians, offers the following sage advice:

The guide I use is very simple and yet I have not seen it written anywhere. I tell my residents that it is a guide and not a rule: The greater the number of mucosal surfaces in the tract which are seen to be inflamed simultaneously or in rapid succession, i.e., rhinitis, pharyngitis, bronchitis, and perhaps conjunctivitis, antibiotics need *not* be considered. In contrast, bacterial infections are usually more localized and spread less rapidly and in a different way — a lobar pneumonia to the overlying pleura, a bacterial tonsillitis to the related lymph nodes.

Using this guide I have often persuaded a resident to withhold antibiotic treatment (usually penicillin or ampicillin) until, to his [or her, (Ed.)] surprise, temperature subsides without active intervention.

Reference: Lightwood, R.: Pediatrics, *58:*775, 1976.

> *Influenza* — Italian for influence, this term probably alludes to the alleged influence that the stars had on the origin and course of this epidemic disease.

DIAGNOSIS OF ACUTE EXANTHEMATOUS DISEASES

6

A sick child with a rash presents a diagnostic challenge to the physician. A careful description of the lesions and their distribution coupled with a knowledge of the patient's history and associated findings will usually enable you to make the correct diagnosis.

Diseases characterized by a maculopapular eruption

> Measles
> Rubella
> Scarlet fever
> Exanthema subitum (roseola infantum)
> Infectious mononucleosis
> Erythema infectiosum
> Infectious hepatitis
> Mucocutaneous lymph node syndrome
> Drug eruptions
> Sunburn
> Miliaria
> *Mycoplasma pneumoniae* *
> Meningococcemia*
> Typhus and tick-bite fever*
> Typhoid fever

---

*Vesicles also may be seen

Diseases characterized by a papulovesicular eruption

Chickenpox

Smallpox

Eczema herpeticum

Eczema vaccinatum

Herpes zoster

Rickettsialpox

Impetigo

Papular urticaria

Drug eruptions

Molluscum contagiosum

Dermatitis herpetiformis

Sorting these out may be a problem. A picture is worth many thousands of words in these circumstances. Saul Krugman and Robert Ward in their classic text *Infectious Diseases of Children* have provided clear-cut illustrations of the clinical course and distribution of the rashes that will enable you to recognize the most common maculo-papular eruptions — measles, rubella, scarlet fever, and exanthema subitum — as well as to distinguish chickenpox from smallpox easily. These are illustrated on the following pages for both your pleasure and your edification.

Reference: Krugman, S., and Ward, R.: Infectious Diseases of Children, 1st ed. St. Louis, Mo., C.V. Mosby Company, 1958.

*THE EXANTHEMATOUS FAMILY TREE—DISEASES
ONE, TWO, THREE, AND FIVE?*

*Exanthems from an ancient family of five
Achieved great fame; though now just four remain alive.
Rubella, Measles, Scarlet Fever are the three
First christened, since the fourth succumbed in infancy.
Yet little Fifth Disease cannot assume Fourth's name,
Just as the "junior" would not then the "senior" claim.*

*Instead, a new fourth member we might now adopt,
And for the orphan, Roseola, I would opt.
    (Though it was called the Sixth disease by just a few,
    Procedures for adoption were not carried through.)
Or should the fourth become that diagnostic cache—
The MD's sage pronouncement, "It's a 'Viral Rash'. . . ."?*

Caroline Breese Hall, M.D.

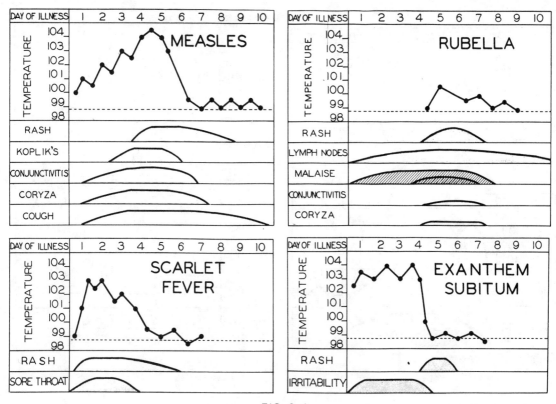

FIG. 6-1

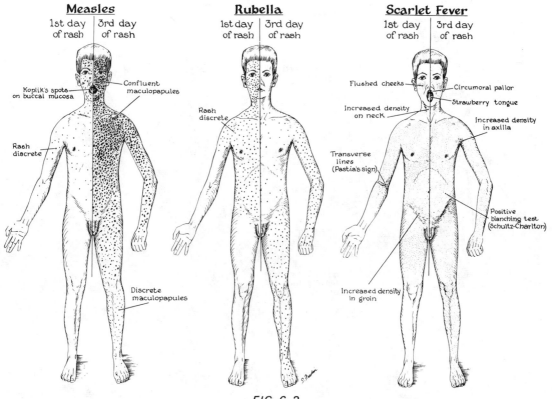

FIG. 6-2

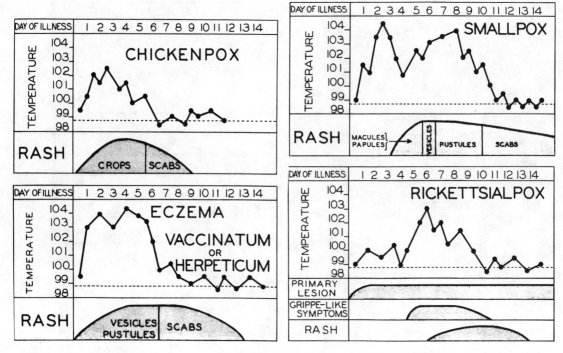

FIG. 6-3

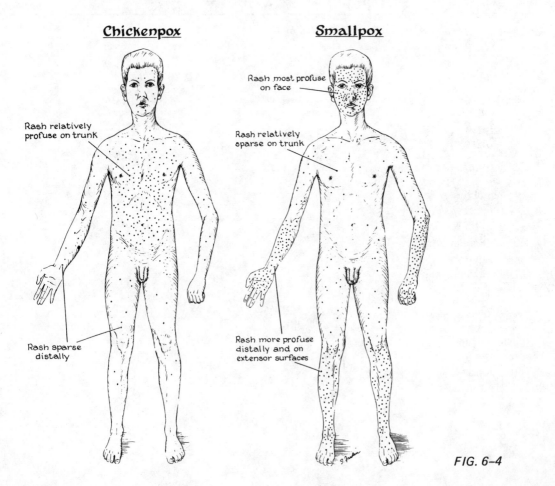

FIG. 6-4

ATYPICAL MEASLES

Shortly after the introduction of killed measles vaccine in the early 1960s, cases of atypical measles began appearing in vaccine recipients. Although atypical measles differs clinically in many respects from ordinary measles, it can be confirmed by serologic tests. It should be considered in any child whose illness has some of the clinical features described below:

The History

Received killed measles vaccine in past
Recent exposure to measles-like illness

The Prodrome

High fever that responds poorly to antipyretics
Headache
Cough
Abdominal symptoms, sometimes severe

The Rash

Begins two to three days after onset of illness
Begins on wrists and feet and usually involves the palms and soles
Progresses toward the trunk and head
Is most dense on distal limbs and in skin folds
Character of rash may be any combination of maculopapular,
   vesicular, or hemorrhagic lesions
Is often intensely pruritic

Respiratory Involvement is characteristic

Roentgenogram may show lobar or segmental pneumonia
Hilar adenopathy is consistently present
Pleural effusion is common
Ill-defined nodular lesions may persist on roentgenogram
   for up to two years
Arterial hypoxemia may be seen

Other Symptoms and signs may be seen. They include:

Peripheral edema
Myalgia
Hypertension
Strawberry tongue

Laboratory Findings often include:

Elevated WBC with neutrophilia and marked shift to the left
Appreciable rise in measles HI antibody titers

The illness runs a self-limited course of two to three weeks. No mortality or long-term morbidity has been noted. A few patients have had this illness after having received the live attenuated vaccine now in use.

References: Editorial: Br. Med. J., *1*:235, 1971. St. Geme, J.W., and George, B.L.: Pediatrics, *57*:148, 1976.

INFECTIOUS MONONUCLEOSIS — FREQUENCY OF SIGNS AND SYMPTOMS

Infectious mononucleosis has two basically different presentations. The young (preschool) child who contracts infectious mononucleosis usually does so without developing typical clinical signs or symptoms. The adolescent and young adult who develop infectious mononucleosis will manifest the usual signs and symptoms and laboratory findings noted in the first two tables below. Sometimes it is very difficult without specific serologic testing to differentiate infectious mononucleosis from other common and uncommon disorders. The third table will provide some assistance in this differential diagnosis.

FREQUENCY OF VARIOUS SIGNS AND SYMPTOMS IN YOUNG ADULTS

Symptom or Sign	%
Adenopathy	100
Malaise and fatigue	90–100
Fever	80–95
Sweats	80–95
Sore throat, dysphagia	80–85
Pharyngitis	65–85
Anorexia	50–80
Nausea	50–70
Splenomegaly	50–60
Headache	40–70
Chills	40–60
Bradycardia	35–50
Cough	30–50
Periorbital edema	25–40
Palatal enanthema	25–35
Hepatic or splenic tenderness	15–30
Myalgia	12–30
Hepatomegaly	15–25
Rhinitis	10–25
Ocular muscle pain	10–20
Chest pain	5–20
Jaundice	5–10
Arthralgia	5–10
Diarrhea or soft stools	5–10
Photophobia	5–10
Skin rash	3–6
Conjunctivitis	<5
Abdominal pain	<5
Gingivitis	<3
Pneumonitis	<3
Epistaxis	<3

6

LABORATORY FEATURES

Laboratory Findings	% Positive
Lymphocytosis, relative and absolute	100
Atypical lymphocytosis, definite*	100
Epstein-Barr virus (EBV) antibody in serum	100
Heterophile antibody	80–100
Liver enzyme abnormalities	80–100
Leukocytosis	60–80
Neutropenia	60–80
Hyperbilirubinemia	30–50
Bone marrow granulomata	50
Slight thrombocytopenia	25–50
Increased cold agglutinins	10–50†
Occult hemolysis	20–40†
Hyperuricemia	15–20†
Leukopenia	10–20
Severe thrombocytopenia with bleeding	Rare
Positive direct Coombs' test	Rare
Significant anemia (usually due to hemolysis)	Rare

*20 per cent or more of white blood cells in peripheral blood.
†Tentative values based on scanty information.

DIFFERENTIAL DIAGNOSIS OF INFECTIOUS MONONUCLEOSIS

Diagnosis	Fever, Fatigue, Chills, Sweats	Sore Throat (Pharyngitis)	Headache, Myalgia	Skin Rash	Jaundice	Splenomegaly	Cervical Adenopathy	Atypical Lymphocytosis	Abnormal Liver Function Tests
Streptococcal pharyngitis	+	+	+	±	−	−	+	−	−
Viral pharyngitis	+	+	+	−	−	−	+	±	−
Influenza, adenovirus, URI, etc.	+	±	+	±	±	−	+	±	±
Rubella and other viral exanthemata	+	±	+	+	−	−	+	±	−
Viral (and toxic) hepatitis	+	−	±	−	±	±	−	+	+
Leukemia, lymphoma	+	+	+	±	+	+	+	+	+
Brucellosis	+	−	+	−	+	+	+	±	±
Cytomegalovirus infection	+	−	±	−	±	+	−	+	+
Leptospirosis	+	−	+	±	+	±	−	−	+
Toxoplasmosis	+	−	+	±	−	+	+	±	−
Tuberculosis	+	−	+	−	±	+	+	±	+
Secondary syphilis	+	+	+	+	±	+	+	±	±
Serum sickness	+	−	+	+	−	+	+	+	±
Drug hypersensitivity reaction (PAS, phenytoin)	+	−	+	+	−	+	+	+	±
Diphtheria	+	+	+	−	−	−	+	−	−
Agranulocytosis	+	+	±	−	−	±	+	±	−
Infectious lymphocytosis	+	−	±	±	−	−	−	−	−

Reference: Carter, R. L., and Penman, H.G.: *In* Infectious Mononucleosis. Oxford, Blackwell Scientific Publications, 1969, p. 31.

INFECTIOUS MONONUCLEOSIS IN YOUNG CHILDREN

Until recently, it has been assumed that infectious mononucleosis was a rare disease in early childhood. This was a consequence of the fact that children under the age of 5 years generally do not produce a heterophile antibody in response to this infection. With the identification of the Epstein-Barr virus as the responsible etiologic agent in this disease and the development of techniques for both viral isolation and the measurement of antibody titers, it is now appreciated that infections with Epstein-Barr virus are very common in early childhood. By the age of 4 years, between 30 and 70 per cent of children have acquired antibodies to this agent.

Symptoms and signs in young children may include fever, diarrhea, pharyngitis, tonsillitis, otitis media, pneumonia, lymphadenopathy, hepatomegaly, and splenomegaly.

The total white count and differential are of little help in suspecting the diagnosis. The presence of 10 per cent or more atypical lymphocytes, however, should alert you to the possibility of infectious mononucleosis. Acute and convalescent titers demonstrating a rise in antibody to Epstein-Barr virus will confirm the diagnosis.

Reference: Tamir, D., Benderly, A., Levy, J., et al.: Pediatrics, *53*:330, 1974.

COMPLICATIONS OF INFECTIOUS MONONUCLEOSIS

Although most children with infectious mononucleosis experience a typical illness with an uncomplicated course, exceptions do exist. It is important to recognize the many complications of this common disease. They include the following:

Neurologic

Guillain-Barre syndrome
Facial nerve palsy
Meningoencephalitis
Aseptic meningitis
Transverse myelitis
Seizures
Peripheral neuritis
Optic neuritis
Acute psychosis
Diplopia
Reye's syndrome
Subacute sclerosing panencephalitis

Hepatic

>Hepatitis
>Multiple granulomas

Cardiac

>Pericarditis
>Myocarditis

Hematologic

>Hemolytic anemia
>Thrombocytopenia
>Aplastic anemia
>Hemolytic-uremic syndrome
>Disseminated intravascular coagulation

Splenic Rupture

Pulmonary Infiltration

Airway Obstruction

Glomerulonephritis

Reference: Karzon, D.T.: Adv. Pediatr., *22*:231, 1976.

"It seems impossible that children should ever grow to be men, and drag the heavy artillery along the dusty road of life."

H. W. Longfellow

EPSTEIN-BARR VIRAL ANTIBODY TITERS

Although the heterophile antibody test is sometimes positive in young children with infection caused by the Epstein-Barr virus, heterophile positivity is certainly not as reliable in pediatric patients as it is in adults. But don't despair. More specific antibody assays are soon to be available. They should allow you to determine on a single serum sample whether a patient is currently infected or has had the infection at some time in the past. The three most helpful tests are the following:

ANTIBODY DIRECTED AGAINST	RELATIONSHIP TO CLINICAL ILLNESS
Viral capsid antigen	Develops during clinical illness and persists for life
Early antigen	Develops along with clinical illness and disappears once the patient is well
Epstein-Barr nuclear antigen	Develops 30 to 60 days after the initial infection and persists for life

The timing of these antibody rises is depicted in Figure 6–5.

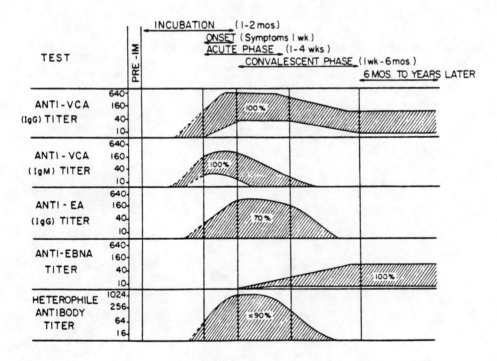

FIG. 6–5

Heterophile antibodies are nonspecific and not directed against the virus. They cause agglutination of sheep, horse, beef, and goat red blood cells. Since other antibodies may cause such agglutination, care should be taken to avoid false-positive reporting. Testing sera with horse RBCs is the most sensitive method, while the beef cell hemolysin test gives the most specific results. The most reliable method for single slide tests is to absorb the sera with guinea pig kidney cells before adding horse RBCs. When the antibody is due to EBV infection, the test should remain positive after such absorption. Many of the rapid test kits include guinea pig kidney cells for this purpose. Rapid test kits may be accurate and helpful, but experienced personnel and fresh testing material are essential for best results.

The list below provides a summary of the contents of some of the commercially available kits.

TRADE NAME	RED BLOOD CELL USED	USE OF GUINEA PIG KIDNEY ABSORPTION	MANUFACTURER
Mono-test	Horse	No	Wampole Labs.
Mono-Diff	Horse	Yes	Wampole Labs.
Monospot	Horse	Yes	Ortho Diagnostics
Diagluto	Horse	Yes	Beckman Instruments, Inc.
Monosticon	Sheep	Yes	Organon Diagnostic Products
Mono-Stat	Native and papain-treated sheep	Not needed	Colab Labs., Inc.
Confirmikit	Native and enzyme-treated horse	Not needed	BBL-BioQuest, Div. of Becton, Dickinson & Co.
Heterol	Native and enzyme-treated horse	Not needed	Difco

Reference: Andiman, W.A.: J. Pediatr., *95:*171, 1980. Figure 6–5 courtesy of Dr. John Sullivan, X-Linked Lymphoproliferative Syndrome Registry. Department of Pathology, University of Massachusetts Medical Center, Worcester, MA.

"ALICE IN WONDERLAND" SYNDROME AND INFECTIOUS MONONUCLEOSIS

Central nervous system involvement is estimated to occur in anywhere from 0.7 to 20 per cent of patients with infectious mononucleosis. The 20 per cent figure includes electroencephalographic abnormalities as a sole manifestation of central nervous system disease. The neurologic abnormalities may range from acute meningo-encephalitis to facial diplegia, retinal abnormalities, mononeuritis, and the Guillian-Barré syndrome.

To this list of neurologic complications should be added the presence of metamorphopsia or the "Alice in Wonderland" syndrome. Metamorphopsia refers to the complaints of distortions in the apparent sizes, shapes, and spatial relations of objects seen. This symptom has previously been recognized in some patients with migraine, epilepsy, or drug-induced hallucinations.

When it occurs in infectious mononucleosis, as a manifestation of central nervous system involvement, it may last from three weeks to three months.

When the patient begins to see things peculiarly, be sure you see correctly the peripheral blood smear, the Mono Spot Test, and, if necessary, the Epstein-Barr virus titers.

References: Copperman, S. M.: Clin. Pediatr., *16:*143, 1977. Schnell, R. G.: Medicine, *45:*51, 1966.

THE ATYPICAL LYMPHOCYTE

Atypical lymphocytes do not always mean that the patient has infectious mononucleosis. Do not forget to consider some of the other diseases listed below.

More than 20 per cent of the white blood cells may be atypical lymphocytes in:

Infectious mononucleosis
Viral hepatitis
The "post-transfusion" syndrome
PAS hypersensitivity
Dilantin and Mesantoin hypersensitivity
Cytomegalovirus

Less than 20 per cent of the white blood cells are atypical lymphocytes in:
  Infections
    Mumps
    Varicella
    Rubeola
    Rubella
    "Primary atypical pneumonia"
    Herpes simplex
    Herpes zoster
    Roseola infantum
    Influenza
    Mycoplasma
    Nonspecific upper respiratory infection
    Many other viral illnesses
    Tuberculosis
    Rickettsialpox
  Radiation
  Other
    Letterer-Siwe disease
    Agranulocytosis
    Lead intoxication
    Stress
  Uncommon causes of atypical lymphocytosis:
    Tertiary syphilis
    Congenital syphilis
    Smallpox
    Bullis fever
    Tetrachlorethane poisoning
    TNT poisoning
    Organic arsenical hypersensitivity
    Severe dermatitis herpetiformis

Reference: Modified from Wood, T.A., and Frenkel, E.P.: Am. J. Med., *42*:929, 1967.

CLINICAL CLUES TO THE ETIOLOGY OF VIRAL MENINGOENCEPHALITIS

The chart on the following page lists the clinical features of the most common agents that cause viral encephalitis. Western equine encephalitis occurs primarily in young children, while St. Louis encephalitis is seen mostly in adults. Focal seizures or focal neurologic signs should immediately suggest herpes simplex infection or possibly infection with the La Crosse virus. Enteroviral infection is always a good bet under any circumstance since it may occur at any time of the year (although peaks are in summer and fall).

Reference: Menkes, J. H.: Hosp. Pract., *12:*73, 1977.

Clinical Features of CNS Disease Associated with Viral Infection

AGENT	AGES AFFECTED	SEASONAL OCCURRENCE	CLINICAL MANIFESTATIONS	FOCAL FINDINGS	SEQUELAE
California encephalitis (La Crosse virus)	Almost always children in rural areas; 2/3 are between 5 and 9 years	June to October only	About 50% of children have a mild meningoencephalitis; 50% present with seizures	Present in 15 to 40% of patients	Present in 15 to 20% usually behavioral problems
St. Louis encephalitis	Adults more often involved than children	July to October	Usually asymptomatic in children	Uncommon	Less common than in Eastern or Western equine encephalitis
Western equine encephalitis	Primarily a disease of infancy (20 to 30% are under 1 year)	July to October	Sudden high fever in infants, focal or generalized seizures, coma	Uncommon	Major sequelae in more than 50% of children affected in first year of life
Herpesvirus hominis	Peak incidence <1 year and >15 years; uncommon between 5 and 15 years	Year-round	Usually a severe and progressive encephalitis with stupor and seizures; about 50% of cases are fatal	Present in 50 to 75% of patients	Found in 75% of survivors; often severe motor and mental deficits
Mumps	All ages; more common in children 2 to 14 years	Year-round	Often occurs in epidemics; a mild-to-moderate meningoencephalitis; 50% have parotitis	Not described	Rare
Enteroviral infection	All ages; more common in children <12 years	Year-round; peak incidence in summer and fall	Most common viral neurologic infection often occurs in epidemics; usually a mild meningoencephalitis; children may have rash	Rare	Uncommon

PROLONGED AND/OR RECURRENT FEVER IN MENINGITIS

Persistent or recurrent fever in a child under treatment for meningitis is a common yet distressing problem. Data from two large studies provide reassurance as to its significance. Bacteriologic persistence or relapse is an uncommon cause.

The table below displays the first afebrile day (defined as the first day during which a rectal temperature remained below 100° F/38.6° C) for the common pediatric cerebrospinal fluid pathogens.

6

First Afebrile Day in Meningitis

ORGANISM	PERCENTAGE OF PATIENTS AFEBRILE BY HOSPITAL DAY					
	Hospital Day					
	1–3	4	5	6–7	8–9	⩾10
Hemophilus influenzae	40	52	59	73	82	100
Neisseria meningitidis	52	68	78	92	94	100
Streptococcus pneumoniae	25	44	62.5	81	87.5	100

Prolonged fever (<10 days) was noted in 9 per cent of children with these and other meningitide . *Persistent infection was not a cause in any case.* Drug fever and nosocomial infection were the most common definable causes No cause was found in the majority of patients.

Recurrence of fever was found in 24 per cent of the children. No recurrence was due to bacteriologic relapse. *Phlebitis was the single most common cause*, as indicated in the table below.

Cause of Recurrent Fever in Children with Meningitis

	PER CENT
Phlebitis	32
Undetermined	28
Drug	19
Viral infection	19
Urinary tract infection	2
All causes	100

References: Lipiridou, O., Lazaridou, S., and Manios, S.: Scand. J. Infect. Dis., *5:*23, 1973. Balagtas, R.C., Levin, S., Nelson, K.E., et al.: J. Pediatr., *77:*957, 1970.

PERSISTENT PLEOCYTOSIS IN ADEQUATELY TREATED BACTERIAL MENINGITIS

Often more questions are raised than answered when the spinal tap is repeated during or following antibiotic therapy for bacterial meningitis. The WBC count may still be elevated even at the conclusion of therapy, especially if the meningitis was due to *H. influenzae*. The following table lists the CSF findings in 30 patients with bacterial meningitis who had sequential lumbar punctures. None of the 30 suffered a relapse of meningitis.

Sequential Spinal Fluid Changes in Bacterial Meningitis

Day of Therapy	H. INFLUENZAE (21 PATIENTS)				S. PNEUMONIAE (9 PATIENTS)			
	Cells (mm³)	Glucose (mg/dl)	Protein (mg/dl)	No. of Patients	Cells (mm³)	Glucose (mg/dl)	Protein (mg/dl)	No. of Patients
0	3162 ± 905* (0–15, 250)	36 ± 7 (0–104)	126 ± 22 (20–330)	21	3496 ± 934 (7–7535)	28 ± 10 (0–100)	261 ± 57 (13–530)	9
1	3925 ± 1477 (135–9300)	52 ± 8 (27–76)	88 ± 29 (40–260)	8	6940 ± 6629 (330–13,500)	56 ± 16 (40–71)	—	2
2	1948 ± 732 (162–6100)	45 ± 6 (16–58)	97 ± 16 (70–140)	9	2006 ± 715 (495–3580)	52 ± 6 (42–70)	142 ± 44 (56–196)	3
3	544 ± 252 (51–1368)	50 ± 7 (23–61)	108 ± 37 (34–218)	5	—	—	—	—
4–7	305 ± 164 (48–1617)	42 ± 4 (22–64)	107 ± 22 (42–240)	11	346 ± 208 (65–1172)	58 ± 3 (55–63)	79 ± 12 (56–110)	5
8–10	44 ± 8 (11–77)	47 ± 3 (32–55)	38 ± 3 (29–54)	11	42 ± 6 (5–98)	61 ± 2 (56–65)	42 ± 6 (23–56)	5
11–15	76 ± 10 (3–160)	51 ± 7 (32–63)	51 ± 7 (23–122)	18	17 ± 5 (3–24)	44 ± 3 38–50	49 ± 10 (20–66)	4
>15	94 ± 20 (4–176)	48 ± 3 (38–61)	40 ± 3 (22–54)	11	6 ± 1 (5–7)	57 ± 3 (54–60)	10 ± 5 (5–15)	3

Numbers in parentheses represent the range.
*Mean ± standard error.
– = data insufficient.

Reference: Chartrand, S.A., and Cho, C.T.: J. Pediatr., 88:424, 1976.

CAUSES OF CSF EOSINOPHILIA

Eosinophils are reported in CSF cell counts only if the laboratory does Wright or Giemsa stains to aid in the differential count. It is unusual, even in the face of CSF pleocytosis, to find more than one or two eosinophils in spinal fluid. If you receive a report stating that your patient has CSF eosinophilia, here are some conditions to consider.

Parasitic infection
Neurosyphilis
Coccidioides immitis meningitis
Postrabies vaccination
Candida albicans meningitis
Pneumococcal meningitis
Hodgkin's disease
Lymphoma
Foreign protein in the CSF
Rubber ventriculoatrial shunt
Multiple sclerosis-like illness
Lymphocytic choriomeningitis

Reference: Chesney, P.J., Katcher, M.L., Nelson, D.B., et al.: J. Pediatr., *94:*750, 1979.

SKIN LESIONS AND PROGNOSIS IN MENINGOCOCCAL INFECTIONS

The presence, type, and location of skin lesions in meningococcal infections can serve as a useful, immediate indicator of prognosis.

The skin manifestations may be of three types:

1. No lesions or other abnormalities.
2. Erythematous, macular, and/or petechial lesions in a generalized distribution over the trunk and extremities.
3. Large purpuric or ecchymotic lesions, usually on the extremities, in association with petechiae.

The clinical manifestations of the disease vary little in groups with no lesions or in those with the generalized macular or petechial eruption, although the incidence of meningitis tends to be increased in those with no skin manifestations.

In contrast, patients with ecchymotic and purpuric lesions have a greater incidence of hyperpyrexia, coagulation abnormalities, shock, and death. The table below illustrates these differences.

Type of Skin Lesions Related to Various Clinical and Laboratory Factors and Mortality

CLINICAL AND LABORATORY FACTORS	SKIN MANIFESTATIONS	
	No Lesion or Generalized Macular/Petechial Lesion (%)	*Peripheral Purpuric/ Ecchymotic Lesion (%)*
Meningitis	54	21
Leukocytosis	85	53
Hyperpyrexia	27	57
Shock	8	62
Bleeding diathesis	7	62
Mortality	3	44

Reference: Toews, W.H., and Bass, J.W.: Am. J. Dis. Child., *127*:173, 1974.

"Each generation makes its own accounting to its children."

Robert F. Kennedy

BACTERIAL INFECTION AND THE WBC

Elevated total white counts frequently provide evidence for bacterial infection. Data now show that the absolute number of neutrophils or neutrophil precursors/mm^3 (percentage neutrophils or bands X total WBC/mm^3) may more accurately predict infection. Eighty per cent of patients presenting with an absolute band count greater than 500/mm^3 or an absolute neutrophil count greater than 10,000/mm^3, or both, will have a bacterial infection. The nature of the bacterial infection may also be inferred from analysis of neutrophil values.

NEUTROPHIL COUNT	BAND COUNT	
	>500	*<500*
>10,000	Either gram-positive or gram-negative	Gram-positive
<10,000	Gram-negative	Infection less likely

The absence of the above values should not be used to exclude infection in a child whose clinical picture indicates its presence, and treatment should not be based on these criteria alone. Commonly, children with osteomyelitis, septic arthritis, or lymphangitis due to streptococcal or staphylococcal infections will have total neutrophil counts that fall within the normal range.

Pertussis—From the Latin *per*, meaning intensive, and *tussis*, or cough.

The blood smear may also provide evidence for bacterial infection. Toxic granules and Döhle bodies are often seen, but vacuolization of the neutrophils is most specific for bacterial infection.

Some bacterial infections present with unusual WBC pictures:

DISEASE	CHARACTERISTIC WBC PICTURE	COMMENTS
Tuberculosis, typhoid fever, and para-typhoid fever	Absence of leukocytosis and neutrophilia	Presence of neutrophilia is suggestive of complications or localization, such as tuberculous meningitis
Scarlet fever and brucellosis	Eosinophilia	
Pertussis	Absolute lymphocytosis; 75 per cent of children will have absolute lymphocyte count $> 10,000/mm^3$	Total WBC count may vary from leukocytosis and is not very helpful; adenovirus infections, which mimic pertussis, can also produce high WBC counts with absolute lymphocytosis
Shigellosis	85 per cent of children with shigellosis will have more band forms than neutrophils	Stool examination for leukocytes is helpful; children with *Shigella, Salmonella,* and invasive *Escherichia coli* gastroenteritis often exhibit fecal neutrophils, whereas children with viral diarrhea, noninvasive toxigenic *E. coli* diarrhea, and diarrhea secondary to parasites rarely exhibit fecal leukocytes

The WBC count and differential may be less useful when it is altered by drugs or noninfectious conditions.

CONDITION	EFFECT ON PERIPHERAL WBC PICTURE	COMMENTS
Epinephrine adminis- tration, stress, or strenuous activity	Leukocytosis and increased absolute number of neutro- phils; no shift to left	Changes in WBC picture occur within minutes
Corticosteroid administration, Cushing's syndrome	Leukocytosis and increased absolute number of neutro- phils; shift to left occurs with eosinopenia	Changes in WBC picture occur within 4 hours of oral corti- costeroid administration and return to normal within 24 hours of administration of last dose
Addison's disease or panhypopituitarism	Neutropenia, eosinophilia, lymphocytosis	
Diabetic ketoacidosis	Leukocytosis as high as 25,000/mm^3 with increased absolute neutrophil count and shift to left	
Burns, operation, crush injuries, fractures, neoplasms	Leukocytosis, increased absolute neutrophil count, and shift to left	
Acute hemorrhage	Leukocytosis, increased absolute neutrophil count, and shift to left	Leukocytosis and shift to left are greater if bleeding is against serous membrane than if it is external
Acute hemolysis	Leukocytosis, increased absolute neutrophil count, and shift to left	Children with sickle cell anemia, erythroblastosis fetalis, auto- immune hemolytic anemia, or any other hemolytic process often exhibit profound leukocytosis and shift to left in absence of infection

Reference: Weitzman, M.: Am. J. Dis. Child., *129*:1183, 1975.

BACTEREMIA AND FEVER

Nature often works against the pediatrician. One of the clear manifestations of that fact is the finding that the children most likely to have positive blood cultures are those under 2 years of age. These infants, their veins hidden under layers of adiposity, may appear only slightly ill. Of 600 febrile children under 24 months of age studied by Teele and coworkers, 19 were found to be bacteremic, but only two were judged to be sufficiently ill to warrant hospitalization before the culture results were known. Other important observations by this group were:

1. No bacteremic child had a rectal temperature less than 38.9° C (102° F).

2. Fifteen of the 19 bacteremic patients had a total WBC of greater than 15,000/mm³.

3. The pathogen in 15 of the 19 children was pneumococcus.

4. Clinical diagnosis of 14 of the 19 bacteremic children was upper respiratory infection/fever of unknown origin or pneumonia.

Conclusion: Suspect bacteremia in febrile infants under 2 years of age. Increase your suspicion if the child has a fever of greater than 38.9° C, a WBC of greater than 15,000/mm³, and symptoms of upper respiratory infection or pneumonia.

Reference: Teele, D.W., Pelton, S.I., Grant, M.J.A., et al.: J. Pediatr., *87*:227, 1975.

FEVER OF UNKNOWN ORIGIN

Prolonged episodes of fever without an apparent explanation are an uncommon diagnostic problem in pediatrics. Because of their rarity, they represent an exacting challenge and provide the clinician with an unequaled opportunity to demonstrate his skills in both careful history taking and physical examination. At least 50 per cent of "fevers of unknown origin" can be diagnosed by thoughtful attention to details and very simple laboratory studies. Unfortunately, the designation "fever of unknown origin" often prompts a myriad of tests and radiographic procedures in a nonsystematic fashion.

What are the usual causes of obscure, prolonged fevers in children and how do they differ in etiology from those observed in adults? The accompanying table summarizes the findings in two studies involving infants and children and contrasts them with a representative study of adult patients. Fever was defined as the presence of a rectal temperature of 38.5°C (99.8°F) on at least four occasions over a minimum period of two weeks.

Causes of Fever of Unknown Origin

INFANTS AND CHILDREN		ADULTS
Pizzo and Associates	*McClung*	
Infections (52%)	*Infections* (29%)	*Infections* (40%)
Viral syndromes	Respiratory	Tuberculosis
Respiratory	Central nervous system	Endocarditis
Central nervous system	Salmonella	Localized to peritoneum,
Urinary tract	Endocarditis	urinary tract, or liver
Osteomyelitis	Histoplasmosis	
Endocarditis	Brucellosis	
Tuberculosis	Epstein-Barr infection	
Herpes simplex, generalized		
Sinusitis		
Salmonella		

Collagen-Vascular (20%)	Collagen-Vascular (11%)	Collagen-Vascular (15%)
Rheumatoid arthritis	Rheumatoid arthritis	Rheumatoid arthritis
Vasculitis	Lupus	Rheumatic fever
Anaphylactoid purpura	Unclassified	Lupus
Lupus erythematosus		Polyarteritis
		Temporal arteritis
		Wegener's granulomatosis
Neoplastic (6%)	Neoplastic (8%)	Neoplastic (20%)
Leukemia	Leukemia	Leukemia
Lymphoma	Lymphoma	Lymphoma
	Neuroblastoma	Multiple myeloma
	Reticulum cell sarcoma	Colonic, pancreatic, and renal tumors
		Metastatic disease to bone and liver
Miscellaneous (10%)	Miscellaneous (10%)	Miscellaneous (20%)
Agranulocytosis	Regional enteritis	Granulomatous disease
Lamellar ichthyosis	Thyroiditis	Sarcoid
Milk allergy	Salicylate toxicity	Hepatitis
Agammaglobulinemia	Diencephalic syndrome	Regional enteritis
Behcet's syndrome	Dehydration fever	Ulcerative colitis
Anicteric hepatitis	Immunodeficiency	Thrombophlebitis
Ruptured appendix		Factitious fever
Central nervous system fever		Mediterranean fever
Aspiration pneumonia		Cirrhosis
		Whipple's disease
	Physically well children (9%)	
Undiagnosed (12%)	Undiagnosed (32%)	Undiagnosed (5%)

6

The Diagnostic Evaluation

1. *Initial studies* should be determined by clues provided by the history and physical examination. One must particularly search for a history of recent immunizations, transfusions, travel, exposure to animals, or other sick individuals.

2. *Initial diagnostic procedures* should include a complete blood count, urinalysis, erythrocyte sedimentation rate, chest film, and serum protein electrophoresis in addition to more specific studies indicated from the history and physical examination.

3. If sedimentation rate is elevated, if serum electrophoresis reveals a reversed albumin-globulin ratio or increase in the alpha globulin fraction, or if leukocytosis exists, these should all be considered evidence of an active disease process.

4. If initial studies fail to provide a diagnosis, other useful studies might include:

        Blood cultures, urine cultures, stool cultures
        Liver function tests
        Bone marrow biopsy and culture
        Antinuclear antibodies
        Latex fixation test
        Lupus erythematosus preparations
        Upper gastrointestinal films
        Barium enema
        Intravenous pyelogram
        Bone scan
        Sinus films

5. Ultimately, the diagnosis may require a biopsy of skin, muscle, and/or liver.

6. It is useful to establish an orderly timetable for the pursuit of the diagnosis. All too often the investigation proceeds in an aimless fashion without a logical schedule.

References: Pizzo, P.A., Lovejoy, F.H., Jr., and Smith, D.H.: Pediatrics, *55*:468, 1975. McClung, J.: Am. J. Dis. Child., *124*:544, 1972. Jacoby, G.A., and Swarts. M.N.: N. Engl. J. Med., *289*:1407, 1972.

FECAL LEUKOCYTES IN DIARRHEA

The presence (or absence) of leukocytes in a methylene blue stain of stool may help delineate the cause of diarrhea. In general, the presence of fecal leukocytes appears to indicate a disruption of distal intestinal mucosa.

The stain is prepared by spreading a small fleck of diarrhea mucus (or stool, if no mucus in specimen) on a clean glass slide. The mucus or stool is then mixed with two drops of methylene blue and covered with a coverslip. A microscopic examination is performed after a two to three minute delay, which allows for good nuclear staining.

Diarrheas Associated with Fecal Leukocytes

ILLNESS	PREDOMINANT LEUKOCYTE	NUMBER OF LEUKOCYTES PER HIGH POWER FIELD
E. coli, enteropathogenic	Polymorphonuclear	>25 in 68% of patients
Shigella	Polymorphonuclear	
Salmonella		
Typhoid	Mononuclear	<3 in over 50% of patients
Nontyphoid	Polymorphonuclear	
Ulcerative colitis	Polymorphonuclear	>25

Diarrheas not Associated with Fecal Leukocytes

E. coli, enterotoxigenic	*Giardia lamblia*
Vibrio cholerae	*Entamoeba histolytica*
Viral	"Nonspecific"

Reference: Harris, J.C., Dupont, H.L., and Hornick, R.B.: Ann. Intern. Med., *76*:697, 1972.

SHIGELLOSIS—THE BAND COUNT—A CLUE TO EARLY DIAGNOSIS

It is often difficult to decide whether patients with diarrhea have bacterial or viral gastroenteritis. The table on page 330 should prove of some value in this decision. The white count and differential may also prove to be a helpful diagnostic test.

Approximately 85 per cent of patients with shigellae in their stools will have more band forms than segmented neutrophils in their peripheral blood smears. In contrast, only 17 to 20 per cent of patients with other forms of infectious diarrhea will display this finding.

Lesson — do not rely on the total white count; always request a differential.

Reference: Poh, S.: Pediatrics, *39*:119, 1967.

PERTUSSIS AND THE WHITE BLOOD CELL COUNT

A marked leukocytosis (WBC $> 25,000/mm^3$) with a differential demonstrating the presence of 50 to 90 per cent lymphocytes is usually considered presumptive evidence of pertussis in infants and children with a cough.

Unfortunately, it is not generally appreciated that infants under 6 months of age often do not display this degree of leukocytosis and that the white cell count may be normal during the prodromal phase of the illness.

The table below illustrates the range of white cell counts by age in patients with pertussis.

TOTAL WBC	0 TO 6 MONTHS %	6 MONTHS TO 2 YEARS %	2 TO 5 YEARS %	5 YEARS %	TOTAL GROUP %
5,000 to 15,000	38	6	14	31	23
15,000 to 25,000	31	49	32	31	36
25,000 to 50,000	29	33	45	31	34
>50,000	2	12	9	7	7

The percentage of lymphocytes in this group of patients varied from 27 to 99 per cent with a mean of 70.4 per cent.

Patients with a leukemoid reaction (WBC >50,000) are more likely to have pulmonary complications such as atelectasis and pneumonia.

The relation of the total white cell count to the stage of the illness is illustrated in the table below.

WHITE CELL COUNT	CATARRHAL STAGE (WEEKS 1-2) (%)	PAROXYSMAL STAGE (WEEKS 3-5) (%)
5,000 to 15,000	28	12
15,000 to 25,000	42	34
>25,000	30	54

Reference: Brooksaler, F., and Nelson, J. D.: Am. J. Dis. Child., *114:*389, 1967.

PRESEPTAL OR ORBITAL CELLULITIS?

When a patient presents with a red and swollen eye, the diagnosis of orbital cellulitis must always by entertained. The table below provides some guidelines in reaching a clinical decision. Unfortunately the eye may be swollen shut, and it may be impossible to perform an adequate examination of the eye. Under these circumstances computerized axial tomography will rapidly determine the etiology of the process and localize the orbital abscess if it is present.

Distinguishing Features of Bacterial Preseptal Cellulitis, Orbital Cellulitis Secondary to Sinusitis, and Cavernous Sinus Thrombosis

FINDING	BACTERIAL PRESEPTAL CELLULITIS	ORBITAL CELLULITIS SECONDARY TO SINUSITIS	CAVERNOUS SINUS THROMBOSIS
Lid edema	Moderate to marked	Marked	Marked
Color of lids	Red	Red	Blue-purple
Increased warmth of lids	Present	Present	Absent
Proptosis	Absent or slight	Marked	Marked
Chemosis	Moderate	Marked	Moderate
Sensation			
V–1	Normal	May be reduced	Reduced
V–2	Normal	Normal	Reduced
Vision	Normal	May be reduced	Generally reduced
Pupil	Normal	Normal	Dilated, sluggish reaction to light (III paresis)
Motility	Normal	Restricted in proportion to orbital edema	III, IV, VI paresis
Pain on motion	Absent	Present	Absent
Intraocular pressure	Normal	May be elevated	May be elevated
Ophthalmoscopy	Normal	May be normal	Venous congestion; disc edema
Temperature	Normal or slightly elevated	Elevated (102–104° F)	Elevated (102–104° F or above)
White blood cell count	10,000–12,000/mm^3	15,000–20,000/mm^3	Above 15,000/mm^3
Other features	Evidence of trauma	X-ray changes of sinusitis	Bilateral involvement
	Purulent drainage	Unilateral	Progressive loss of consciousness
			Intracranial complications

Reference: Jones, D.B., Duane, T. (Ed.: In Clinical Ophthalmology. Vol. 4, Chapter 25, New York, Harper & Row, 1976.

6

DIFFERENTIAL DIAGNOSIS OF THE INFLAMED EYE

Red eyes in children are usually due to one of three causes: conjunctivitis, iritis, or corneal trauma or infection. Conjunctivitis, of course, is usually bacterial, viral, or allergic. The following two tables will aid in distinguishing the causes of red eyes.

	CONJUNCTIVITIS	IRITIS	CORNEAL TRAUMA OR INFECTION
Lids	Normal or slightly swollen	Normal	Normal or slightly swollen
Conjunctival injection	Diffuse	Circumcorneal	Circumcorneal
Cornea	Normal	Normal	Abrasion, ulcer, or foreign body
Pupil	Normal	Miotic	Normal
Discharge	Watery, mucoid, or purulent	Absent	Present
Vision	Normal	Slightly blurred	Usually blurred
Light sensitivity	None	Moderate to marked	None to moderate

DIFFERENTIAL DIAGNOSIS OF CONJUNCTIVITIS

	Bacterial	Viral	Allergic
Onset	Acute	Acute	Acute, subacute, or chronic
Fever	Rare	Frequent	None
URI symptoms	Rare	Frequent	None
Preauricular node	Only if hyperacute	Frequent	None
Conjunctival reaction	No follicles	Follicles in the anterior fornix	Follicles on the upper tarsus
Discharge	Mucoid or purulent	Watery	Usually none
Symptoms	Mild irritation	Mild irritation	Frequent itching
Allergy history	Infrequent	Infrequent	Common

Reference: Carlson, M.R.: Ophthalmologic emergencies in children. J. Continuing Ed. Pediatr., *21:*31–39, 1979.

THE PARANASAL SINUSES AND THE MASTOID SINUS

Sinusitis is underdiagnosed in infants and children (also frequently misspelled sinisitis, as well). Sinusitis is seen with increased frequency in patients with cyanotic heart disease, in leukemia and aplastic anemia while patients are neutropenic, in cystic fibrosis, and in patients with a history of nasal allergies.

It is useful to remember the ages at which the sinuses are pneumatized. Once a true sinus is present, the possibility of infection exists.

6

| Sinuses present at birth | Anterior and posterior *ethmoid*.
Maxillary antra. |
| Two to four years | Pneumatization of *frontal*
sinuses begins — complete by
5 to 9 years of age.
Sphenoid sinus becomes visible
by age 3. |

The *mastoid antrum* is present at birth, and pneumatization of the temporal bone starts in early infancy. The *mastoid process* is not present at birth, but begins to grow during the first year. Pneumatization is a slow, irregular process, but is generally complete prior to adolescence.

RATE OF FALL OF THE ESR
IN OSTEOMYELITIS

The erythrocyte sedimentation rate (ESR) is elevated in approximately 95 per cent of patients with osteomyelitis and/or septic arthritis; the rate with which the ESR falls during therapy is extremely variable, as can be seen in Figure 6-6. The level of ESR is plotted against the number of days of therapy. The patients included in this figure had either uncomplicated osteomyelitis or osteomyelitis complicated by septic arthritis. Many patients had a rapid fall in ESR; however, in some the level remained elevated for over a month. The moral to this story is: expect the ESR to fall with adequate therapy, but don't be surprised if it doesn't return to normal quickly.

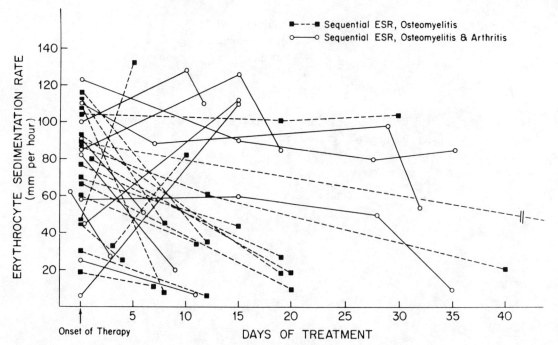

Sequential erythrocyte sedimentation rates (ESRs) in 17 cases of uncomplicated osteomyelitis and in 11 patients with associated arthritis.

FIG. 6-6

Reference: Dich, V.Q., Nelson, J.D., and Haltalin, K.C.: Am. J. Dis. Child., *129:*1273, 1975. Copyright 1975, American Medical Association.

AGE AND SYMPTOMS OF URINARY TRACT INFECTION

Pediatricians are well aware of the fact that the manifestations of many diseases vary as a function of the age of the patient. One striking example of this is illustrated in the table below, which describes the relationship between the presenting symptom of urinary tract infection and the age of the patient.

PRESENTING SYMPTOM	PERCENTAGE OF PATIENTS WITH VARIOUS SYMPTOMS BY AGES			
	Newborn–1 Mo	*1 Mo–2 Yr*	*2–6 Yr*	*6–18 Yr*
Failure to thrive, feeding problem	65	40	7	0
Diarrhea/vomiting	42	42	16	3
Unexplained fever	30	36	22	50
CNS*	29	7	9	5
Purulent meningitis	8	–	–	–
"Sepsis," jaundice	47	0	0	0
Colic, irritability, screaming attacks	0	15	5	0
Discolored or malodorous urine	0	9	14	0
Urgency, frequency, dysuria	0	8	44	41
Abdominal or flank pain	0	0	10	66
Enuresis	0	0	38	29

*Central nervous system disorders—including convulsions, hypotonicity, irritability, sluggishness, respiratory irregularities.

Reference: Boineau, F.G., and Lewy, J.E.: Pediatr. Ann., *64:*515, 1975.

TOXIC SHOCK

At this writing the toxic shock syndrome has been related to toxin-producing *Staphylococcus aureus* and tampons. Young women, including adolescent females, are most often affected. Most develop the syndrome during or shortly following menstruation. The syndrome has also been reported in males and nonmenstruating females, and in such cases *Staphylococcus aureus* has been isolated from focal lesions of the skin, bone, or lung.

Since fever, rash, and diarrhea are not infrequently encountered in pediatric patients with viral infections, the following is included to aid in recognition of this syndrome. All of the six criteria listed must be present if a diagnosis of toxic shock syndrome is to be made.

Toxic Shock Syndrome Case Definition

1. Fever (temperature ≥38.9°C [102°F]).
2. Rash (diffuse macular erythroderma).
3. Desquamation, 1–2 wk after onset of illness, particularly of palms and soles.
4. Hypotension (systolic blood pressure ≤90 mm Hg for adults or <5th percentile by age for children <16 years of age, or orthostatic syncope).
5. Involvement of 3 or more of the following organ systems:
   a. Gastrointestinal (vomiting or diarrhea at onset of illness).
   b. Muscular (severe myalgia or creatine phosphokinase level ≥2 X ULN*).
   c. Mucous membrane (vaginal, oropharyngeal, or conjunctival hyperemia).
   d. Renal (blood urea nitrogen level or creatinine level ≥2 X ULN or ≥5 white blood cells per high-power field–in the absence of a urinary tract infection).
   e. Hepatic (total bilirubin, serum glutamic oxaloacetic transaminase level, or serum glutamic pyruvic transaminase level ≥2 X ULN).
   f. Hematologic (platelets ≤100,000/mm³).
   g. Central nervous system (disorientation or alterations in consciousness without focal neurologic signs when fever and hypotension are absent).
6. Negative results on the following tests, if obtained: Serologic tests for Rocky Mountain spotted fever, leptospirosis, or measles.

---

*Twice upper limits of normal for laboratory.

Management of patients in whom the diagnosis is made includes aggressive fluid replacement and treatment with beta-lactamase resistant antistaphylococcal antibiotics. Careful vaginal examination should be made in female patients so that any retained tampon may be removed.

It is important to remember that 30 per cent of patients who have developed this syndrome have experienced at least one recurrence.

Reference: Morbidity and Mortality Weekly Report, *29:*441, 1980.

DOG BITES AND THE RISKS OF INFECTION

Dog bite is an extremely common problem in this country, with an estimated 0.5 to 1 million people being bitten each year. Surprisingly, there is little objective information available to make rational decisions concerning suturing, prophylactic antibiotics, and other forms of treatment. The following table illustrates the risk of wound infection from dog bites with respect to the location of the bite, time of initial treatment, type of wound, and whether the wound was sutured, debrided, or irrigated. Certain risk factors are clear. An age greater than 50 years, puncture wounds, hand or arm wounds, and delay of more than 24 hours in seeking treatment all increase the risk of infection. Facial wounds are very low risk. Debridement and adequate high pressure irrigation (at least 150 ml of saline) are crucial to good results. The more meticulously this is carried out, the better the result. *Except for* puncture wounds, most lacerations may be sutured after debridement and irrigation. Wounds of the hand, because of the risk of infection in the deep spaces, present a special problem. Punctures here must never be closed, and what appears to be a simple laceration may have a puncture wound underlying it. Thus far, there is no controlled evidence that prophylactic antibiotics are of any benefit. If infection does occur, treatment should be directed toward the more likely offending organisms. About one-half of all infections are caused by *Pasteurella multocida.* Most dogs carry this organism on their tonsils. As a matter of fact, 3 per cent of veterinary students carry *Pasteurella* in their throats. The remainder of infections are caused by a wide variety of organisms, including beta-hemolytic *Streptococcus, Streptococcus viridans,* and *Staphylococcus aureus.* Only about 5 per cent of dog bite infections would not be responsive to simple penicillin. Unfortunately, cultures of uninfected wounds are of little help, since organisms present do not correlate well with subsequent infection.

When treating dog bites, don't forget the need for tetanus immunization.

Dog Bite Wound Infections

A. **LOCATION OF BITE** — **PER CENT INFECTED**

LOCATION OF BITE	PER CENT INFECTED
Scalp	12.5
Face	4
Torso	0
Leg	15
Foot	1
Arm	27
Hand	30

B. **TIME TO TREATMENT**

<24 hours	8.8
>24 hours	66.6

C. TYPE OF WOUND
Puncture — 22
Laceration — 11

D. EFFECT OF SUTURING
Sutured (excluding puncture wounds) — 2.9
Left open — 25

E. EFFECT OF DEBRIDING
Debrided — 7.1
Not debrided — 17

F. EFFECT OF IRRIGATION
Irrigated — 12
Not irrigated — 69

Reference: Callaham, M.L.: JACEP, 7:83, 1978

ANIMALS AS DISEASE SOURCE

It is 4:00 A.M. You are just completing an admission note on a child with a confusing constellation of signs and symptoms. Suddenly, the third year student announces that he has learned that the child recently returned from a summer at a grandmother's goat farm and that several of the goats were ill.

The accompanying table may help you to handle such situations constructively by suggesting or ruling out various zoonoses once a careful environmental history has been obtained.

Potential Host Distribution of Selected Zoonoses

| | DOMESTIC ANIMALS | | | | | | | | | | | | WILD ANIMALS | | | | | | |
| | | | | | | | | | | | | | | | MAMMALS | | | |
VIRUS DISEASES	Horses	Cattle	Sheep	Goats	Swine	Dogs	Cats	Lab rodents	Poultry	Invertebrates	Fish	Amphibians	Reptiles	Birds	Rodents	Primates	Carnivores	Ungulates	Other
Arbovirus encephalitis	X	X	X	X	X					X	X		X	X	X			X	X
Cat-scratch disease (virus suspected)							X										X		
Lymphocytic choriomeningitis						X		X							X				
Newcastle									X					X					
Rabies	X	X	X	X	X	X	X	X	X						X	X	X	X	X
Vesicular stomatitis	X	X			X						X								
Yellow Fever											X				X	X			X

6

Disease	DOMESTIC ANIMALS									WILD ANIMALS					MAMMALS				
	Horses	Cattle	Sheep	Goats	Swine	Dogs	Cats	Lab rodents	Poultry	Invertebrates	Fish	Amphibians	Reptiles	Birds	Rodents	Primates	Carnivores	Ungulates	Other
RICKETTSIAL DISEASES																			
Q fever		X	X	X										X	X				
Rocky Mountain spotted fever			X	X		X				X					X				
SPIROCHETAL DISEASES																			
Leptospirosis	X	X	X	X	X	X	X	X							X	X	X	X	X
Rat-bite fever						X			X						X	X			
BACTERIAL DISEASE																			
Anthrax	X	X	X	X	X	X	X	X	X						X	X	X	X	X
Brucellosis	X	X	X	X	X	X	X	X	X						X		X	X	X
Erysipelas					X				X	X		X			X	X			
Hemorrhagic septicemia	X	X	X	X	X	X	X	X	X										
Listeriosis	X	X	X	X	X	X				X					X	X	X		
Melioidosis	X	X	X	X	X	X	X	X							X				
Plague		X	X			X	X	X							X	X	X		X
Pseudotuberculosis		X	X	X	X		X	X											
Psittacosis										X					X				
Salmonellosis	X	X	X	X	X	X	X	X	X	X	X	X	X	X	X	X	X	X	X
Scarlet fever		X			X														
Septic sore throat		X																	
Staphylococcosis		X																	
Tetanus	X												X				X		
Tuberculosis	X	X	X	X	X	X	X	X	X			X			X		X	X	X
Tularemia		X	X	X	X	X	X								X	X	X	X	X
Vibriosis		X	X	X															
FUNGUS DISEASES																			
Actinomycosis	X	X	X	X	X	X	X								X		X	X	X
Aspergillosis	X	X	X	X	X	X		X	X						X				
Coccidioidomycosis	X	X	X	X	X										X	X	X	X	
Cryptococcosis	X	X	X	X	X	X	X				X				X	X	X	X	
Epizootic lymphangitis	X																		
Histoplasmosis	X	X	X	X	X	X	X	X	X						X	X	X		X
Nocardiosis	X	X	X	X	X	X	X								X				X
North American blastomycosis	X					X													
Rhinosporidiosis	X	X																	
Ringworm	X	X	X	X	X	X	X	X	X						X	X	X	X	X
Sporotrichosis	X	X				X		X											
Streptothricosis	X	X	X	X		X												X	
PROTOZOAN																			
Amebiasis																X			
Balantidiasis					X											X			
Leishmaniasis						X									X		X		
Plasmodium (malaria)																X			
Sarcocystis	X	X	X	X						X					X				X
Toxoplasmosis		X				X	X	X							X	X	X		X
Trypanosomiasis	X	X	X	X	X	X	X	X		X							X	X	

Reference: Fowler, M.E.: Curr. Probl. Pediatr., *4*:3, 1974.

ZOONOSES

It is often difficult to remember which animals may be responsible for which diseases in humans. The list below is not complete, but it describes the major bacterial, viral, and rickettsial diseases that may be transmitted from animals to your patient.

Review of Bacterial, Viral, and Rickettsial Diseases of Animals That Can Be Transmitted to Humans

DISEASE	ETIOLOGIC AGENT	COMMON ANIMAL HOST	USUAL METHOD OF HUMAN INFECTION
Anthrax	*Bacillus anthracis*	Cattle, horses, sheep, swine, goats, dogs, cats, wild animals, birds	Inhalation or ingestion of spores; direct contact
Brucellosis	*Brucella melitensis, B. abortus, B. suis*	Cattle, goats, swine, sheep, horses, mules, dogs, cats, fowl, deer, rabbits	Milk; direct or indirect contact
Cat-scratch fever	Unknown	Cats, dogs	Cat or dog scratch
Colorado tick fever	Arbovirus	Squirrels, chip-munks, mice, porcupines	Tick bite
Cowpox	Cowpox virus	Cattle, horses	Skin abrasions
Herpes B viral encephalitis	*Herpesvirus simiae*	Monkeys	Monkey bites; con-tact with material from monkeys
Encephalitis (California)	Arbovirus	Rats, squirrels, horses, deer, hares, cows	Mosquito
Encephalitis (St. Louis)	Arbovirus	Birds	Mosquito
Encephalomyelitis (eastern equine)	Arbovirus	Birds, ducks, fowl, horses	Mosquito
Encephalomyelitis (Venezuelan equine)	Arbovirus	Rodents, horses	Mosquito
Encephalomyelitis (western equine)	Arbovirus	Birds, snakes, squirrels, horses	Mosquito
Glanders	*Pseudomonas mallei*	Horses	Skin contact; inhalation
Listeriosis	*Listeria monocytogenes*	Sheep, cattle, goats, guinea pigs, chick-ens, horses, rodents, birds, crustaceans	Unknown

DISEASE	ETIOLOGIC AGENT	COMMON ANIMAL HOST	USUAL METHOD OF HUMAN INFECTION
Lymphocytic choriomeningitis	Arbovirus	Mice, rats, dogs, monkeys, guinea pigs	Inhalation of contaminated dust; ingestion of contaminated food
Mediterranean fever (boutonneuse fever, African tick typhus)	*Rickettsia conorii*	Dog	Tick bite
Melioidosis	*Pseudomonas pseudomallei*	Rats, mice, rabbits, dogs, cats	Arthropod vectors, water, food
Orf (contagious ecthyma)	Virus	Sheep, goats	Through skin abrasions
Pasteurellosis	*Pasteurella multocida*	Fowl, cattle, sheep, swine, goats, mice, rats, rabbits	Animal bite
Plague (bubonic)	*Yersinia pestis*	Domestic rats, many wild rodents	Flea bite
Q fever	*Coxiella burnetii*	Cattle, sheep, goats	Inhalation of infected soil and dust
Rabies	Rabies virus (rhabdovirus group)	Dogs, bats, opossums, skunks, foxes, cats, cattle	Bite of rabid animal
Rat bite fever	*Spirillum minus*	Rats, mice, cats	Rat bite
Rat bite fever	*Streptobacillus moniliformis*	Rats, squirrels, weasels, turkeys	Rat bite
Relapsing fever (borreliosis)	*Borrelia* sp.	Rodents, porcupines, opossums, armadillos, ticks, lice	Tick or louse bite
Rickettsialpox	*Rickettsia akari*	Mice	Mite bite
Rocky Mountain spotted fever	*Rickettsia rickettsii*	Rabbits, squirrels, rats, mice, groundhogs	Tick bite
Salmonellosis	*Salmonella* sp. (except *S. typhosa*)	Fowl, swine, sheep, cattle, horses, dogs, cats, rodents, reptiles, birds, turtles	Direct contact; food
Scrub typhus	*Rickettsia tsutsugamushi*	Wild rodents, rats	Mite bite
Tuberculosis	*Mycobacterium bovis*	Cattle, horses, cats, dogs	Milk; direct contact

6

DISEASE	ETIOLOGIC AGENT	COMMON ANIMAL HOST	USUAL METHOD OF HUMAN INFECTION
Tularemia	*Francisella tularensis*	Wild rabbits, most other wild and domestic animals	Direct contact with infected carcass, usually rabbit; tick bite, biting flies
Typhus fever (endemic)	*Rickettsia mooseri*	Rats	Flea bite
Vesicular stomatitis	Virus (rhabdovirus group)	Cattle, swine, horses	Direct contact
Weil's disease (leptospirosis)	*Leptospira interrogans*	Rats, mice, skunks, opossums, wildcats, foxes, raccoons, shrews, bandicoots, dogs, cattle, swine	Through skin, drinking water, eating food
Yellow fever (jungle)	Yellow fever virus	Monkeys, marmosets, lemurs, mosquitoes	Mosquito

Reference: Youmans, G.P.: *In* Youmans, G.P., Paterson, P.Y., and Sommers, H.M. (eds.): The Biologic and Clinical Basis of Infectious Diseases. Philadelphia, W.B. Saunders Company, 1980, pp. 718–719.

TREATMENT OF SCABIES

The physician who sees children daily as outpatients is familiar with the clinical manifestations of scabies. Treatment will be more effective if parents and physicians understand the details of proper therapy and the results to be anticipated.

All household members and any sexual contacts outside the household should be treated at the same time. The incubation period may vary from less than one month to two months, and the family member who is not treated because of lack of symptoms may transmit the disease to the treated members.

Once therapy is instituted, all intimate articles of clothing should be machine washed or dryed using the hot cycle, boiled, or laundered and ironed. Outerwear and furniture need no special treatment, since the infesting mites survive only briefly away from the human host.

Transmission of scabies is unlikely after 24 hours of treatment with an effective scabicidal agent.

The symptoms and signs of scabies are in part a hypersensitivity response, and the destruction of the mite may not lead to their immediate disappearance. Symptoms and signs may persist for weeks after effective treatment.

Topical corticosteroid therapy may potentiate the infestation and should not be used prior to scabicidal therapy.

Chemical irritation may occur with too frequent use of scabicides. The contact dermatitis that results may be mistaken for resistance to therapy. Overuse should be discouraged. One ounce of a topical preparation is sufficient to adequately cover the trunk and extremities of an average adult, and children will need proportionately less. The prescription should allow for only the amount needed and should specify that no refills be given.

One application of the most commonly used scabicide, gamma benzene hexachloride, is usually sufficient. A second application one week after the first is theoretically justifiable to destroy recently hatched larvae and nymphs from eggs that were present at the time of the initial application. The lotion should be applied after a warm bath or shower and left on for 24 hours. The lotion should not be applied near the eyes or mucous membranes. A second bath or shower should be taken at the conclusion of the 24-hour treatment.

Reference: Orkin, M., Epstein, E., and Maibach, H. I.: J.A.M.A., *236:*1136, 1976.

PARASITES

"Stool for ova and parasites" is often ordered with little thought given to the possible parasitic pathogen in a given clinical situation. Parasitic disease is much less frequent in the United States than in most of the rest of the world, but the pediatrician should be familiar with parasites that may be encountered here and abroad.

The table on the following pages lists parasites that are likely to be encountered in the United States. Some, such as the plasmodia and the tapeworms, are included because of the frequency with which they are found in U.S. citizens who travel abroad or in immigrants from other countries. Treatment regimens are not listed because of the frequency with which treatment recommendations change.

NAME OF PARASITE	ROUTE OF ENTRY INTO HUMAN BODY	MECHANISM OF INFECTION	CLINICAL MANIFESTATIONS	METHOD OF DIAGNOSIS
Enterobius vermicularis (pinworm)	Patient acquires eggs from skin during scratching and transfers them to mouth. Eggs may also be swallowed when inhaled while handling clothes and bedclothes of infected individuals.	Worm inhabits the rectum or colon and emerges onto perianal skin during sleep, causing intense itching.	No systemic manifestations.	Application of transparent adhesive tape to perianal skin and inspection of tape under microscope.
Ascaris lumbricoides (roundworm)	Acquired through ingestion of eggs found in soil contaminated with human feces.	Inhabits the small intestine. Larvae penetrate intestinal villi, enter portal circulation, proceed to lungs. They ascend to oropharynx where they are swallowed, and they inhabit the small intestine and mature to adult worms.	May be asymptomatic. May have fever, malaise, eosinophilia. Large number of worms may cause intestinal obstruction. May migrate to appendix, perforate, and cause peritonitis.	Detection of ova in the stool.
Toxocara canis (dog roundworm)	Acquired through ingestion of eggs found in soil contaminated with dog feces.	Larvae hatched in small intestine, migrate aimlessly through tissue (thus the disease is called visceral larva migrans).	Eosinophilia to 50 per cent of the white blood count. Larvae may enter central nervous system, eye, lung, liver, and so on.	Detection of larvae in liver biopsy and/or high titers of human isohemagglutinins.
Necator americanus and *Ancylostoma duodenale* (hookworm)	Eggs are deposited with stool and become larvae, which penetrate human skin and enter the blood stream. They pass through the lungs to the pharynx where they are swallowed.	Adult worms inhabit small intestine and feed on the villi.	Anemia, hypoproteinemia, malnutrition.	Detection of ova in the stool.

Organism			
Giardia lamblia	Cyst is ingested in water contaminated by human feces.	Inhabit the duodenum.	May be asymptomatic. May cause protracted, severe diarrhea with fever and weight loss.	Detection of trophozoite or cysts in the stool. Stool examination should be done multiply. Examination of duodenal fluid may be required.
Taenia saginata and *Taenia solium* (tapeworm)	Ingested head (scolex) from poorly cooked beef or pork establishes itself in the small intestine.	Generated segments (proglottids) increase length of worm. The proglottid is regurgitated into the stomach and may lead to migration and formation of cysts in the brain or eye.	Cramps, pain.	Detection of proglottids or ova in the stool.
Echinococcus granulosus (dog tapeworm)	Ingestion of eggs contained in dog feces.	Cysts form in liver, lung, and elsewhere.	Cysts act as space-occupying lesions and, if ruptured, may lead to metastatic cysts.	Casoni skin test. Serologic tests.
Entamoeba histolytica	Cysts contained in human feces are ingested in contaminated food or water.	Excystation allows deposit of trophozoites in the colonic mucosa.	May be asymptomatic. May cause protracted colitis. Infrequently leads to hepatic abscess, lung or skin infections.	Detection of trophozoites or cysts in stool. Serologic tests.
Strongyloides stercoralis	Larvae enter the human skin from contaminated soil. Larvae hatched in patient's intestine may reinfect the same patient via penetration of the intestinal wall and travel through the blood stream.	Inhabits the small intestinal mucosa.	May be asymptomatic. May cause protracted mucoid diarrhea and malabsorption.	Detection of larvae in stool.

Continued

6

NAME OF PARASITE	ROUTE OF ENTRY INTO HUMAN BODY	MECHANISM OF INFECTION	CLINICAL MANIFESTATIONS	METHOD OF DIAGNOSIS
Trichuris trichiura	Eggs deposited in soil are ingested. Larvae hatch in the small intestine and migrate to the cecum and large intestine.	Inhabits large intestine. The anterior end is buried in the mucosa.	Usually asymptomatic. No eosinophilia. With heavy infection there may be diarrhea and tenesmus.	Detection of ova in stool.
Trichinella spiralis	Larvae encysted in skeletal muscle of pork or bear. They mature in the small intestine. Larvae pass to the lungs, are shunted to the left side of the heart and the systemic circulation.	Migrating larvae lodge in muscle and sometimes in central nervous system.	Gastroenteritis, periorbital edema, myositis, petechial hemorrhages, fever, eosinophilia.	Skin test, serology, appropriate history.
Schistosoma mansoni	Larvae emerge into water from infected snail. The larvae penetrate human skin and proceed to liver sinusoids. They grow there and migrate to venules throughout the body.	Larvae obstruct the portal circulation. Granulomas are formed in any tissue in which worms are embedded.	Fibrosis of liver, lung; circulatory obstruction, cor pulmonale, pseudopolyps of bladder, neurologic manifestations.	Detection of ova in stool or urine. May have to be done often, since relatively few eggs reach intestinal lumen.
Plasmodium falciparum, Plasmodium malariae	Parasite enters human blood stream via bite of a female anopheline mosquito. Parasite may also be transferred to a patient who receives blood from an infected donor.	Parasites mature in the liver for up to two weeks. They are then able to infect erythrocytes and additional hepatocytes.	Fever during erythrocyte infection. Musculoskeletal pain, headache, diarrhea, anemia. *P. falciparum* may cause hemoglobinuria, coma, convulsions, death. "Induced" malaria contracted from infected blood donor has no erythrocyte phase. Fever is only manifestation.	Detection of parasites in erythrocytes on usual blood smear or "thick smear."

6

Pneumocystis carinii	Person to person contact (?). Asymptomatic carriers (?).	Patients affected are immuno-suppressed, have primary immune deficiency or malignancy.	Dyspnea, fever, unproductive cough, tachycardia, tachypnea, mild anemia. Chest roentgenogram shows bilateral diffuse or patchy interstitial infiltrates.	Lung biopsy, bronchial washings, tracheal aspirate.
Toxoplasma gondii	Acquired: ingestion of raw or poorly cooked meat. Contact with oocysts via cat feces.	Parasite invades host tissues. Usually localized to lymph nodes, but may invade brain, heart, lung, liver, and muscle in immuno-suppressed host.	Clinically evident infection is rare. Lymphadenopathy is usually the only symptom. Immunosuppressed patient may have generalized involvement with hepatitis, pneumonitis, pericarditis, myocarditis, meningo-encephalitis.	Serologic tests.
	Congenital: infection acquired trans-placentally.	Congenital infection is generalized. Infant is more severely affected with acquisition in late gestation.	Hepatosplenomegaly, enlarged lymph nodes, myocarditis, anemia, edema, exudates in the body cavities. The eye is usually involved with white scars visible on the fundus. There may be intracerebral calcifications, hydro-cephalus, convulsions.	

References: Katz, M.: J. Pediatr., *87*:165, 1975. Beverley, J.K.A.: Bri. Med. J., *2*:475, 1973. Walzer, P.D., Perl, D.P., Krogstad, D.J., et al.: Ann. Intern. Med., *80*:83, 1974.

RUBELLA EXPOSURE DURING PREGNANCY

The dangers of maternal rubella infection during pregnancy are well known. The course to take after an expectant mother has been exposed to rubella is outlined as follows:

Management of a Pregnant Female Exposed to Rubella

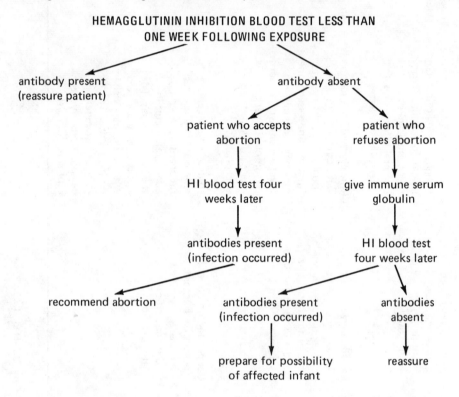

If a blood sample for HI test is obtained more than one week after exposure to rubella, one cannot tell if antibodies present are from a past or the present exposure. Therefore, a second blood specimen taken one or two weeks after the first blood sample is tested for CF, HI, and IgM specific antibody. A rising antibody titer and/or the presence of IgM specific rubella antibody is indicative of current rubella infection.

There is no evidence that immunization of a child whose mother is in the early stages of pregnancy carries any risk of infection to the fetus.

Reference: Honig, P.J., and Tunnessen, W.W.: Clinical Diagnostic Quiz, *1*:7, 1976.

7
ALLERGY/
IMMUNOLOGY

CLASSIFICATION OF IMMUNODEFICIENCY DISORDERS

The evaluation for possible immunodeficiency is predicated upon an understanding of the full spectrum of these disorders. The two tables below illustrate the more important diseases associated with immunodeficiency and provide a suggested approach to the actual evaluation. Secondary immunodeficiencies, such as those that occur with chronic disease, are not included here.

Classification

ANTIBODY (B CELL) IMMUNODEFICIENCY DISEASES

X-linked hypogammaglobulinemia (congenital hypogammaglobulinemia)
Transient hypogammaglobulinemia of infancy
Common, variable, unclassifiable immunodeficiency (acquired hypogamma-
 globulinemia)
Immunodeficiency with hyper-IgM
Selective IgA deficiency
Selective IgM deficiency
Selective deficiency of IgG subclasses

CELLULAR (T CELL) IMMUNODEFICIENCY DISEASES

Congenital thymic aplasia (DiGeorge's syndrome)
Chronic mucocutaneous candidiasis (with or without endocrinopathy)

COMBINED ANTIBODY MEDIATED (B CELL) AND CELL-MEDIATED (T CELL) IMMUNODEFICIENCY DISEASES

Severe combined immunodeficiency disease (autosomal recessive, X-linked,
 sporadic)
Cellular immunodeficiency with abnormal immunoglobulin synthesis
 (Nezelof's syndrome)
Immunodeficiency with ataxia-telangiectasia
Immunodeficiency with eczema and thrombocytopenia (Wiskott-
 Aldrich syndrome)
Immunodeficiency with thymoma
Immunodeficiency with short-limbed dwarfism
Immunodeficiency with enzyme deficiency
Episodic lymphopenia with lymphotoxin
Graft-versus-host disease

PHAGOCYTIC DYSFUNCTION

Chronic granulomatous disease
Glucose-6-phosphate dehydrogenase deficiency
Myeloperoxidase deficiency
Chédiak-Higashi syndrome
Job's syndrome
Tuftsin deficiency
"Lazy leukocyte syndrome"
Elevated IgE, defective chemotaxis, eczema, and recurrent infections

COMPLEMENT ABNORMALITIES AND IMMUNODEFICIENCY DISEASE

C1q, C1r, and C1s deficiency
C2 deficiency
C3 deficiency (type I, type II)
C4 deficiency
C5 dysfunction, C5 deficiency
C6 deficiency
C7 deficiency
C8 deficiency

Initial Screening Evaluation

ANTIBODY-MEDIATED IMMUNITY

Quantitative immunoglobulin levels: IgG, IgM, IgA
Schick test: measures specific IgG antibody response to diphtheria
Isohemagglutinin titer (anti-A and anti-B): measures IgM function

CELL-MEDIATED IMMUNITY

White blood count with differential: measures total lymphocytes
Delayed hypersensitivity skin test: measures specific T-cell and macrophage
   response to antigens

PHAGOCYTOSIS

White blood count with differential: measures total neutrophils
NBT, chemiluminescence: measures neutrophil metabolic function

COMPLEMENT

Hemolytic complement quantitation (CH_{50}): quantitates complement activity
C3 level: measures amount of important complement component

Reference: Ammann, A.J., and Fudenberg, H.H.: Immunodeficiency diseases. *In* Fudenberg, H.H., Stites, D.P., Caldwell, J.L., and Wells, J.V. (eds.): Basic and Clinical Immunology. Los Altos, CA, Lange Medical Publications, 1980, p. 410.

APPROACH TO IMMUNODEFICIENCY

Initial evaluation of the child with frequent or unusual infections is within the capability of any pediatrician and almost any hospital laboratory. Your approach may be streamlined by the use of the following guidelines.

A. Frequent mild respiratory infections without complications (up to 14 per year may be normal) are usually *not* suggestive of immunologic deficit. These are especially common in the preschool child and tend to decrease with age. Similarly, pneumonias that recur (or persist) at a single anatomic site are not likely to be due to immunodeficiency.

B. Several patterns of illness *are* suggestive of immune defect:
1. Family history positive for immunologic problems, lymphoproliferative disorders, or autoimmune disease.
2. Recurrent infections caused by bacteria of high-grade virulence.
3. Those caused by bacteria that are ordinarily nonpathogens.
4. Those caused by fungi.
5. Unusual reaction to live vaccine or to ordinarily mild viral illnesses.
6. Infections at unusual sites.
7. Infections that persist or that resolve unusually slowly.

C. Many patterns of infection that initially appear to suggest immuno-deficiency may be explainable on a nonimmunologic basis, such as:
1. Mechanical or other host factors:
   a. CNS: e.g., cranial or dermal sinuses, neurenteric cysts, post-traumatic skull defect.
   b. Respiratory tract: e.g.,, tracheoesophageal fistula, foreign body, cystic fibrosis.
   c. Urinary tract: e.g., neurogenic bladder, posterior urethral valves, urethral stenosis.
   d. Secondary immunodeficiencies: e.g., malnutrition, malignant diseases, drugs.
   e. Miscellaneous conditions favoring infection, e.g., diabetes mellitus, congenital heart disease, burns, indwelling catheters, eczema, sickle cell anemia, trisomy-21.

7

or by

2. Microbiologic factors:
   a. Inadequately treated infections: e.g., incorrect drug, incorrect dose, occult abscess.
   b. Repeated exposure to pathogens: e.g., streptococcal carrier in family.
   c. Unusual resistance of common organism: e.g., ampicillin-resistant *Hemophilus influenzae.*
   d. Presence of unidentified (and therefore untreated) organism.

D. If the preceding points have been considered and an immunodeficiency is still being sought, the following table provides clinical clues and suggestions for *screening* tests in each area of host defense.

TYPE OF DEFICIT (AND RELATIVE FREQUENCY)	LIKELY PATHOGENS OR PROBLEMS	HISTORY AND PHYSICAL EXAMINATION CLUES	SCREENING TESTS AND EXPECTED RESULTS
T cell (5%)	Viruses, fungi, protozoans, autoimmunity, surveillance against malignancy	Growth failure, vaccinial scar, ataxia-telangiectasia, absence of lymph nodes	1. Lymphocyte count low (<1200) 2. Lymphocyte morphology may be abnormal 3. Absence of thymic shadow on infant roentgenogram 4. No response to standard anergy tests
Combined T and B cell (25%)		Features of T cell (above) and B cell (below) both occur in the combined immunodeficiency	
B cell (50–75%)	Severe bacterial infections	Usually well until 5 to 6 months, then: growth failure, eczema, petechiae, arthritis, absence of lymph nodes	1. Decrease in hemoglobin common 2. Decrease in level of one or more immunoglobulins 3. Absence of expected specific antibodies, e.g., ASO, isohemagglutinins 4. Decreased platelet count in Wiskott-Aldrich 5. Plasma cells in bone marrow or periphery, if present, suggest *some* B cell function
Phagocytes (1%)	Recurrent bacterial infections and/or abscesses	Mouth ulcers, impalpable spleen, abscesses, draining sinuses	1. Abnormal appearance and/or low number of neutrophils. Repeat weekly for one month if cyclic neutropenia is considered 2. Howell-Jolly bodies 3. Low NBT in some defects
Complement (1%)	Recurrent bacterial infections and/or abscesses; auto-immune disease	Mouth ulcers, abscesses, impalpable spleen, draining sinuses	1. Low C_3 2. Low CH_{50}

References: Norman, M.E., and South, M.A.: Clin. Pediatr., *13*:644, 1974. Ammann, A.J., and Wara, D.W.: Curr. Probl. Pediatr., Vol. 5, 1975.

TESTING FOR DELAYED HYPERSENSITIVITY

Skin testing for delayed hypersensitivity is becoming more and more common as patients are evaluated for possible immunologic defects. Interpretation of such tests has been hampered by the fact that many apparently normal children are anergic. The table below provides some figures on the percentage of positive reactions, of varying sizes, in patients of different ages, employing four different skin testing agents.

	No.	CANDIDA ALBICANS					DIPHTHERIA-TETANUS					MUMPS					SK/SD				
		Induration†			Erythema†		Induration			Erythema		Induration			Erythema		Induration			Erythema	
		≥2	≥5	≥10	≥10	≥15	≥2	≥5	≥10	≥10	≥15	≥2	≥5	≥10	≥10	≥15	≥2	≥5	≥10	≥10	≥15
Newborn infant	2	0	0	0	0	0	0	0	0	0	0	0	0	0	0	0	0	0	0	0	0
0–6 mo	18	27	5	0	0	0	53*	7	0	15	0	100	61	0	44	16	0	0	0	0	0
7–12 mo	14	50	42	7	21	7	100	50	0	28	7	100	84	0	76	53	7	0	0	0	0
1–5 yr	26	65	46	3	23	3	88*	73	3	42	19	100	92	7	88	53	20	16	7	20	16
6–10 yr	18	66	50	22	44	16	100	88	16	50	16	100	100	50	100	94	51	55	33	50	44
11–15 yr	19	63	47	15	36	15	100	73	21	68	36	100	100	31	84	74	73	73	63	73	68
16–20 yr	17	88	76	23	70	35	88*	82	23	58	41	100	94	11	82	82	82	76	76	82	64

*Includes patients not receiving DPT immunization.
†Induration and erythema expressed in millimeters.

The following reagents were used:

1. Oidiomycin (*Candida albicans*) 1/100 (Hollister-Stier).
2. Mumps skin test antigen — undiluted (Eli Lilly).
3. Streptokinase/streptodornase — diluted with buffered saline to 40 units SK and 10 units SD/ml (Lederle).
4. Diphtheria and tetanus toxoids, adsorbed (pediatric DT) — diluted 1/100 with buffered saline (Dow).

Reference: Franz, M.L., Carella, J.A., and Galant, S.P.: J. Pediatr., *88*:975, 1976.

CLINICAL CONDITIONS ASSOCIATED WITH ANERGY

Delayed hypersensitivity skin testing is of relatively little value in establishing the diagnosis of defective cellular immunity in the first year of life. In this circumstance, in vitro assay for T-cell numbers and function is much more useful in the diagnosis of congenital immuno-deficiency disease. After this age, the detection of anergy may be elicited in a wide variety of clinical conditions. The causes of anergy are multiple (see the table) but broadly fall into errors of testing, infections, and immunodeficiency syndromes (either primary or secondary).

I. TECHNICAL ERRORS IN SKIN TESTING

Improper dilutions
Bacterial contamination
Exposure to heat or light
Adsorption of antigen on container walls
Faulty injection (too deep, leaking)
Improper reading of reaction

II. IMMUNOLOGIC DEFICIENCY

Congenital
    Combined deficiencies of cellular and humoral immunity
        Ataxia-telangiectasia
        Nezelof's syndrome
        Severe combined immunodeficiency
        Wiskott-Aldrich syndrome
    Cellular immunodeficiency
        Thymic and parathyroid aplasia (DiGeorge's syndrome)
        Mucocutaneous candidiasis

Acquired
- Sarcoidosis
- Chronic lymphocytic leukemia
- Carcinoma
- Immunosuppressive medication
- Rheumatoid diseases
- Uremia
- Alcoholic cirrhosis
- Biliary cirrhosis
- Surgery
- Hodgkin's disease and lymphomas

III. INFECTIONS

Influenza
Mumps
Measles
Viral vaccines
Typhus
Miliary and active tuberculosis
Disseminated mycotic infection
Lepromatous leprosy
Scarlet fever

Reference: Heiss, L.I., and Palmer, D.L.: Am. J. Med., *56:*323, 1974.

THE FUNGAL SKIN TEST— A DIAGNOSTIC HINDRANCE

A common error of clinical practice is the reliance on a fungal skin test to make a diagnosis of an acute fungal infection. Test results are misleading. The following points should be remembered.

1. *Cross reactions* can occur because of shared antigens.
2. *Elevations of antibody titers* may be produced by the introduction of small amounts of antigen via the intradermal route.
3. *False-negative skin test* reactions are very common during the acute phase of fungal infections.

Measuring changes in complement-fixing antibodies is of far greater significance in establishing a diagnosis in patients suspected of having coccidioidomycosis, histoplasmosis, or blastomycosis. A titer of 1:16 or greater should be considered as presumptive evidence of a recent infection with one of these agents and should result in intensive efforts to isolate the organism by culture of sputum, urine, bone marrow, or other body fluids.

Blastomycin, as a skin test antigen, may elevate histoplasmosis antibodies and usually produces a negative result in patients with active blastomycosis.

Histoplasmin can elevate the complement-fixing antibody titer to histoplasmin, and will produce elevations of antibody titer to blastomycin as well.

Coccidioidin is the most specific of the skin test antigens but frequently may be negative during the acute phase of the illness.

These three skin tests should not be applied in the evaluation of patients with fevers of undetermined origin. These skin tests can be of more value as prognostic indicators in patients with culture-proved fungal disease, as epidemiologic tools in community studies, as antigens for in vivo determination of cellular immunity, and as indicators of past fungal exposure in patients in whom immunosuppressive therapy is to be instituted.

Reference: Levin, S.J.: J. Infect. Dis., *122*.343, 1970.

PROPERTIES OF
HUMAN IMMUNOGLOBULINS

Which immunoglobulin is the lightest, fixes complement, has the highest serum concentration, crosses the placenta, and has some antibacterial as well as antiviral activity? Which immunoglobulin has the most antiviral activity? Which causes the greatest bacterial lysis? Which causes the greatest complement fixation? Maybe some of us carry this sort of information in our hip pockets, but most people probably do not. For those in the latter group who wear pocketless jeans, the following table should prove of some usefulness.

	IgG	IgA	IgM	IgD	IgE
H chain class	γ	α	μ	δ	ϵ
H chain subclass	$\gamma1, \gamma2, \gamma3, \gamma4$	$\alpha1, \alpha2$	$\mu1, \mu2$		
L chain type	k and λ	k and λ	k and λ	k and λ	k and λ
Molecular formula	$\gamma2L2$	$\alpha2L$ * or $(\alpha2L2)_2 SC^\dagger J^\ddagger$	$(\alpha2L2) 5J^\ddagger$	$\delta2L2$	$\epsilon2L2$
Sedimentation coefficient (S)	6–7	7	19	7–8	8
Molecular weight (approximate)	150,000	160,000* 400,000§	900,000	180,000	190,000
Electrophoretic mobility (average)	γ	Fast γ to β	Fast γ to β	Fast γ	Fast γ
Complement fixation (classic)	+	0	++++	0	0
Serum concentration (approximate; mg/dl)	1000	200	120	3	0.05
Placental transfer	+	0	0	0	0
Reaginic activity	?	0	0	0	++++
Antibacterial lysis	+	+	+++	?	?
Antiviral activity	+	+++	+	?	?

*For monomeric serum IgA.
†Secretory component.
‡J chain.
§For secretory IgA.

Reference: Goodman, J.W., and Wang, A–C.: Immunoglobulins: structure, diversity and genetics. *In* Fudenberg, H.H., Stites, D.P., Caldwell, J.L., and Wells, J.V. (eds.): Basic and Clinical Immunology. Los Altos, CA, Lange Medical Publications, 1980, p. 33.

NORMAL LEVELS OF IMMUNE GLOBULINS

The level of serum IgG is relatively static in any one individual over time, while the levels of total γ-globulin, IgM, and IgA increase with age. Figure 7–1 demonstrates the relationship between serum IgG and age over the first nine months of life.

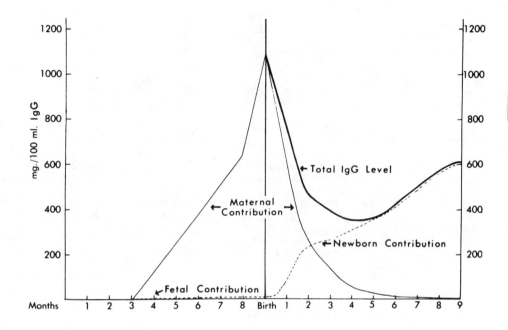

FIG. 7–1

References: Allansmith, M., McClellan, B.H., Butterworth, M., and Maloney, J.R.: The development of immunoglobulin levels in man. J. Pediatr., *72:*276, 1968. Stiehm, E.R., and Fudenberg, H.H.: Serum levels of immune globulins in health and disease: a survey. Pediatrics, *37:*715, 1966.

SERUM IMMUNOGLOBULINS AND ISOHEMAGGLUTININS

A frequently occurring question is, "Are these immunoglobulin levels normal for the patient's age?" Another frequent question is, "At what age is the failure to detect isohemagglutinins, anti-A or anti-B, of diagnostic significance?" The table on the following page attempts to provide you with these answers.

Relation of Age to Serum Immunoglobulin (Ig) Levels and Isohemagglutinin Activity (IHA)

	IgG (mg/100 ml) (Mean + 1 SD and Range)	IgA (mg/100 ml) (Mean + 1 SD and Range)	IgM (mg/100 ml) (Mean + 1 SD and Range)	IHA Titer (Mean and Range)
Cord blood	1086 ± 390 (740 – 1374)	2 ± 2 (0 – 15)	14 ± 6 (0 –22)	0*
1–3 months	512 ± 152 (280 – 950)	16 ± 10 (4 – 36)	28 ± 14 (15 – 86)	1:5 0 – 1:10†
4–6 months	520 ± 180 (240 – 884)	22 ± 14 (11 – 52)	36 ± 18 (21 – 74)	1:10 0 – 1:160†
7–12 months	742 ± 226 (281 – 1280)	54 ± 17 (22 – 112)	76 ± 27 (36 – 150)	1:80 0 – 1:640‡
13–24 months	945 ± 270 (290 – 1300)	67 ± 19 (9 – 143)	88 ± 36 18 – 210)	1:80 0 – 1:640‡
26–36 months	1030 ± 152 (546 – 1562)	89 ± 34 (21 – 196)	94 ± 23 (43 – 115)	1:160 1:10 – 1:640 §
3–5 years	1150 ± 244 (546 – 1760)	126 ± 31 (56 – 284)	87 ± 24 (26 – 121)	1:80 1:5 – 1:640
6–8 years	1187 ± 289 (596 – 1744)	147 ± 35 (56 – 330)	108 ± 37 (54 – 260)	1:80 1:5 – 1:640
9–11 years	1217 ± 261 (744 – 1719)	146 ± 38 (44 – 208)	104 ± 46 (27 – 215)	1:160 1:20 – 1:640
12–16 years	1248 ± 221 (796 – 1647)	168 ± 54 (64 – 290)	96 ± 31 (60 – 140)	1:160 1:10 – 1:320

*IHA is rarely detectable in cord blood.
†50% of normal infants have no isohemagglutinins at age 6 months.
‡10% of normal infants have no isohemagglutinins at age 1 year.
§Beyond age 2, all normal individuals (except those with blood type AB) have isohemagglutinins.

Reference: Johnson, R.B., Jr., and August, C.S.: *In* Kampe, C.H., Silver, H.K., and O'Brien, D. (eds.): Current Pediatric Diagnosis and Treatment, 5th ed. Los Altos, California, Lange Medical Publications, 1978, p. 428.

TREATMENT OF IMMUNODEFICIENCY

The management of immunodeficiency syndromes depends on the specific nature of the defect and can extend from gamma globulin injections all the way to transplantation with bone marrow or fetal thymus. The accompanying table indicates a current management approach to these problems.

TREATMENT	B-CELL DISORDERS	T-CELL DISORDERS	PHAGOCYTIC DISORDERS	COMPLEMENT DISORDERS
Gamma globulin	X-linked hypogammaglobulinemia; acquired hypogammaglobulinemia; secondary hypogammaglobulinemia when associated with infection; do not use in selective IgA deficiency	Use only when absent antibody response is demonstrated; not recommended for Wiskott-Aldrich syndrome	Not recommended	Not recommended
Hyperimmune gamma globulin	Use in above disorders when specific exposure has occurred	May be used when specific exposure has occurred	May be used when specific exposure has occurred	May be used when specific exposure has occurred
Frozen plasma by intravenous infusion	X-linked hypogammaglobulinemia and acquired hypogammaglobulinemia when intramuscular administration is not tolerated or is ineffective	Use only when absent antibody response is demonstrated; irradiate to prevent GVH	Not recommended	Use with caution; plasma may exacerbate autoimmune disease
Infusions of white cells	Not recommended	Not recommended	Questionable value	Not recommended
Infusions of red cells	Not recommended	May be of benefit in certain enzyme deficiencies associated with immunodeficiency (adenosine deaminase, purine nucleoside phosphorylase); irradiate to prevent GVH	Not recommended	Not recommended
Bone marrow transplant	Not recommended	Use only when impaired T-cell function is present; must have histocompatible donor	Not recommended	Not recommended

Continued

7

TREATMENT	B-CELLS DISORDERS	T-CELL DISORDERS	PHAGOCYTIC DISORDERS	COMPLEMENT DISORDERS
Fetal thymus transplantation	Not recommended	DiGeorge's syndrome; severe combined immunodeficiency without suitable bone marrow donor; selective use in other combined immunodeficiency disorders	Not recommended	Not recommended
Cultured thymus epithelium	Not recommended	Selective cases of T-cell disorders where no suitable bone marrow donor is available	Not recommended	Not recommended
Fetal liver transplantation	Not recommended	Sometimes used in severe combined immunodeficiency in absence of suitable bone marrow donor	Not recommended	Not recommended
Transfer factor	Not recommended	May be successful in chronic candidiasis when combined with antifungal agent; highly debatable effect in other disorders	Not recommended	Not recommended
Thymosin and other thymic factors	Not recommended	Limited evaluation to date; may enhance T-cell function in a variety of T-cell disorders, including DiGeorge's syndrome; no effect in chronic candidiasis or severe combined immunodeficiency	Not recommended	Not recommended

Reference: Ammann, A.J., and Fudenberg, H.: Immunodeficiency diseases. *In* Fudenberg, H.H., Stites, D.P., Caldwell, J.L., and Wells, J.V. (eds.): Clinical and Basic Immunology. Los Altos, CA, Lange Medical Publications, 1980, p. 411.

PRIMARY IMMUNIZATIONS OF CHILDREN NOT IMMUNIZED IN INFANCY

Not infrequently, the pediatrician is faced with a child who is over 1 year of age and who has not been immunized. The following schedules should be used to accomplish immunization as rapidly as possible.

If the child is 1 to 5 years of age:

First visit — DPT, TOPV, tuberculin test
1 month later — measles, rubella, mumps
2 months later — DPT, TOPV
4 months later — DPT, TOPV
6 to 12 months later or preschool — DPT, TOPV
Age 14–16 years — Td; continue every 10 years

If the child is 6 years of age and over:

First visit — Td, TOPV, tuberculin test
1 month later — measles, rubella, mumps
2 months later — Td, TOPV
6 to 12 months later — Td, TOPV
Age 14–16 years — Td; continue every 10 years

DPT = Diphtheria, Pertussis, Tetanus; TOPV = Trivalent Oral Polio Vaccine; Td = adult type diphtheria tetanus toxoid.

Reference: American Academy of Pediatrics: Report of the Committee on Infectious Diseases. 1974, p. 9.

COW'S MILK ALLERGY

Many physicians still remain skeptical about the diseases that may be produced by allergy or sensitivity to whole cow milk protein. Careful observations do indicate, however, that from 7 to 25 per cent of infants may manifest symptoms upon exposure to whole cow milk. As a general rule, the earlier the introduction of the whole cow milk into the diet, the more likely the adverse symptoms are likely to develop. Diseases that may be produced by whole cow milk include:

Gastrointestinal Bleeding

Approximately one-half of all infants and children found to have iron deficiency anemia have associated whole cow milk–induced gastrointestinal bleeding. Removal of whole cow milk from the diet results in the disappearance of occult fecal blood loss within 48 hours.

Malabsorption Syndrome

In its most severe form, these children demonstrate diarrhea and failure to thrive. Vomiting, recurrent respiratory infections, and eczema are also commonly present. Serum IgA levels are increased; milk antibodies are present. Jejunal mucosa shows alterations and may be flat. Elimination of cow milk produces improvement in days to several months. Reintroduction of cow milk reproduces symptoms in hours or may take three to four weeks. Some of these infants also manifest sensitivity to soy and wheat as well.

Exudative Enteropathy

Patients manifest edema, hypoproteinemia, and anemia. Symptoms frequently are first observed when cow milk has been fed during a diarrheal disease. Some, but not all, children will have diarrhea. Many will have eosinophilia and eosinophils in the stool. Stool often contains milk antibodies.

Recurrent Serous Otitis Media, Bronchiolitis, Bronchitis, Skin Rashes and Vomiting

These may occur as individual illnesses, or the child may manifest multiple symptoms. Because of the common nature of such symptoms, strict criteria must be applied before allergy to cow milk can be claimed to be the cause. Clinical criteria should include the following:

1. Symptoms subside after dietary elimination of milk.
2. Symptoms recur within 48 hours after milk challenge.
3. Reactions to three such challenges must be positive and have a similar onset, duration, and clinical features.

It is important to remember that about 20 per cent of children allergic to cow milk protein will also be allergic to soy protein.

Other diseases in which cow milk protein allergy may play a role include idiopathic pulmonary hemosiderosis, enuresis, steroid-dependent nephrosis, and the "tension-fatigue" syndrome. This latter entity is probably on the shakiest ground in terms of its relationship to cow milk. Its symptoms and signs include:

Tension	overactivity, restlessness
	clumsiness
	inability to relax
	irritability
	oversensitivity
	insomnia
	hypersensitivity to pain
Fatigue	tiredness
	achiness
	sluggishness
	torpor

and

pallor
nasal stuffiness
infraorbital circles
infraorbital edema
abdominal pain
headache
enuresis
arthralgias

Only a scrupulously administered elimination diet with careful observation of symptoms can establish this constellation of signs and symptoms as a manifestation of milk allergy.

References: Walker-Smith, J.: Arch. Dis. Child., *50*:347, 1975. Crook, W.C.: Pediatr. Clin. North Am., *22*:227, 1975.

HYPERSENSITIVITY PNEUMONITIS

Organic dust inhalation or chemical or drug exposure may cause a puzzling acute or chronic lung disease. The agents that have been incriminated appear in the following chart.

Antigens Causing Hypersensitivity Pneumonitis

AGENTS	TYPICAL EXPOSURES
Molds	
Thermophilic actinomycetes *(Micropolyspora faeni, Thermoactinomyces vulgaris)*	Dairy farming, bagasse processing, mushroom growing, air conditioners, humidifiers
Maple bark *(Cryptostroma corticale)*	Paper making, sawmills
Penicillium casei	Cheese washing
Aspergillus clavatus and *A. fumigatus*	Malt processing
Other plant antigens	
Wood dust*	Carpentry
Sisal dust*	Sisal processing
Legumes, especially lentils*	Aspiration
"Blackfat" tobacco*	Smoking of moldy tobacco
Cotton dust	Cotton processing
Animal dusts	
Bird droppings	Pigeon breeding, parakeet breeding, pet birds, chickens
Fur dust	Sewing furs
Pituitary powder (snuff)	Teatment of diabetes insipidus
Smallpox virus*	Nursing
Grain weevil *(Sitophilus granarius)*	Laboratory exposure

Continued

---

*Suspected but not proved.

AGENTS	TYPICAL EXPOSURES
Bacterial antigens	
Tuberculin*	Laboratory exposure
Bacillus subtilis enzymes*	Detergent manufacture
Chemicals and drugs*	
Epoxy resins	Plastics manufacture, painting
Antituberculosis therapy (?PAS)	Medications
Busulfan	
Hexamethonium	
Hydralazine	
Hydrochlorothiazide	
Mecamylamine	
Methysergide	
Nitrofurantoin	
Sulfonamides	

*Suspected but not proved.

The diagnosis of this symptom complex is most often made on the basis of clinical presentation. A summary of signs, symptoms, and laboratory data to be expected is included below.

Signs and Symptoms

Acute form — follows heavy exposure
Fever (101–104°F)
Chills
Dyspnea
Malaise
Aches and pains
Inspiratory rales loudest at the bases
Marked weight loss may occur

(The chills and fever usually occur within 4 to 6 hours of exposure, while rales, dyspnea, and other complaints may last for weeks.)

Chronic form — due to chronic or frequent limited exposure
Dyspnea
Decreased exercise tolerance
Chronic cough
Anorexia
Weight loss

(The onset may be insidious.)

Laboratory Data

Chest x-ray
May show infiltrates with interstitial pattern that is indistinguishable from other interstitial pneumonias. With continued exposure increased bronchial markings may persist.

Pulmonary function tests

A restrictive defect is noted with arterial oxygen desaturation, especially with exercise. Occasionally an obstructive pattern is seen. Chronic disease leads to decreased pulmonary function identical to that seen in emphysema. The impairments resolve with withdrawal of antigen exposure.

Hypergammaglobulinemia

Increases are primarily in IgA and IgG fractions. When hypergammaglobulinemia exists, a search should be made for precipitating antibody to a specific antigen. Commercial kits are available to test for precipitating antibody using only the patient's serum. This test is not diagnostic, however, since some patients show no antibody, and other persons with no disease may show a positive test.

Skin tests

An intradermal test may give rise to an Arthus-like reaction with local hemorrhage, edema, and pain in 7 to 8 hours.

White blood cell count

There is usually a mild neutrophilia. Eosinophilia is unusual.

Lung biopsy

This is not usually considered necessary for diagnosis; however, when available, it shows granulomatous interstitial pneumonia without caseation. In chronic cases there may be collapsed alveoli with thickened fibrotic septi and fragmentation of elastic fibers.

It is of interest that patients with hypersensitivity pneumonitis may or may not have a history of atopy.

Other terms for this disorder include farmer's lung, bird-fancier's or bird-breeder's lung, bagassosis, and pituitary snuff taker's lung.

Allergic bronchopulmonary aspergillosis is a somewhat different disease from that described above. Clinically there is wheezing with purulent sputum containing brown flecks or mucous plugs with fungal mycelia. The chest x-ray in allergic aspergillosis may show consolidation or collapse, and eosinophilia is usually present. Progressive pulmonary destruction includes proximal bronchiectasis. The immediate skin test to *Aspergillus* is positive, and the precipitating antibody response to *Aspergillus* antigen is present. Treatment for allergic aspergillosis involves administration of corticosteroids.

A differential diagnosis of hypersensitivity pneumonitis appears in the chart below.

Differential Diagnosis of Hypersensitivity Pneumonitis

ACUTE ONSET	INSIDIOUS ONSET
Asthma	Chronic obstructive lung disease
Infectious processes	Effects of noxious agents
Bronchopneumonia	Asbestos
Influenza	Talc
Other viral pneumonias	Silica
Varicella	
Miliary tuberculosis	Radiation pneumonitis
Miliary fungous infection	
	Generalized disease of unknown etiology
Acute diffuse interstitial fibrosis	Sarcoidosis
(Hamman-Rich syndrome)	Rheumatoid arthritis, polymyositis,
	disseminated lupus erythematosus,
Effects of noxious agents	scleroderma, etc.
Irritating gases such as chlorine,	Necrotizing granulomatosis
phosgene, sulfur dioxide, and	Pulmonary histiocytosis
oxides of nitrogen (silo-filler's	Lymphogenous carcinomatosis,
disease)	including lymphomas and pulmonary
Bordeaux mixture	adenomatosis
Epoxy resins	Pulmonary alveolar microlithiasis
	Primary pulmonary hemosiderosis
Generalized systemic disease	Hamman-Rich syndrome
Uremia	Desquamative interstitial pneumonitis
	Chronic eosinophilic pneumonia
Acute disseminated lupus erythematosus	
Acute polyarteritis nodosa	

The treatment for hypersensitivity pneumonitis is strict avoidance of the offending antigen. The diagnosis and treatment depend on a careful and accurate history and a high level of suspicion.

References: Feldman, G., and Gordon, V.H.: South Med. J., *68*:952, 1975. Rosenberg, M., Patterson, R., and Roberts, M.: J. Pediatr., *91*:914, 1977.

POLLENS OF NORTH AMERICA

Your child starts sneezing mid-March each year only to stop by mid-April. Is he allergic to alder trees, maples, beeches, or ragweed? The seasonal variations for common allergens are listed below and should help answer this question:

Pollen Seasons of North America

	January	February	March	April	May	June	July	August	September	October	November	December
Hazel			xxxxx									
Alder			xxxxx									
Elm				xxx								
Maple (Box-elder)				xxxxxxx								
Poplar				xxxxx								
Birch				xxx								
Oak					xxx							
Ash					xxx							
Beech					xxx							
Hickory (Pecan)					xxx							
Sweet vernal grass					xxxxx							
English plantain					xxxxxxxx							
Sorrel					xxxxx							
June grass					xxxxx							
Orchard grass					xxxxx							
Timothy						xxxxx						
Ragweed								xxxxxxx				

Reference: Sherman, W.B.: Hypersensitivity Mechanisms and Management. Philadelphia, W.B. Saunders Company, 1968.

7

As it takes two to make a quarrel, so it takes two to make a disease, the microbe and its host.

Charles V. Chapin
Papers, "The Principles of Epidemiology"

CHRONIC GRANULOMATOUS DISEASE (CGD) OF CHILDHOOD

What are its manifestations and what are the organisms that produce most of the problems?

Signs and Symptoms

FINDING	PER CENT OF PATIENTS
Marked lymphadenopathy	92
Pneumonitis	87
Male sex	87
Suppuration of nodes	86
Hepatomegaly	84
Dermatitis	84
Onset of signs by 1 year of age	78
Splenomegaly	74
Hepatic-perihepatic abscess	45
Death before age 7 years	37
Osteomyelitis	33
Onset with dermatitis	30
Onset with lymphadenitis	30
Persistent rhinitis	25
Conjunctivitis	23
Persistent diarrhea	22
Perianal abscess	18
Ulcerative stomatitis	16

Infecting Organisms

Most organisms that produce infections in patients with CGD are catalase-positive and are capable of destroying their own hydrogen peroxide, thus protecting themselves.

Common bacterial infecting agents, in order of frequency, include:

Staphylococcus aureus
Klebsiella-Aerobacter organisms
Escherichia coli
Staphylococcus albus
Serratia marcescens
Pseudomonas and *Proteus* species
Salmonella organisms
Paracolobactrum organisms

Fungal agents that also produce disease include:

Candida albicans
Aspergillus organisms
Nocardia organisms
Actinomyces

Note that pneumococci, beta-hemolytic streptococci, and *Hemophilus influenzae* do not cause infections in these patients with increased frequency.

Reference: Johnston, R.B., Jr., and Baehner, R.L.: Pediatrics, *48*:733, 1971.

8
BLOOD/TUMORS

ANEMIA IN EARLY INFANCY

During the first months of life there are many causes of anemia. Anemia during the first three months of life is rarely a result of nutritional iron deficiency. The accompanying table is intended to call your attention to the more likely causes of anemia that occur at birth and at two or three months of age as well as provide you with leads to establishing the diagnosis.

Common Causes of Anemia in Early Infancy

AGE	DIAGNOSIS	SUPPORTING DATA
At birth	Hemorrhage	
	Obstetric accidents (placenta previa, abruptio placentae, incision of placenta, rupture of cord, rupture of anomalous placental vessel)	History and visual inspection of placenta and cord
	Occult hemorrhage	
	Fetomaternal	Demonstration of fetal cells in maternal circulation
	Twin-to-twin	Demonstration of significant difference in hemoglobin values of identical twins
	Internal hemorrhage (intracranial, retroperitoneal, intrahepatic, intrasplenic, cephalhematoma)	Physical examination
	Isoimmunization	Blood groups of mother and infant; evidence of antibody on infant's red cells
	Inherited defect of red cell (includes G-6-PD deficiency, pyruvate kinase deficiency, hereditary spherocytosis, elliptocytosis, stomatocytosis, etc.)	Red cell morphology, family history, and appropriate screening tests
	Acquired defect (generally in association with hypoxemia, acidosis, or infection)	Physical findings, red cell morphology, coagulation disturbance, blood and urine cultures, and serologic studies and gamma-M determination
	Red cell hypoplasia (Blackfan-Diamond syndrome, congenital leukemia, osteopetrosis)	Rare disorders; bone marrow aspirate
2–3 months	Iron deficiency as a consequence of previous hemorrhage	Obstetric history when available
	Late manifestation of previous isoimmunization	Blood types of mother and infant; maternal antibody titers

Continued

AGE	DIAGNOSIS	SUPPORTING DATA
2–3 months	Hereditary defects of the red cell	Persistence of hemolytic anemia; red cell morphology and laboratory tests
	Thalassemia major	Red cell morphology, splenomegaly, persistence of fetal hemoglobin elevation, family studies
	Sickle cell anemia	Red cell morphology, hemoglobin electrophoresis
	Vitamin E deficiency	Infant of low birth weight; red cell morphology, low serum E level, positive hydrogen peroxide hemolysis test
	Folic acid deficiency	Premature infant, history of infections or diarrhea, red cell and marrow morphology, response to folic acid
	Persistent infection	Elevated titers to rubella, cytomegalovirus, toxoplasmosis
	Renal tubular acidosis	Acidosis, hypochloremia, mild azotemia, urine pH of 6.0 or greater in presence of acidosis

ANEMIA—A DIAGNOSTIC APPROACH

The child with anemia is either overlooked or overstudied on many occasions. The accompanying flow diagram suggests a means of arriving at a probable diagnosis with a minimum of laboratory studies. The evaluation begins with a careful history that should include information regarding age, sex, color, ethnic background, birth weight and neonatal course, diet, drugs, diarrhea, infections, history of other family members with anemia, and a statement about the presence or absence of pica. The initial laboratory studies should include a calculation of *red cell indices, a reticulocyte count,* and *examination of a well-prepared peripheral blood smear*. With these facts in hand, proceed to determine if your patient has a hypochromic-microcytic anemia, a normocytic anemia, or a macrocytic anemia. Follow the logical steps to diagnosis.

A Diagnostic Approach to Anemia

MICROCYTIC–HYPOCHROMIC

6 mos – 2 yrs – MCV <70
2 yrs – 5 yrs – MCV <73
5 yrs – 12 yrs – MCV <76

Iron deficiency
Thalassemia syndromes
  alpha
  beta
Lead poisoning
Chronic infection
Severe protein deficiency
Siderocrestic
  pyridoxine–responsive

Studies:
  Serum iron, TIBC, FEP,
  Hb electrophoresis
  Brilliant cresyl blue prep
  Fetal hemoglobin
  Marrow iron stain

HISTORY

Age		*Drugs*
Sex		Diarrhea
Color	and	*Infection*
Ethnic		Inheritance
Neonatal		*Pica*
Diet		

MACROCYTIC

(MCV >96 μ^3)

Macrocytosis
Reticulocytosis
Liver disease
Hypothyroidism
Down's syndrome
Normal newborn

Macro-ovalocytosis with anemia
Bone marrow

MEGALOBLASTIC

Folic Acid
Dietary
Malabsorption
Dilantin

B_{12} *Deficiency*
Pernicious anemia
  Juvenile
  Adult
  Grasbock
  Ileal disease

OROTIC ACIDURIA

Continued

8

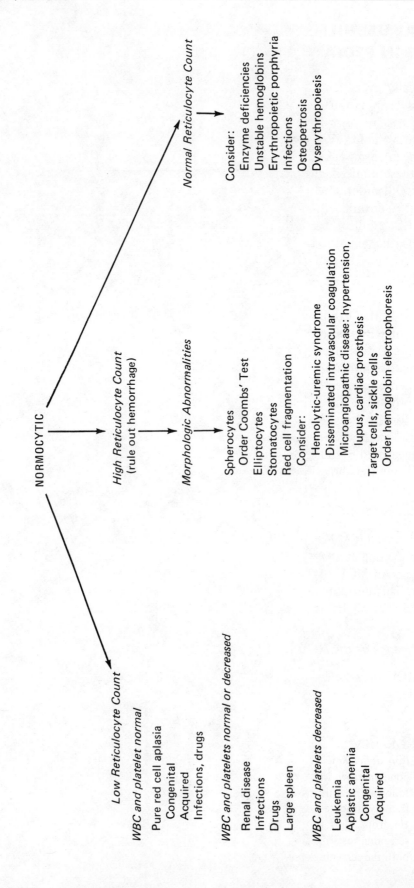

NORMOCYTIC

High Reticulocyte Count
(rule out hemorrhage)

Morphologic Abnormalities

Spherocytes
  Order Coombs' Test
Elliptocytes
Stomatocytes
Red cell fragmentation
  Consider:
    Hemolytic-uremic syndrome
    Disseminated intravascular coagulation
    Microangiopathic disease: hypertension,
      lupus, cardiac prosthesis
  Target cells, sickle cells
    Order hemoglobin electrophoresis

Normal Reticulocyte Count

Consider:
  Enzyme deficiencies
  Unstable hemoglobins
  Erythropoietic porphyria
  Infections
  Osteopetrosis
  Dyserythropoiesis

Low Reticulocyte Count

WBC and platelet normal

Pure red cell aplasia
  Congenital
  Acquired
  Infections, drugs

WBC and platelets normal or decreased

Renal disease
Infections
Drugs
Large spleen

WBC and platelets decreased

Leukemia
Aplastic anemia
  Congenital
  Acquired

CLINICAL USEFULNESS OF RED BLOOD CELL INDICES IN PEDIATRICS

Practically every laboratory utilizes electronic counting equipment for CBC determinations and in so doing, red blood cell (RBC) indices are automatically provided. These include the RBC count, the mean corpuscular volume (MCV), the mean corpuscular hemoglobin (MCH), and the mean corpuscular hemoglobin concentration (MCHC). Properly utilized, these indices aid greatly in the characterization of many hematologic disorders.

Before electronic equipment became available less then 10 years ago, the RBC indices calculated after directly measuring the hemoglobin (Hb), the hematocrit (Hct), and the RBC count were:

$$MCV = \frac{Hct}{RBC} \qquad MCH = \frac{Hb}{RBC} \qquad MCHC = \frac{Hb}{Hct}$$

Now with the Coulter Counter type of automated equipment, a suspension of RBCs in a metered volume of electrolyte solution simply passes through a small orifice which is electrically charged. Since each RBC is a relative nonconductor, a change in the electrical charge occurs, which is then expressed as an RBC count. The magnitude of the charge change is proportional to the cell volume, and thus an MCV is derived as well. Finally, a hemoglobin is determined by an automated colorimetric method. Thus, only the Hb, MCV, and RBC count are actually measured, while the Hct, MCH, and MCHC are computed internally using the above equations.

Normal Values for MCV, MCH, MCHC (see table on p. 245)

The normal MCV in newborns is higher than at any other time of life, but beginning at a few months of age the MCV becomes lower than adult values. An MCV of 70, for example, may be normal for a 1 year old infant. This developmental change in MCV is paralleled by changes in the MCH. The MCHC is fairly constant throughout life.

The Significance of the MCV

The MCV may be low, normal, or high in various disorders, and specific diagnostic tests for anemia should be based on clues provided by the MCV.

A. The Low MCV
   1. *Iron deficiency.* The earliest changes in iron deficiency are a fall in bone marrow iron and a concomitant fall in serum ferritin. This is followed by a decrease in serum iron and a rise in the quantity of RBC free erythrocyte porphyrin (FEP). The MCV then falls, and finally the Hb drops. Currently, the MCV and the FEP are the most widely used screening tests for iron deficiency, but the serum ferritin may soon be both the screening and the diagnostic test.

2. *Lead (Pb) poisoning.* Microcytosis may be seen in lead poisoning but is not uniformly present, while a rise in FEP is almost invariably found. The FEP is now the standard screening test for Pb poisoning. The FEP tends to be much higher in Pb poisoning than in iron deficiency, although some overlap may exist.

3. *Thalassemia minor.* A low MCV is the hallmark of thalassemia minor, and the MCV may be used as a screening test of high sensitivity in the detection of beta thalassemia minor. In our own series of children and adults with thalassemia minor, the MCV was 62 ± 4 fl. In alpha thalassemia, the MCV on the average is slightly higher than in beta thalassemia. A Hb electrophoresis is best considered a confirmatory test for thalassemia.

A very simple calculation may be used to distinguish iron deficiency and lead poisoning from thalassemia minor based on the MCV and RBC count. The RBC count falls in iron deficiency and Pb poisoning but is normal in thalassemia minor. If the MCV is divided by the RBC count, a discriminate index is obtained where:

$$\frac{MCV}{RBC} < 12 = \text{Thalassemia minor}$$

$$\frac{MCV}{RBC} > 14 = \text{Iron deficiency or Pb poisoning}$$

Values between 12-14 are indiscriminate. Since these formulas are correct 95% of the time, a more rational selection of confirmatory tests is possible.

4. *Miscellaneous.* Other causes of microcytosis are much less common but include the anemia of chronic disorders (this is usually normocytic, but 10 per cent are microcytic), severe protein malnutrition, sideroblastic anemia, and copper deficiency.

B. Normocytic Anemia

Anemia with a normal MCV is usually caused by bone marrow failure, recent blood loss, or hemolysis.

C. The High MCV

Unlike in adults, macrocytosis in a child should not call B_{12} deficiency to mind first. The causes of a high MCV include:

1. *Normal newborn.* All normal newborns are macrocytic. In fact, an MCV of 94 or less should suggest a diagnosis of alpha thalassemia minor, the most common cause of microcytosis in newborns.

2. *Reticulocytosis.* Reticulocytes are very large and, when averaged with more mature RBCs, may produce a high MCV. A review of the peripheral blood smear will show that an elevated MCV is merely a reflection of young RBCs.

3. *Down's syndrome.* In Down's syndrome, the MCV averages 10 fl higher than normal.

4. *Liver disease.* This will deposit excessive lipids on the RBC, producing enlargement.

5. *Hypothyroidism.* A low T_4 commonly produces large spiculated or targeted RBCs.

6. *Drugs.* Any drug (such as methotrexate) which alters DNA synthesis may cause macrocytosis.

7. *Folate deficiency.*

8. *B_{12} deficiency.* B_{12} and folate deficiency, in addition to producing macrocytosis, will cause hypersegmentation of neutrophils, distinguishing them from other causes of macrocytosis.

9. *Miscellaneous.* Other causes include preleukemic states and congenital pure RBC aplasia (Blackfan-Diamond syndrome).

Alterations of MCH and MCHC

Since the MCH falls as the Hb falls, relatively little information is obtained from the MCH itself. The same is somewhat true of a low MCHC, which adds nothing to what is already known from the MCV.

A *high* MCHC is important to recognize, since it indicates that the hemoglobin content of the RBC is being very tightly packaged. A high MCHC almost invariably means spherocytes are present and suggests such diagnoses as hereditary spherocytosis, ABO incompatibility, autoimmune hemolytic anemia, and occasionally microangiopathic hemolytic anemias.

	MCV (fl)	MCH (pg/RBC)	MCHC
Normal adult	90 ± 10	31 ± 4	34 ± 3
Normal newborn	119 ± 9.0	36 ± 2	32 ± 2
Ages 10–17 mo	77 ± 7	26.1 ± 2.8	34.2 ± 1.6
18–48 mo	80 ± 6	27.0 ± 3.0	33.6 ± 1.4
4–7 yr	81 ± 5	27.6 ± 2.4	33.6 ± 1.6

"Children, blessings seem, but torments are."

Otway

FREE ERYTHROCYTE PROTOPORPHYRIN AS A DIAGNOSTIC AID

With the development of a simple, rapid, and inexpensive method for the measurement of free erythrocyte protoporphyrin (FEP), screening for both iron deficiency and lead poisoning has become simplified and can be performed on capillary samples of blood.

Normal values for FEP may vary from laboratory to laboratory, but in general the following values can be applied:

Upper limit of normal:
90 micrograms/100 ml RBCs
or
30 micrograms/100 ml whole blood

Modest elevations of the FEP (30 to 190 micrograms/100 ml of whole blood) may be observed in iron deficiency, while values in excess of 190 signify lead poisoning or the rare patient with erythropoietic protoporphyria.

Pica—From the Latin *pica*, meaning magpie. The magpie picks up and eats and hoards odd objects. A scavenger bird of prey.

Iron Deficiency and Thalassemia Minor

When the FEP is used in conjunction with the measurement of erythrocyte mean corpuscular volume (MCV), a very accurate means of distinguishing iron deficiency from thalassemia minor is provided. The FEP is normal in patients with thalassemia minor unless they have associated iron deficiency anemia. The accompanying diagram illustrates a suggested approach to the initial diagnosis of these disorders employing the MCV, derived from the Coulter Counter, and the FEP.

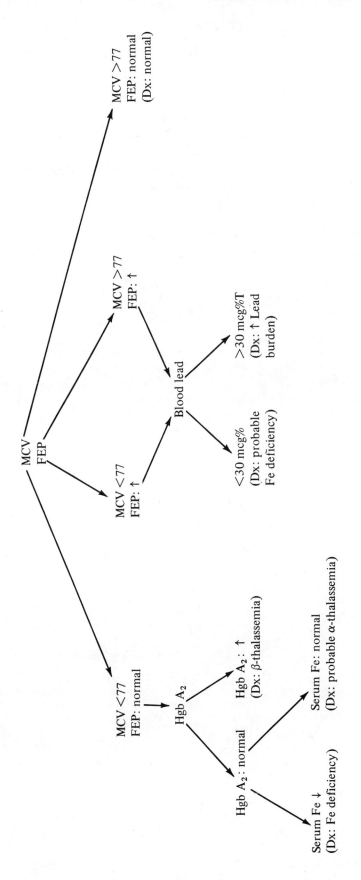

Lead Poisoning

The Center for Disease Control has provided the following guidelines for the use of the FEP in the diagnosis and management of patients with lead poisoning:

1. The FEP should be used for the initial screening for lead poisoning.
2. Children with an elevated FEP should have a blood lead determination performed.
3. With the results of the FEP and blood lead, the patients may be classified into four major categories:

TEST	CLASS I Normal	CLASS II Minimally Elevated	CLASS III Moderately Elevated	CLASS IV Extremely Elevated
Pb (mcg/100 ml)	29	30–49	50–79	80
FEP (mcg/100 ml whole blood)	59	60–109	110–189	190

4. In situations where there is a discrepancy between the blood lead and the FEP, the FEP is more likely to reflect the true status of the patient.
5. Some Class I children may be placed into two additional categories. Class Ia would include those children with iron deficiency anemia. Class Ib children appear, on the basis of present experience, to have transient or declining blood lead elevations. The anticipated combinations of blood lead and FEP as a suggested guideline to estimate the most likely degree of risk are:

TEST RESULTS	FEP ≤59	FEP 60–109	FEP 110–189	FEP ≥190
Pb ≤29	I	Ia	Ia	EEP+
Pb 30–49	↓Ib	II	↑III	↑IV
Pb 50–79	*	↓II	III	↑IV
Pb ≥80	*	*	*	IV

EEP+ = Erythropoietic protoporphyria.
* = Combination of results is not generally observed in practice; when blood lead is repeated, the results will generally indicate contamination of the first specimen.
↓ = Downgrading of the estimate of risk of lead intoxication suggested by blood lead is altered on the basis of the FEP results.
↑ = Upgrading of the estimate of risk of lead intoxication suggested by blood lead is altered on the basis of the FEP results.

6. Guidelines for management are as follows:

Class I   Routine rescreening until age 6 years.

Class Ia   Diagnosis and treatment of iron deficiency anemia.

Class Ib   Reevaluation at monthly intervals until it is certain that the child does not have undue body lead burden.

Class II   Should be considered to have increased lead absorption if there is no iron deficiency. Both conditions may exist. Look for other evidence of lead poisoning (long bone films, urinary coproporphyrin, EDTA mobilization test). If mobilization is abnormal, perform chelation. If no evidence of lead poisoning, evaluate at three-month intervals after it is determined that patient is no longer exposed to lead. If lead exposure continues, evaluate at monthly intervals.

Class III   If asymptomatic, perform EDTA mobilization test. If test is positive, then chelate. If patient is symptomatic, then hospitalize immediately and begin chelation therapy. If chelation is unnecessary, follow at monthly intervals.

Class IV   These children, regardless of lack of symptoms, should be hospitalized for evaluation and chelation therapy.

References: Piomelli, S.: Pediatrics, *51*:254, 1973. Stockman, J.A., Weiner, L.S., Simon, G.E., et al.: J. Lab. Clin. Med., *85*:113, 1975. Center for Disease Control: J. Pediatr., *87*:824, 1975.

IRON DEFICIENCY —
A PROGRESSION OF FINDINGS

The development of iron deficiency anemia is preceded by a sequence of abnormalities that may exist some time before the anemia. With the recognition that iron deficiency is a multisystem problem and that symptoms may occur well in advance of the onset of anemia, screening tests have been devised to detect iron deficiency before anemia is present. The sequential changes are indicated in the table.

Sequential Changes in the Development of Iron Deficiency

		STAGE I IRON DEPLETION	STAGE II IRON-DEFICIENT ERYTHROPOIESIS	STAGE III IRON DEFICIENCY
Serum ferritin	E A R L Y	Decreased levels	Decreased levels	Decreased levels
Bone marrow iron		Decreased staining	Decreased staining	Decreased staining
Total serum iron binding capacity (TIBC)	I N T E R M E D I A T E	Normal	Elevated	Elevated
Serum iron		Normal	Decreased levels	Decreased levels
Erythrocyte proto-porphyrins		Normal	Increased levels	Increased levels
Hemoglobin	L A T E	Normal	Normal	Low
Hematocrit		Normal	Normal	Low
Mean corpuscular volume (MCV)		Normal	Normal or low	Low
Red cell morphology		Normal	Normal	Microcytosis Hypochromia

Reference: Bates, H.M.: Lab. Management, *18:*9, 1980.

THE RISE IN HEMOGLOBIN WITH IRON THERAPY

How fast should the hemoglobin rise when you start treating your iron deficient patient with oral iron?

Two important factors must be considered when judging the adequacy of the hematologic response. They are the initial hemoglobin value and the duration of the period of observation. The lower the initial hemoglobin, the greater is the hemoglobin rise per day. The shorter the observation period, the greater is the calculated hemoglobin rise per day. As one gets closer to a normal hemoglobin value, the daily rise in hemoglobin is much less. In our own experience in treating patients with hemoglobin values of less than 8.0 gm/100 ml, one may anticipate a hemoglobin rise of 0.2 to 0.3 gm per day during the first 7 to 10 days of therapy. During the period of 10 to 24 days, the hemoglobin rises at a rate of 0.15 gm per day and slows after that point to a rate of 0.10 per day until a normal level is achieved. Normally, the reticulocyte count begins to increase in 48 to 72 hours and reaches a peak 7 to 10 days after the initiation of therapy.

Listed below is another guide to the expected response as a function of the initial hemoglobin level.

INITIAL HEMOGLOBIN (gm/dl)	HEMOGLOBIN RISE IN ONE WEEK (gm/dl)
2.0 – 5.0	1.61
5.1 – 6.0	1.53
6.1 – 7.0	1.17
7.1 – 8.0	1.11
8.1 – 9.0	0.98
9.1 – 10.0	0.57
10.1 – 11.0	0.72
11.1 – 12.0	0.40

Optimal responses to oral iron therapy are achieved by treating the patient with ferrous sulfate. A patient should receive 2 to 3 mg of elemental iron per kg three times per day. The iron should be given between meals and never administered with milk.

Reference: Mehta, B.C., Lotliker, K.S., and Patel, J.C.: Indian J. Med. Res., *61*:1818, 1973.

FAILURE TO RESPOND TO IRON THERAPY

There are many reasons why anemic children do not respond to iron. The most common reason is *failure to take the iron* prescribed. Other reasons include:

1. *Wrong diagnosis:* Thalassemia minor and lead poisoning are often confused with iron deficiency.
2. *Improper administration:* If administered with milk or other products high in phosphorus or phytate content, iron may not be well absorbed.
3. *Improper dosages:* Most iron preparations are only 20 per cent elemental iron and calculations should be based on this. The proper dose of iron is 2 to 3 mg/kg of elemental iron given three times daily.
4. *Malabsorption of iron:* As many as 20 per cent of children may fail to absorb iron efficiently in the face of iron deficiency.
5. *Inability to utilize iron:* In the presence of concomitant lead poisoning or certain chronic disease states (especially those associated with inflammation), iron may be absorbed but not incorporated into hemoglobin.
6. *Ongoing blood losses.*

Since compliance is the leading cause of this problem, a simple diagnostic test for the detection of iron in the stools is often indicated.

Step 1. Ask the mother to bring in a small specimen of stool without telling her specifically why.

Step 2. Mix a small amount of stool with a 2N HCl and take one drop of this suspension and place on Whatman #1 filter paper.

Step 3. Add one drop of 0.25 per cent potassium ferricyanide to the rim of clear fluid around the sample. The immediate development of a blue color (ferrous ferricyanide) is a positive test for iron and indicates that the child has been ingesting medicinal doses of iron.

This test is simple, reliable and quick (less than two minutes). If the test is positive, a stool guaiac should also be performed to rule out blood in the bowel movement. The potassium ferricyanide test will be positive with both GI bleeding (detecting hemoglobin iron) and the administration of iron. A stool guaiac will be positive with blood in the stool but will be negative with iron administration.

Reference: Afifi, A.M., Bunwell, G.S., Benneson, R.J., et. al.: Br. Med. J., *1*:1021, 1966.

BEETURIA

Beeturia is a term applied to the deep red or pink coloration of urine which may occur after the ingestion of beetroot. The color is due to the presence of betanin, a red pigment which is chemically different from the anthocyanins, the reddish violet pigments of most plant species.

Beeturia occurs commonly in infants with iron deficiency anemia. Ingestion of as little as·six tablespoons of pureed beets is enough to discolor the urine that is voided following the meal.

Think of iron deficiency when a mother tells you that her child has had a pink urine following a meal containing beets. She will think you are a genius—so will your unsuspecting friends. Beeturia quickly disappears with iron therapy.

Reference: Tunnessen, W., Smith, C., and Oski, F.: Am. J. Dis. Child., *117*:424, 1969.

8

IRON DEFICIENCY OR THALASSEMIA TRAIT?

Children with mild microcytic anemias are commonly encountered in the practice of pediatrics. Most of these patients have either iron deficiency or thalassemia trait. The use of red cell indices can provide a simple means of making a presumptive diagnosis without requiring serum iron determinations or hemoglobin electrophoresis.

Two formulas employing these indices have been proposed. They are as follows:

1. The Mentzer Formula $= \dfrac{\text{MCV}}{\text{Red Cell Count}}$

Interpretation: Values in excess of 13.5 strongly suggest that the patient has iron deficiency anemia, while values below 11.5 indicate that thalassemia trait is the most likely diagnosis.

2. The Discriminant Function = MCV − RBC − (5 × Hb) − 3.4

> *Thalassemia*—From the Greek *thalassa*, meaning sea, and *haima*, meaning blood. So named because the originally recognized patients all lived around the Mediterranean Sea.

Interpretation: Positive values suggest a diagnosis of iron deficiency, while negative values indicate that thalassemia trait is the cause of the microcytic anemia.

Caution: These formulas are useful only in uncomplicated situations. Confusing answers may be obtained in patients with associated hemolytic anemias or in patients with thalassemia minor who have hemorrhage or are pregnant, or in patients who are polycythemic secondary to chronic hypoxemia.

These formulas are useful in initial evaluation of patients. If iron deficiency is suggested by the formula and the patient does not respond to iron therapy, then further evaluation is indicated. A diagnosis of thalassemia trait should be confirmed in at least one family member.

References: Mentzer, W.C., Jr.: Lancet, *1*:882, 1973. England, J.M., and Fraser, P.: Lancet, *1*:449, 1973.

THALASSEMIA SYNDROMES — A SPECTRUM OF DISORDERS

A great deal is now known about the thalassemias that was not known just a few years ago. The table below is intended to help the clinician sort out this extremely heterogeneous group of disorders. As a point of reference, the a-thalassemias are that variety in which the a chain of hemoglobin is not produced owing to absence of one or more of the four structural genes that control a globin production (1 gene deletion = silent carrier, 2 gene deletion = heterozygous or trait, 3 gene deletion = Hgb H disease, 4 gene deletion = homozygous or hydrops fetalis). In the β-thalassemias, the structural genes are present but no β globin synthesis occurs, for unknown reasons. This presents in a heterozygous (trait) or homozygous (major) state with some (β^+) or no (β^0) globins being made. The thalassemia syndromes also include two other rare disorders, hereditary persistence of fetal hemoglobin (HPFH) and hemoglobin Lepore (which is due to an unequal crossing over of the δ and β chain globin genes).

Differential Diagnosis of Thalassemia Syndromes

DISORDER	HgB A$_2$ (%)	HgB F (%)	MCV (fl)	HgB (mg/dl)	MORPHOLOGY
α-Thalassemia					
Silent carrier	Normal	Normal	Normal	Normal	Normal
Heterozygous	Normal	Normal	Low/normal	Low/normal	Normal or microcytic target cells
HbH (∼5%)	Low/normal	Normal	Low	Low/normal	Supravital stain of peripheral blood inclusion (Heinz) bodies
Homozygous α-thal (hydrops fetalis)					Marked abnormality or RBC, pronounced erythroblastemia, anisopoikilocytosis
β-Thalassemia					
Heterozygous β^0 or β$^+$	3.5 – 8.0	2 – 4	64 ± 4	Low/normal	Microcytosis, anisocytosis, poikilocytosis, hypochromia, target cells, basophilic stippling
Homozygous					
β^0/β^0 (no HbA)	1 – 6	95	Low	Very low	Severe anemia, reticulocytosis, nucleated RBC, basophilic stippling, target cells, extreme poikilocytosis, anisocytosis
β$^+$/β$^+$ (variable)	2 – 8	Variable			
β$^+$/β^0	1 – 3	Variable			Supravital stain—bone marrow—inclusions in RBC precursors
Lepore heterozygous 5–15% Lepore homozygous 10–20%	Low/normal	2 – 4	Low	Low/normal	Poikilocytosis, hypochromia, anisocytosis, microcytic target cells
HPFH					
Greek	1 – 3	10 – 20	Normal	Normal	Hypochromia, microcytosis, anisocytosis and poikilocytosis
Swiss		3 – 13			
Black		17 – 33	Low/normal	Low/normal	Normal, few target cells

Reference: Lubin, B., Kleman, K., and Pennathur-Das, R.: Lab. Management, *18*:38, 1980.

8

DIFFERENTIAL DIAGNOSIS OF
COMMON HEMOGLOBINOPATHIES

The most common hemoglobinopathies observed in the United States include the sickling disorders, the thalassemia syndromes, and HbC. The most significant highlights of these are as follows:

8

DIAGNOSIS	FREQUENCY	CLINICAL SEVERITY	HGB (gm/dl)	HCT (%)	MCV (μ^3)	% RETIC	RBC MORPHOLOGY	SOLUBILITY TEST	ELECTRO-PHORESIS	DISTRIBUTION HbF
SS	1:625	Moderate–Severe	7.5 (6–10)	22 (18–30)	93	11 (4–30)	Many ISCs, target cells, nucleated red cells	Positive	80–90%S 2–20%F <3.6%A_2	Uneven
SC	1:833	Mild–Moderate	10 (9–14)	30 (26–40)	80	3 (1.5–6)	Many target cells, rare ISCs	Positive	45–55%S 45–55%C 0.2–8%F	Uneven
S/B⁰ Thal		Moderate–Severe	8.1 (7–12)	25 (20–36)	69	8 (3–18)	Marked hypochromia, microcytosis and target cells, variable ISC	Positive	50–85%S 2–30%F >3.6%A_2	Uneven
S/B⁺ Thal	1:1667	Mild–Moderate	11 (8–13)	32 (25–40)	76	3 (1.5–6)	Mild microcytosis, hypochromia, rare ISCs	Positive	55–75%S 15–30%A 1–20%F >3.6%A_2	Uneven
S/HPFH	1:25,000	Asymptomatic	14 (11–15)	40 (32–48)	84	1.5 (0.5–3)	No ISCs, occasional target cells, and mild hypochromia	Positive	60–80%S 16–35%F 1–3%A_2	Even
AS	1:17	Asymptomatic	Normal	Normal	Normal	Normal	Normal	Positive	38–45%S 60–55%A 1–3%A_2	Uneven
ASα Thal	1:300	Asymptomatic	Low/Normal	Low/Normal	70	Normal	Microcytic	Positive	29–35%S 71–75%A	Uneven

SS = Homozygous sickle cell disease.
S = Sickle trait.
C = C hemoglobin.
B⁰, B⁺ = β-Thalassemias.
HPFH = Hereditary persistence of fetal hemoglobin.
ISC = Irreversible sickle cells.

Reference: Lubin, B., Kleman, K., and Pennathur-Das, R.: Lab. Management, *18*:38, 1980.

Yet who would have thought the old man to have had so much blood in him?

William Shakespeare
Macbeth, V, i, 43

CLASSIFICATION OF RED CELL HEMOLYTIC DISORDERS BY PREDOMINANT MORPHOLOGY

In the following lists, nonhemolytic disorders of similar morphology are enclosed in parentheses for reference.

SPHEROCYTES

Hereditary spherocytosis
ABO incompatibility in neonates
Immunohemolytic anemias with IgG- or C3-coated red cells
Acute oxidant injury (hexose monophosphate shunt defects during hemolytic crisis, oxidant drugs and chemicals)
Hemolytic transfusion reactions
Clostridium welchii septicemia
Severe burns, other red cell thermal injury
Spider, bee, and snake venoms
Severe hypophosphatemia
Hypersplenism*

BIZARRE POIKILOCYTES

Red cell fragmentation syndromes (micro- and macroangiopathic hemolytic anemias)
Acute oxidant injury*
Hereditary elliptocytosis in neonates
Hereditary pyropoikilocytosis

ELLIPTOCYTES

Hereditary elliptocytosis
Thalassemias
(Other hypochromic-microcytic anemias)
(Megaloblastic anemias)

STOMATOCYTES

Hereditary stomatocytosis
Rh$_{null}$ blood group
Stomatocytosis with cold hemolysis
(Liver disease, especially acute alcoholism)
(Mediterranean stomatocytosis)

IRREVERSIBLY SICKLED CELLS

Sickle cell anemia
Symptomatic sickle syndromes

---

*Disease sometimes associated with this morphology.

INTRAERYTHROCYTIC PARASITES

Malaria
Babesiosis
Bartonellosis

SPICULATED OR CRENATED RED CELLS

Acute hepatic necrosis (spur cell anemia)
Uremia
Red cell fragmentation syndromes*
Infantile pyknocytosis
Embden-Meyerhof pathway defects*
Vitamin E deficiency*
Abetalipoproteinemia
Heat stroke*
McLeod blood group
(Postsplenectomy)
(Transiently after massive transfusion of stored blood)
(Anorexia nervosa)*

TARGET CELLS

Hemoglobins S, C, D, and E
Hereditary xerocytosis
Thalassemias
(Other hypochromic-microcytic anemias)
(Obstructive liver disease)
(Postsplenectomy)
(Lecithin:cholesterol acyltransferase deficiency)

PROMINENT BASOPHILIC STIPPLING

Thalassemias
Unstable hemoglobins
Lead poisoning*
Pyridine 5'-nucleotidase deficiency

NONSPECIFIC OR NORMAL MORPHOLOGY

Embden-Meyerhof pathway defects
Hexose monophosphate shunt defects
Unstable hemoglobins
Paroxysmal nocturnal hemoglobinuria
Dyserythropoietic anemias
Copper toxicity (Wilson's disease)
Cation permeability defects
Erythropoietic porphyria
Vitamin E deficiency
Hemolysis with infections*
Rh hemolytic disease in neonates
Paroxysmal cold hemoglobinuria*

*Disease sometimes associated with this morphology.

NONSPECIFIC OR NORMAL MORPHOLOGY *(Continued)*

 Cold hemagglutinin disease
 Hypersplenism
 Immunohemolytic anemia*

---

*Disease sometimes associated with this morphology.

Reference: Lux, S.: Disorders of the red cell membrane. *In* Nathan, D.G., and Oski, F.A. (eds.): Hematology of Infancy and Childhood, Vol. I. Philadelphia, W.B. Saunders Company, 1981, p. 483.

THE RATIONAL USE OF BLOOD PRODUCTS

Transfusion of blood or blood products is a frequent need on a busy pediatric service. The most scientific use of this procedure requires an estimation of the blood product requirement of the patient. The following pages outline methods for such estimations.

Simple Transfusion (With Packed Red Cells)

Assuming a packed cell hemoglobin (Hgb) content of 22 gm/100 ml and a postneonatal blood volume of 75 ml/kg, this formula states:

$$\frac{\text{Volume of packed}}{\text{cell transfusion (ml)}} = \frac{\text{Wt (in kg)} \times 75 \text{ ml/kg} \times \text{desired rise in Hgb (gm/100 ml)}}{22 \text{ gm/100 ml}}$$

Example: To raise the Hgb of an 11 kg child from 4 gm/100 ml to 10 gm/100 ml, one would calculate:

$$\frac{\text{Transfusion}}{\text{volume (ml)}} = \frac{11 \text{ kg} \times 75 \text{ ml/kg} \times 6 \text{ gm/100 ml}}{22 \text{ gm/100 ml}} = 225 \text{ ml}$$

If for some reason whole blood must be used, or if packed cell Hgb differs from that assumed, substitution of the correct value in the denominator will still provide an accurate estimate of transfusion needs.

Reference: Oski, F.A., and Naiman, J.L.: Hematologic Problems in the Newborn. Philadelphia, W.B. Saunders Company, 1972.

Partial Exchange Transfusion

In situations when time or volume considerations suggest use of partial exchange transfusion (e.g., anemia with heart failure), a modification of the previous formula may be useful:

$$\frac{\text{Exchange}}{\text{volume (ml)}} = \frac{\text{Wt (in kg)} \times 75 \text{ ml/kg} \times \text{desired rise in Hgb}}{22 \text{ gm/100 ml} - \text{Hgb}_R}$$

Hgb_R = mean of the initial and final hemoglobin. This represents the Hgb content of blood *removed* during the exchange.

$$\frac{(Hgb \; initial + Hgb \; desired)}{2}$$

Example: To raise the Hgb of a 17 kg child from 3.0 gm/100 ml to 7.0 gm/100 ml using a partial exchange transfusion with packed cells, one could calculate:

$$\frac{Exchange}{volume \; (ml)} = \frac{17 \; kg \times 75 \; ml/kg \times 4 \; gm/100 \; ml}{22 \; gm/100 \; ml - \dfrac{(3 \; gm/100 \; ml + 7 \; gm/100 \; ml)}{2}} = 300 \; ml$$

Reference: Nieburg, P.I., and Stockman, J.A.: Am. J. Dis. Child. (in press).

Exchange Transfusion with Plasma

Neonates or older children with significant polycythemia may benefit from a partial exchange transfusion designed to reduce their hemoglobin.

This can be accomplished by using plasma in the exchange transfusion as indicated in the following formula:

$$\frac{Exchange}{volume \; (ml)} = \frac{Wt \; (kg) \times 100 \; ml/kg* \times desired \; fall \; in \; Hgb \; (gm/100 \; ml)}{Hgb_R}$$

Hgb_R = mean of initial and desired hemoglobin = $\dfrac{(Hgb \; initial + Hgb \; desired)}{2}$

Example: To lower the Hgb of a 4 kg neonate from 24 gm/100 ml to 16 gm/100 ml, one would calculate:

$$\frac{Exchange}{volume} = \frac{4 \; kg \times 100 \; ml/kg \times 8 \; gm/100 \; ml}{20 \; gm/100 \; ml} = 160 \; ml$$

*Neonatal blood volume.

Reference: Oski, F.A., and Naiman, J.L.: Hematologic Problems in the Newborn. Philadelphia, W.B. Saunders Company, 1972.

Platelet Transfusion

Infusion of 0.2 units/kg of fresh platelets will provide a post-infusion rise in platelet count of approximately 60,000 to 90,000 platelets/mm^3.

Example: To raise the platelet count by 60,000 to 90,000/mm^3 in a 15 kg child, the following calculation would be made:

$$Platelet \; units = 0.2 \; units/kg \times 15 \; kg = 3 \; units$$

COMPATIBILITY OF IV SOLUTIONS
AND BLOOD TRANSFUSIONS

In regard to the question of which crystalloids should be infused concomitantly with red blood cell transfusions, the following guidelines are offered. Normal saline is the ideal solution to infuse with blood or to start a blood transfusion. Most solutions containing dextrose and water [5 per cent aqueous dextrose (D5/W), 5 per cent dextrose in 0.9 per cent saline (D5/NS), 5 per cent dextrose in 0.225 per cent saline (D5/0.2S)] are inappropriate, since aggregation of erythrocytes occurs, and the osmotic concentration may lead to lysis of erythrocytes in vivo. Dextrose 5 per cent in 0.225 per cent saline is not suitable for starting blood transfusions because it is associated with hemolysis and because of the lengthy retention of this solution in intravenous tubing after transfusion has begun. Blood warming devices enhance erythrocyte alterations and thus make these conditions even less optimal.

Lactated Ringer's solution is a physiological solution, but it contains a high concentration of calcium, which may neutralize anticoagulant activity of the citrate anticoagulant used in the blood preservative solution and lead to clot formation in the lines.

Clotting in intravenous tubing may be enhanced where flow rate is slow and the ambient temperature is high. Hence, small fibrin clots may be produced in intravenous tubing and be administered to patients when transfusions are started using lactated Ringer's solution. Ringer's solution is thus less than ideal for starting a transfusion or for simultaneous administration with blood.

In summary, only physiologic saline should be infused concomitantly with blood. Furthermore, lactated Ringer's solution and dextrose 5 per cent in 0.225 per cent saline should *not be used* to start blood transfusions.

Reference: Ryden, S.E., and Oberman, H.A.: Transfusion, *15*:250, 1975.

PORPHYRIA

The next time you see a patient with photosensitivity or abdominal pain, you may be fortunate enough to remember that these may be symptoms of porphyria. The chart below lists the six recognized forms of porphyria and their clinical and biochemical findings.

Manifestations of Different Types of Porphyrias in Man

FORM	INHERITANCE	CLINICAL MANIFESTATIONS	BIOCHEMICAL FINDINGS
Acute intermittent porphyria (AIP) (Swedish type)	Autosomal dominant with variable expression	Acute attacks of abdominal colic, hypertension, nervous system involvement, no photo sensitivity; usually after puberty	Increased urinary excretion of ALA and PBG during attacks and usually also during remission
Congenital erythropoietic porphyria	Autosomal recessive	Photosensitivity, severe dermatitis, hemolytic anemia, splenomegaly, erythrodontia; observed in early infancy and persistent through childhood and adult life	Increased amount of uroporphyrin and coproporphyrin, mainly trypsin 1, in bone marrow, erythrocytes, plasma, urine, and feces
Erythropoietic protoporphyria	Autosomal dominant with variable expression	Photosensitivity, mild dermatitis; usually first observed	Increased amount of protoporphyrin bone marrow, erythrocytes, plasma, and feces
Porphyria cutanea tarda		Photosensitivity and dermatitis; hepatic toxin required, especially alcohol	Increased excretion of urinary uroporphyrin; urinary coproporphyrin; protoporphyrin normal or slightly increased
Porphyria variegata (South African type)	Autosomal dominant with variable expression	Photosensitivity and dermatitis, acute attacks of abdominal and neurologic manifestations; usually after puberty	Increased amount of coproporphyrin and protoporphyrin in feces during attacks and remission; and increased urinary excretion of ALA and PBG and porphyrins during acute attacks
Hepatic coproporphyria	Autosomal dominant with variable expression	Photosensitivity (rare), gastrointestinal, neurologic, and psychiatric manifestations similar to those in AIP; any age group	Increased amounts of coproporphyrin III in feces and urine; excessive urinary excretion of ALA and PBG during acute attacks

8

In general, of the porphyrias that are associated with excretion of excessive amounts of porphyrin precursors, only acute intermittent porphyria is associated with abdominal pain. Those porphyrias in which the latter part of the heme synthesis pathway is affected are associated with excretion and accumulation of porphyrins. These forms of the disease include congenital erythropoietic porphyria, erythropoietic protoporphyria, and porphyria cutanea tarda. Dermatologic manifestations predominate in these forms.

The forms of the disease in which both porphyrias and their precursors are excreted are associated with both abdominal pain and dermatologic manifestations. These forms include porphyria variegata and hepatic coproporphyria.

Reference: Kaplan, B.H.: *In* Rudolph, A.M. (Ed.): Pediatrics. New York, Appleton-Century-Crofts, 1977, p. 758.

THE SLOW SEDIMENTATION RATE

All of the factors responsible for determining the rate at which erythrocytes sediment have not been identified. Factors that are known to influence the sedimentation rate include the quantity of fibrinogen, alpha$_1$-globulin, the gamma-M globulin, and the serum cholesterol, with the quantity of fibrinogen perhaps playing the most important role. In addition, alterations in the morphologic characteristics of the red cell or in cell surface charge that hinder rouleau formation will affect the erythrocyte sedimentation rate.

Everyone is familiar with the long and nondescript list of diseases that produce an increase in the erythrocyte sedimentation rate. It is generally not appreciated that certain disorders or drugs characteristically produce a slow sedimentation rate or a rate that is slower than would be anticipated. Disorders that produce a slow sedimentation rate include:

Anorexia nervosa
Hypofibrinogenemia, congenital or acquired
Abetalipoproteinemia (acanthocytosis)
Sickle cell anemia (if many sickled forms are present)
Pyruvate kinase deficiency (usually postsplenectomy if associated with
  marked morphologic alterations of the erythrocytes)
Hereditary spherocytosis
Congestive heart failure
Nephrotic syndrome
Steroid therapy
Aspirin administration
Serum sickness

In patients with the nephrotic syndrome in whom an infection is suspected, the measurement of the C-reactive protein provides a useful alternate screening test.

EOSINOPHILIA

The presence of more than 700 eosinophils per mm³ is defined as eosinophilia. A heterogeneous group of disorders may be associated with eosinophilia. The mnemonic NAACP may help you to categorize them (Neoplasia, Allergy, Addison's disease, Collagen-vascular disease, Parasites). More specific causes include the following.

Neoplasms

 Hodgkin's disease*
 Any neoplasm
 Eosinophilic leukemia*
 Myeloproliferative disorders

Allergy

 Asthma
 Hay fever
 Urticaria
 Eczema
 Drug sensitivity*

Adrenal insufficiency

Collagen-vascular diseases

 Periarteritis nodosa*
 Rheumatic fever

Parasites

 Helminthic: Trichinosis, ascariasis, hookworm, strongyloidiasis*
 Toxocara (visceral larva migrans)*
 Malaria

Miscellaneous

 Fanconi's aplastic anemia
 Cirrhosis
 Dermatitis herpetiformis
 Radiation therapy
 Peritoneal dialysis
 Congenital heart disease
 Hereditary familial eosinophilia
 Idiopathic hypereosinophilic syndrome*

 *Marked eosinophilia

References: Lukens, J.N.: Pediatr. Clin. North Am., *19*:969, 1972. Muido, L.: Supplied the mnemonic.

CAUSES OF BASOPHILIA

Basophils are the smallest of the blood granulocytes. Their granules stain metachromatically and contain histamine, heparin, and 5-hydroxytryptamine. Virtually all the histamine in the blood is contained within basophils. Basophils bind IgE. Contact with antigen will release IgE, which causes degranulation of the basophil with the release of histamine.

Since normal basophil counts are so low, factors that depress the basophil count (corticosteroid, thyroxin, and progesterone) are not usually clinically obvious in the peripheral blood smear.

Chronic myelocytic leukemia is the most common cause of a raised basophil count. The finding of basophilia can imply significant serious illness such as:

1. Certain blood disorders, including chronic myelocytic leukemia, polycythemia vera, myelofibrosis, hemolytic anemia, basophilic leukemia, and mast cell disease.
2. Hypersensitivity states.
3. Miscellaneous diseases such as ulcerative colitis, tuberculosis, diabetes, influenza, and carcinoma.

THROMBOCYTOSIS

Often the report of a peripheral blood smear contains the observation "platelets appear increased." Often this is disregarded. Elevations in platelet count frequently have diagnostic significance. Just recently it provided the clue to the fact that one patient had a neuroblastoma. The causes of thrombocytosis (platelet count in excess of 400,000/mm^3) are listed below. Those in italics are the most common.

Hereditary
  Asplenia
  Myeloproliferative disorder in Down's syndrome

Nutritional deficiency
  Iron deficiency
  Megaloblastic anemia
  Vitamin E deficiency

Metabolic
  Hyperadrenalism

Immume
  Graft vs. host reaction
  Nephrotic syndrome

Infectious
  Virus
  Bacteria
  Mycobacteria

Drug response
  Vinca alkaloids
  Citrovorum factor
  Corticosteroid therapy

Neoplastic
  Chronic myelogenous leukemia
  Histiocytosis
  Carcinoma
  Lymphoma
  Megakaryocytic leukemia
  Neuroblastoma

Traumatic
  Surgery
  Fractures
  Hemorrhage

Miscellaneous
  Splenectomy
  Caffey's disease
  Inflammatory bowel disease
  Pulmonary embolism
  Thrombophlebitis
  Cerebrovascular accident
  Sarcoidosis
  Idiopathic

Reference: Addiego, J.E., Jr., Mentzer, W.C., Jr., and Dallman, P.R.: J. Pediatr., *85:*805, 1974.

DIAGNOSTIC APPROACH TO THE BLEEDING PATIENT

The patient admitted for surgery who has a history of prolonged bleeding following dental extractions, the very ill patient who suddenly begins leaking blood from IV sites, and the child with a history of easy bruisability should each have immediate screening tests to determine if a coagulation defect exists. The results of the prothrombin time (PT), partial thromboplastin time (PTT), and platelet count are telephoned from the lab, and the most logical next step must be chosen. Logical steps are not always easy to come by, but reference to the chart below may provide the appropriate one.

A Diagnostic Approach to the Bleeding Patients

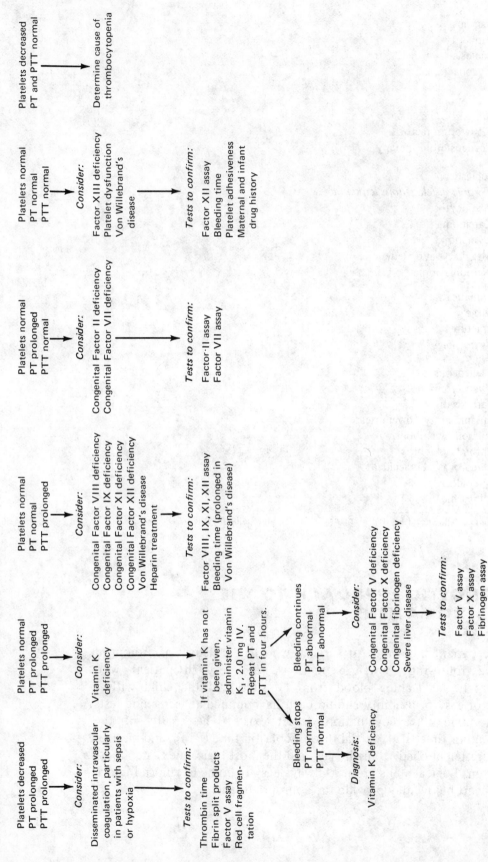

Platelets decreased
PT prolonged
PTT prolonged

Consider:

Disseminated intravascular
coagulation, particularly
in patients with sepsis
or hypoxia

Tests to confirm:

Thrombin time
Fibrin split products
Factor V assay
Red cell fragmen-
tation

Platelets normal
PT prolonged
PTT prolonged

Consider:

Vitamin K
deficiency

If vitamin K has not
been given,
administer vitamin
K₁, 2.0 mg IV.
Repeat PT and
PTT in four hours.

Bleeding continues
PT abnormal
PTT abnormal

Consider:

Congenital Factor V deficiency
Congenital Factor X deficiency
Congenital fibrinogen deficiency
Severe liver disease

Tests to confirm:

Factor V assay
Factor X assay
Fibrinogen assay

Bleeding stops
PT normal
PTT normal

Diagnosis:

Vitamin K deficiency

Platelets normal
PT normal
PTT prolonged

Consider:

Congenital Factor VIII deficiency
Congenital Factor IX deficiency
Congenital Factor XI deficiency
Congenital Factor XII deficiency
Von Willebrand's disease
Heparin treatment

Tests to confirm:

Factor VIII, IX, XI, XII assay
Bleeding time (prolonged in
Von Willebrand's disease)

Platelets normal
PT prolonged
PTT normal

Consider:

Congenital Factor II deficiency
Congenital Factor VII deficiency

Tests to confirm:

Factor II assay
Factor VII assay

Platelets normal
PT normal
PTT normal

Consider:

Factor XIII deficiency
Platelet dysfunction
Von Willebrand's
disease

Tests to confirm:

Factor XII assay
Bleeding time
Platelet adhesiveness
Maternal and infant
drug history

Platelets decreased
PT and PTT normal

Determine cause of
thrombocytopenia

Along with the information included in the chart, it may be helpful to remember that the most common cause of congenital coagulation abnormality is von Willebrand's disease, inherited in an autosomal dominant pattern.

PURPURA AND PETECHIAE—WHAT DOES IT ALL MEAN?

Listed below are some clues to the significance of various forms of purpura.

Thrombocytopenic purpura	Petechiae are *nonpalpable*. Platelet count < 20,000/ml.
Thrombocytopathic purpura	Easily bruised. Petechiae are *rare*.
Vasculitic purpura (+/− thrombocytopenia)	Petechiae are *palpable*.
Drug purpura (+/− thrombocytopenia)	Often associated with *hemorrhagic bullae* in the mouth.
Allergic purpura (Henoch-Schöenlein)	*Pruritic* crops of symmetrical purpura on proximal extremities (4+ lower) associated with *urticarial* and erythematous lesions.
Purpura fulminans (skin manifestation of D.I.C.)	Large symmetrical ecchymoses particularly on distal extremities complicated by *acral gangrene*. Petechiae are *rare*.
"Devil's pinches" (autoerythrosensitization vs. factitious)	Females. "Spontaneous" *painful* ecchymoses (+/− erythematous base) on anterior-lateral aspect of thigh and abdomen in a stepladder distribution.
Hyperglobulinemic purpura	Lower extremities (after exercise or prolonged standing). Tendency for skin to develop *brownish pigmentation*. Identical to idiopathic nonhyperglobulinemic syndrome, called Schamberg's disease, except that the latter has normal serum globulin levels.
Cryoglobulinemic purpura	Purpura (+/− gangrene) on *exposed acral areas* (fingers, nose, ears, face).
Amyloid purpura	Spontaneous *periorbital* purpura (usually post Valsalva maneuver). "Touch purpura."
Scorbutic purpura	Purpura around hair *follicles* (perifollicular petechiae). Characteristically associated with corkscrew hairs. Saddle distribution.

8

Senile purpura	Purple *flat* ecchymotic spots on extensor surface of *forearms*, dorsum of *hands*, and neck in the *elderly*. Identical lesions are found in *cachectic states* and chronic *hypercortisonism*.
Embolic purpura	A. Septic embolic *White centered* petechial lesion often located on mucous membranes and conjunctivae (e.g., bacterial endocarditis). B. Fat emboli Petechiae limited to upper one-half of body, particularly to *anterior chest*. *Never seen on the face or back* (skimming effect).
Palatine petechiae	Infectious mononucleosis. Sepsis. Trauma (e.g., dentures).
Petechiae (lesion $\leq$ 3 mm)	Almost always indicates a disturbance of platelets or a vasculopathy. Rarely do they indicate an abnormality of coagulation.

Reference: Seckler, S.G.: Hospital Practice, 5:36, 1977.

EFFECTS OF DRUGS ON PROTHROMBIN TIME

The prothrombin time that is unexpectedly high or low may be a manifestation of the effect of any number of drugs. The following table lists drugs that increase or decrease the prothrombin time. The mechanism of prothrombin time increase is listed, while the mechanism for a shortened test is not known.

Drugs that Increase Prothrombin Time

By causing a decrease in vitamin K synthesis or absorption:

Cathartics	Neomycin
Chlortetracycline	Streptomycin
Cholestyramine	Succinylsulfathiazole
Kanamycin	Sulfamethoxazole
Mineral oil	

By decreasing clotting factor synthesis:

Acetaminophen	L-Asparaginase
Acetylsalicylic acid (large doses)	6-Mercaptopurine
	Quinidine
Aminosalicylic acid	Quinine

By altering liver function (bile salt excretion, cholestasis, hepatotoxicity):

Acetohexamide	Methotrexate	Sulfisoxazole
Chlordiazepoxide	Methyltestosterone	Tetracycline
Chlorpromazine	Niacin	Thiazides
Chlorpropamide	Oral contraceptives	Tolazamide
Halothane	Prochlorperazine	Tolbutamide
Mepazine	Promazine	Trifluoperazine

By decreasing prothrombin concentration or activity:

Chloramphenicol	Doxycycline
Cremomycin	Pyrazinamide
Cyclophosphamide	Sulfachlorpyridazine
Demeclocycline	

Drugs that Shorten the Prothrombin Time

Acetylsalicylic acid (small doses)
Anabolic steroids
Azathioprine
Edetic acid (early in therapy)
Kanamycin (early in therapy)
Vitamin K

TIP-OFFS TO MALIGNANT DISEASE

A significant number of both congenital malformations and acquired diseases are now recognized to be associated with an increased incidence of malignancy. Detection of a condition listed below should occasion a high index of suspicion, regular observation, and appropriate studies for early detection of malignancy.

CONDITION	ASSOCIATED MALIGNANCY
Agammaglobulinemia	Lymphoma, lymphosarcoma
Albinism	Basal cell carcinoma, squamous cell carcinoma
Aniridia (non-familial)	Wilms' tumor
Ataxia telangiectasia	Leukemia, lymphoma, lymphosarcoma
Beckwith's syndrome	Wilms' tumor, liver carcinoma, adrenal cortical carcinoma, nesidioblastosis of pancreas
Bloom's syndrome	Leukemia
Chédiak-Higashi syndrome	Lymphoma, lymphosarcoma, leukemia
D-trisomy	Leukemia

Continued

CONDITION	ASSOCIATED MALIGNANCY
Down's syndrome	Leukemia
Familial polyposis of colon	Colonic carcinoma
Family history (first degree) of malignancy	Same or other malignancy
Genitourinary anomalies	Wilms' tumor
Giant cell hepatitis	Carcinoma of liver
Hemihypertrophy	Wilms' tumor, adrenal cortical carcinoma, liver carcinoma, hepatoblastoma
Hippel-Lindau disease	Pheochromocytoma
Horner syndrome	Neuroblastoma
Irradiation:	
in utero	Leukemia
of head and neck in early life	Thyroid carcinoma, brain and parotid tumors
for retinoblastoma	Osteosarcoma
for Wilms' tumor	Osteosarcoma, osteochondroma
for neuroblastoma	Osteosarcoma, osteochondroma
Klinefelter's syndrome	Leukemia
Multiple mucosal neuromas	Medullary thyroid carcinoma
Maternal stilbestrol during pregnancy	Vaginal adenocarcinoma
Neurofibromatosis	Pheochromocytoma, sarcoma, schwannoma, leukemia
Nevus sebaceous	Basal cell carcinoma
Poland's syndrome	Leukemia
Thyroid cancer (medullary)	Pheochromocytoma
Ulcerative colitis/regional ileitis	Colonic carcinoma
Wiskott-Aldrich syndrome	Lymphoma, lymphosarcoma
Xeroderma pigmentosa	Basal cell or squamous cell carcinoma

References: Craven, E.M.: J.A.M.A., *215*:795, 1971. Feman, S.S., and Apt, L.: J. Pediatr. Ophthalmol., *9*:224, 1972.

ENVIRONMENTAL CARCINOGENS

There are a number of agents that are unequivocally linked to an increased risk of cancer, and an even greater number suspected of such a relationship. Among the more prominent of these are the following:

TARGET ORGAN	CONFIRMED	SUSPECTED
Bone		Beryllium
Brain	Vinyl chloride	
Gastrointestinal tract	Asbestos	Smoked meats
Hematopoietic tissue (leukemia)	Benzene, styrene butadiene, other synthetic rubbers	
Kidney	Coke oven emissions	Lead
Larynx	Asbestos, chromium	
Liver	Vinyl chloride	Aldrin, dieldrin, heptachlor, Kepone, mirex, DDT, carbon tetrachloride, chloroform, PCBs, trichlorethylene
Lung	Arsenic, asbestos, bis (chloromethyl) ether, chloromethyl methyl ether, chromates, nickel, coke oven emissions, mustard gas, soots and tars, uranium, vinyl chloride	Beryllium, cadmium, chloroprene, lead
Lymphatic tissue		Arsenic, benzene
Nasal mucosa	Chromium, nickel, wood dust	
Pancreas		Benzidine, PCBs
Pleural cavity	Asbestos	
Prostate		Cadmium
Scrotum	Soots and tars	Chloroprene
Skin	Arsenic, cutting oils, coke oven emissions, soots and tars	
Urinary bladder	4-Aminobiphenyl, benzidine, β-naphthylamine	Auramine, magenta, 4-nitrodiphenyl

Reference: Key, M.M., et al.: Occupational Diseases. A Guide to Their Recognition. No. 77-181, U.S. Dept. HEW (NIOSH), 1977.

TOXICITY OF CANCER CHEMOTHERAPY

Longer survival of children with malignancies and an ever increasing number of chemotherapeutic agents given to these children mean that pediatricians will need to be alert to both the early and the late side-effects of these agents. The following list suggests the possible side-effects that could be anticipated for each agent. (L) = late effect only.

Adriamycin. Nausea, vomiting, stomatitis, alopecia, cardiac toxicity, red urine, bone marrow depressions, hyperpigmentation of dermal creases and nails, and cellulitis at injection site (total dose–related).

Arabinosylcytosine (Ara-C, Cytarabine). Nausea, vomiting, abdominal pain, diarrhea, hepatic toxicity (rarely), fever, alopecia, conjunctivitis, epithelial ulceration, keratitis, megaloblastosis, and bone marrow depression (leukopenia and thrombocytopenia).

Asparaginase (Elspar). Nausea, vomiting, fever, anaphylactic reaction, hepatotoxicity, pancreatitis, lethargy, confusion, azotemia, urticaria, hyperglucosemia, hypoproteinemia, hypolipidemia and hyperlipidemia, fatty metamorphosis of the liver, decreased levels of coagulation factors, and pancytopenia.

Bischloroethyl nitrosourea (BCNU). Nausea and vomiting, hepatic toxicity, and bone marrow depression (leukopenia and thrombocytopenia).

Bleomycin. Nausea and vomiting, stomatitis, fever, chills, edema and dermatitis of hands, hyperpigmentation, nail changes, alopecia, pneumonitis, and pulmonary fibrosis. There is no evidence for bone marrow or immunologic depression.

Busulfan (Myleran). Bulbous eruption of the skin, cataracts, glossitis, adrenal insufficiency–like syndrome, skin pigmentation, diffuse pulmonary fibrosis and ossification, and bone marrow depression; menstrual dysfunction (L).

Chlorambucil (Leukeran). Bone marrow depression; menstrual dysfunction (L); azoospermia (L).

Corticosteroids. Cushingoid features, osteoporosis, growth retardation, hypertension, psychosis, peptic ulcers, hyperglucosemia, fluid retention, hypokalemia, myopathy, cataracts, and thromboembolic phenomena.

Cyclohexylchloroethyl nitrosourea (CCNU). Nausea and vomiting, hepatic toxicity, and bone marrow depression (leukopenia and thrombocytopenia).

Cyclophosphamide (Cytoxan). Nausea and vomiting, alopecia, transverse ridging of nails, skin pigmentation, hemorrhagic cystitis, fibrosis of urinary bladder, possibly interstitial pneumonitis, and bone marrow depression (leukopenia, thrombocytopenia, and anemia); primary ovarian failure (L); azoospermia (L).

Dactinomycin (Actinomycin D). Nausea and vomiting, stomatitis, diarrhea, alopecia, irritant at infusion site, and bone marrow depression.

Daunomycin. Nausea and vomiting, alopecia, cardiac toxicity, red urine, irritant at infusion site, and bone marrow depression (leukopenia and thrombocytopenia).

Fluorouracil (5-FU). Nausea, ulcerations of mouth and gastrointestinal tract, maculopapular rash, photophobia, diarrhea, acute cerebellar syndrome, and bone marrow depression.

Hydroxyurea (Hydrea). Nausea, vomiting, stomatitis, maculopapular rash, facial erythema, and bone marrow depression.

Mechlorethamine (Nitrogen mustard). Nausea, vomiting, leukopenia, thrombocytopenia, and strong vesicating effect on skin and veins.

Methotrexate (Amethopterin). Ulcerations of mouth and gastrointestinal tract, diarrhea, hepatic necrosis, cirrhosis, perifolliculitis, acne, pneumonitis, megaloblastosis from folate deficiency, and bone marrow depression; hepatic fibrosis (L); diffuse pulmonary disease (L); osteoporosis with pathologic fractures (L).

Procarbazine (Natulan). Nausea, vomiting, mental depression, stomatitis, constipation, diarrhea, myalgia, and arthralgia, chills and fever, dermatitis, paresthesia, ataxia, and bone marrow depression (leukopenia and thrombocytopenia).

Thioguanine (6-TG). Nausea, vomiting, and bone marrow depression.

Triethylenemelamine (TEM). Nausea, vomiting, abdominal pain, alopecia, cystitis, and bone marrow depression.

Triethylenethiophosphoramide (Thio-Tepa). Nausea, vomiting, headache, and bone marrow depression.

Vinblastine (Velban). Nausea, vomiting, irritant at infusion site, alopecia, areflexia, constipation, stomatitis, and bone marrow depression; menstrual dysfunction (L).

Vincristine (Oncovin). Alopecia, irritant at infusion site, constipation, paralytic ileus, abdominal pain, oral ulcers, bladder atonia, dysuria, muscular weakness, joint pain, jaw pain, fever, hypertension, inappropriate antidiuretic hormone secretion, vocal cord paralysis, peripheral neuritis, ataxia, foot drop, neuralgia, paresthesia of fingers and toes, sensory loss, neuralgia, cranial nerve palsies, depressed to absent deep tendon reflexes, patchy liver necrosis, and mild depression of the bone marrow.

References: Hughes, W.T.: Pediatr. Clin. North Am., *23*:225, 1976. Jaffe, N.: Pediatr. Clin. North Am., *23*:233, 1976.

9
CRITICAL CARE
MEDICINE

TEMPERATURE CONVERSION AND CORRECTION FACTORS FOR ARTERIAL BLOOD GASES

Extremes of body temperature that are sometimes encountered in the critically ill patient can cause significant difference between the actual arterial blood gas values and those that are obtained in the laboratory at room temperature. The tables below can be used to make these temperature corrections for arterial blood gases if your laboratory does not routinely do this. For example, reported blood gases of pH 7.30, Pa_{CO_2} 50 torr, and Pa_{O_2} 100 torr in a patient with a body temperature of 33°C are actually pH 7.36, Pa_{CO_2} 41.2, and Pa_{O_2} 71.2.

	↑ 1°C*†	↓ 1°C*†
pH	↓ .015	↑ .015
P_{CO_2} (mm Hg)	↑4.4%	↓4.4%
P_{O_2} (mm Hg)	↑7.2%	↓7.2%

*Change with reference to 37° C.
†Percentage change of the value measured at standard 37° C.

Reference: Reuler, J.B.: Ann. Intern. Med., *89:*519, 1978.

9

It is customary, but I think it is a mistake, to speak of happy childhood. Children, however, are often over-anxious and acutely sensitive. Man ought to be man and master of his fate; but children are at the mercy of those around them.

Sir John Lubbock, Baron Avebury
The Pleasures of Life, Pt. 1, Ch. 1

RELATIONSHIP OF pH TO Pa$_{CO_2}$ AND BASE CHANGE

Quick calculations are often helpful in assessing a child who is very ill. The two formulas below are estimates, but useful ones.

1. A change of Pa$_{CO_2}$ of 10 torr is associated with a decrease or increase in pH of 0.08 units:

   Pa$_{CO_2}$ 10 torr ↑ ↓ pH 0.08

   For example:

   Pa$_{CO_2}$ 40 torr—pH 7.40—Normal

   Pa$_{CO_2}$ 50 torr—pH 7.32—Respiratory Acidosis—Hypoventilation

   Pa$_{CO_2}$ 30 torr—pH 7.48—Respiratory Alkalosis—Hyperventilation

2. A base change (base excess or base deficit) of 10 mEq/L is associated with a pH change of 0.15.

   For example:

   Pa$_{CO_2}$ 40 torr—pH 7.25

   Normal Pa$_{CO_2}$ — No respiratory component

   Calculated pH 7.40

   Measured pH 7.25

   pH difference—0.15

   Base deficit = 10 mEq/L—Metabolic acidosis

   No respiratory component—Metabolic acidosis only

ALPHABET SOUP

You can expect to encounter a variety of cardiovascular symbols and formulas in the intensive care unit since invasive hemodynamic monitoring is so commonly performed now. The following table should help you understand this area of medical jargon.

When using these parameters in patient management, remember:

1. Analysis of numbers alone is meaningless. They must be correlated with your clinical examination.

2. No one parameter is adequate in all patients at all times. You need to examine the interrelationships among the various factors to get the whole picture.

3. Trends are more useful than isolated values.

4. Think "optimal" rather than "normal." Normal values are generally determined on a normal healthy population. Critically ill patients are far from normal and healthy, and may, in fact, do best at levels of cardiovascular performance that are quite deviant from "normal range."

9

PARAMETER	ABBREVIATION	FORMULA	UNITS	MEANING/USE
Mean arterial pressure	$\overline{MAP}$	$DP + \dfrac{SP^* - DP^*}{3}$	Torr	Useful endpoint for titrating vasoactive agents. Used to calculate systemic vascular resistance.
Central venous pressure	CVP	Directly measured	Torr cm H_2O	Used as index of volume status and right ventricular preload.
Pulmonary artery occlusion pressure ("wedge pressure")	PAo	Directly measured	Torr	Index of volume status and left ventricular preload. More reliable than CVP.
Mean pulmonary artery pressure	$\overline{PAP}$	$DP + \dfrac{SP\dagger - DP\dagger}{3}$	Torr	Used to calculate pulmonary vascular resistance.
Cardiac output	C.O.	Directly measured	Liters/min	Prime measurement of hemodynamic function.
Cardiac index	CI	$\dfrac{C.O.}{Body\ surface\ area}$	Liters/min/ sq meter	
Stroke volume	SV	C.O./Pulse	ml	Provides some information about cardiac performance.
Systemic vascular resistance	SVR	$\dfrac{\overline{MAP} - CVP}{C.O.} \times 80$	dynes/cm/sec^{-5}	Measure of resistance of arterial tree. Useful in differential diagnosis of various shock states.
Pulmonary vascular resistance	PVR	$\dfrac{\overline{PAP} - PAo}{C.O.} \times 80$	dynes/cm/sec^{-5}	Measure of resistance of pulmonary vascular bed. Elevated in pulmonary embolism, chronic obstructive airway disease, acute respiratory failure.

9

PARAMETER	ABBREVIATION	FORMULA	UNITS	MEANING/USE
Left ventricular stroke work	LVSW	SV $\overline{(MAP-PA)}$ 0.0136	gm/meter	Measure of left ventricular performance.
Right ventricular stroke work	RVSW	SV $\overline{(PAP-CVP)}$ 0.0136	gm/meter	Measure of right ventricular performance.
Arteriovenous oxygen difference	$C(a-\bar{v})\ O_2$	Directly measured from arterial and mixed venous blood gases	ml/dl	Index of adequacy of tissue oxygenation.
Oxygen transport	O_2 Trans. (O_2 Del)	$C.O. \times CaO_2$ CaO_2 = arterial oxygen content	ml/min	Amount of oxygen delivered to the tissues.
Oxygen consumption	O_2 Cons.	$C.O. \times C(a-\bar{v})\ O_2$	ml/min	Amount of oxygen extracted by the tissues.
Oxygen utilization coefficient	O_2 Util. Coef.	$\dfrac{O_2\ Cons.}{O_2\ Trans.}$	—	Index of efficiency of oxygen utilization.
Index	I	$\dfrac{Parameter}{Body\ surface\ area}$	—	Eliminates body size as variable, and thus aids in interpreting values of various measurements.

*SP, DP — systolic, diastolic pressure (systemic).
†SP, DP — systolic, diastolic pressure (pulmonary artery).

Reference: Desoutel's, D.A., et al.: Resp. Care, *23*:43, 1978.

DRIPS

The table below should help you in preparing drug solutions for continuous intravenous infusion. These drugs should be administered with a metriset and a constant infusion pump to safeguard against inadvertent administration of a large bolus of the drug. In patients who will need fluid restriction, the final concentration of the drugs may be doubled by halving the amount of solution.

The doses suggested are *starting doses.* They may be increased as needed for clinical response. Please see the table on pp. 288–291 for maximal doses.

It is important to note the concentration of the medication listed. If your pharmacy stocks a different concentration, appropriate adjustments must be made in the recipe used.

MEDICATION	RECIPE	CONCENTRATION	SUGGESTED STARTING DOSE	COMMENTS
Dopamine (40 mg/ml)	60 mg (1.5 ml)/ 100 ml D 5% W	600 μg/ml	0.5–1 ml/kg/hr = 5–10 μg/kg/ min	1. Effects are dose-related. 2. Inactivated by $NaHCO_3$.
Epinephrine 1 : 1000	0.6 mg (3.0 ml)/ 100 ml D 5% W	6 μg/ml	1 ml/kg/hr = 0.1 μg/kg/min	1. Occasionally patients will respond to epinephrine but not to dopamine.
Isoproterenol 1 : 5000	0.6 mg (0.6 ml)/ 100 ml D 5% W	6 μg/ml	1 ml/kg/hr = 0.1 μg/kg/min	1. Chemical pacemaker— use for brady- cardia and shock and for asthma with respiratory failure.
Lidocaine 4%	120 mg (3 ml)/ 100 ml D 5% W	1200 μg/ml	1 ml/kg/hr = 20 μg/kg/min	1. Reduces ventricular irritability. 2. Hypertension may be a side- effect.

Continued

9

MEDICATION	RECIPE	CONCENTRATION	SUGGESTED STARTING DOSE	COMMENTS
Nitroprusside	6 mg/100 ml D 5% W	60 μg/ml	1 ml/kg/hr = 1.0 μg/kg/min	1. Light-sensitive—cover bottle and tape tubing. Change bottle every 4 hr. Patient may get hypotension with new bottle at a previously successful dose.

Reference: Holbrook, P.R., Mickell, J., Polack, M.M., and Fields, A.I.: Crit. Care Med., Dec., 1980, p. 762.

PEDIATRIC EMERGENCY DRUGS

They are all in various handbooks, but we thought you might like to have these medications listed together for easy reference. Please use this list along with the recipes for "Drips" on pp. 285–286. Don't forget to note concentrations of the drugs listed and adjust appropriately if you are not using the same formulation.

A significant part of the discomfort and dysfunction that accompanies illness stems from apprehension, and apprehension is a relievable symptom by human interaction; all else being equal, less fear equals less pain.

Leon Eisenberg

9

DRUG	DOSE	USE/ACTION
Albumin 25%	1 gm/kg or 4 ml/kg IV	Hypotension
Atropine	0.02 mg/kg/dose IV up to 1.0 mg	Sinus bradycardia
Benadryl	2 mg/kg IV slow push	For anaphylaxis or to antagonize oculogyric crisis
Calcium chloride 10%	0.1–0.2 ml/kg slow IV push	Increased myocardial contractility (*Danger:* inhibits sinus node)
Calcium gluconate 10% 9.3 mg Ca++/ml	0.5 ml/kg/dose slow IV push; repeat in 10 min	" "
Cimetidine	20–40 mg/kg/day divided q 6 hr PO/IV max daily dose: 1200 mg	*Toxicities:* include CNS, marrow suppression, and possibly arrhythmias
Dexamethasone	3 mg/kg/IV q 6 hr 0.2 mg/kg IV q 6 hr; adults 4 mg q 6 hr	Septic shock Increased intracranial pressure, croup
Dextrose 50%	1–2 ml/kg/dose IV push	Hypoglycemia
Diazoxide (Hyperstat)	2–5 mg/kg/dose IV push over 30 sec; may repeat if no effect	Hypertension/Immediate arteriolar vasodilation
Digoxin	*Total Digitalizing Dose* <2500 gm: 0.02 mg/kg IV over 24 hr (not p.o.) 2500 gm–2 yr: 0.06 mg/kg p.o., or 0.05 mg/kg IM or IV over 24 hr >2 yr: 0.05 mg/kg p.o., or 0.04 mg/kg IM or IV over 24 hr Maximum: 1.0 mg IV or p.o. over 24 hr	Heart failure, supraventricular tachycardia

9

Drug	*Maintenance Dose* 24 hr after digitalizing dose	
	<2500 gm: 0.005 mg/kg/d ÷ q 12 p.o. or IV 2500 gm–2 yr: 0.015 mg/kg/d p.o. ÷ q 12 hr, or 0.012 mg/kg/d IM or IV ÷ q 12 hr >2 yr: 0.012 mg/kg/d p.o. ÷ q 12 hr, or 0.010 mg/kg/d IM or IV ÷ q 12 hr **Maximum: 0.375 mg over 24 hr**	
Dopamine	2–20 μg/kg/min (ampule = 200 mg/5 ml)	Shock/Dopaminergic and adrenergic effects
Epinephrine	1:1000, 0.01 ml/kg/dose (to 0.3 ml max) 1:10,000, 0.1 ml/kg/dose (to 5 ml max) (Alternate route = ET tube)	Asthma
Glucagon	0.3 mg/kg/dose (do not exceed 1 mg) (1 unit = 1 mg = 1 ml)	Increased myocardial contractility Hypoglycemia
Hydralazine	0.15–0.25 mg/kg IM or IV	Hypertension/Vasodilation
Hydrocortisone	5 mg/kg/dose (physiologic replacement = 25 mg/m^2 /day p.o. or 12 mg/m^2 / day IV 100 mg/m^2 IV	Anaphylaxis, asthma Stress dose
Insulin	0.5–1.0 unit/kg IV with 1.5 gm dextrose/kg	Hyperkalemia
Isoproterenol (Isuprel)	0.1–0.5 μg/kg/min IV infusion, limit 4 gm/min (titrate) (ampule 1 mg/5 ml)	Bradycardia Shock Asthma with respiratory failure
Kayexalate	1 gm/kg q 4–6 hr in 2 ml/kg 70% sorbitol (p.o.) in 10 ml/kg 20% sorbitol (p.r.)	For hyperkalemia
Lasix	1 mg/kg IV, IM, p.o.	Congestive heart failure

Continued

DRUG	DOSE	USE/ACTION
Lidocaine	Loading dose 1 mg/kg IV push (max 100 mg) Then 20–50 μg/kg/min drip repeat loading dose 20 min later regardless—then continue drip	Reduced ventricular irritability (*Danger:* hypertension)
Mannitol	0.25–1 gm/kg IV push May give q 4–6 hr	Temporary control of increased intracranial pressure
Methylprednisolone	30 mg/kg IV q 6 hr 1–2 mg/kg IV q 2 hr	Septic shock Asthma
Morphine	0.1 mg/kg/dose SC, IV, IM q 2–4 hr	Tetralogy cyanotic spell
Naloxone (Narcan)	0.01 mg/kg/dose SC If failure repeat 0.1 mg/kg/dose	Narcotic overdose specific antagonist *Caution:* may induce vomiting
Neostigmine	0.07–0.08 mg/kg	Reversal of nondepolarizing neuromuscular block (give with atropine)
Nitroprusside	0.5 μg/kg/min starting dose Increase to desired response Prepare as: 6 mg/dl D5W = 60 μg/ml 1 ml/kg/hr = 1.0 μg/kg/min	Treatment of hypertension
Pavulon	0.1 mg/kg starting dose 0.01–0.1 mg/kg/dose q 30 min–2 hr	Neuromuscular blockade causes tachycardia Has no analgesic effect
Propranolol	0.05–0.1 mg/kg/dose IV push Max dose: 5 mg	To inhibit supraventricular arrhythmias Tetralogy spells *Caution:* may cause bronchospasm

Drug	Dose	Comments
Sodium bicarbonate 0.9 mEq/ml in 7.5% solution	1–3 mEq/kg/dose IV; repeat q 5–10 min	Metabolic acidosis (*Danger*: hypernatremia)
Syrup of ipecac	10 ml p.o. single dose 15 ml p.o. repeat in 20 min x 1 30 ml p.o.	*Emetic:* for <1 yo for 1–12 yo for >12 yo *Contraindicated if:* Lethargic, seizures, caustic substances or hydrocarbon ingested
Terbutaline	10–40 µg/kg SC	Bronchospasm
THAM E (0.3 M solution)	Base excess x wt (kg) = ml of THAM for IV infusion	Metabolic acidosis (may cause hypoglycemia)
Diazepam (Valium)	0.1–0.2 mg/kg/dose IV push	Seizure (may cause respiratory arrest)
Defibrillation	2 watt-sec/kg. If unsuccessful increase in 50–100% increments. Adult range 200–400 watt-sec.	

9

Administration of Intravenous Antibiotics

(These doses are to be used only for children over 4 weeks of age.)

DRUG	DOSE	MAXIMAL DAILY DOSE	FRE-QUENCY	ROUTE
Amikacin	15–22 mg/kg/d	0.75–1 gm	q 8 hr	IV or IM
Ampicillin	200–400 mg/kg/d	8–12 gm	q 4 hr	IV or IVP*
Carbenicillin	500 mg/kg/d	30–40 gm	q 4 hr	Drip over 1 hr (max conc. 1 gm/5 ml)
Cefamandole	50–150 mg/kg/d	4–6 gm	q 6 hr	Drip over 30 min or IVP*
Cefazolin	50–100 mg/kg/d	4–6 gm	q 6 hr	" "
Cefoxitin	80–160 mg/kg/d	4–6 gm	q 6 hr	Drip over 30 min or IVP*
Cephalothin	100–200 mg/kg/d	4–6 gm	q 6 hr	" "
Chloramphenicol	50–100 mg/kg/d	4–6 gm	q 6 hr	Drip over 30 min
Clindamycin	20–40 mg/kg/d	2–4 gm	q 6 hr	Drip over 30 min (rate not to exceed 30 mg/min; conc. not to exceed 6 mg/ml)
Gentamicin	<3 mo 4–7 mg/kg/d >3 mo 60 mg/m²/d	300 mg	q 8 hr	Drip over 30 min
Kanamycin	15–30 mg/kg/d	0.75–1 gm	q 8 hr	Drip over 30 min (conc. no greater than 2.5 mg/ml and 3–4 ml/min)
Nafcillin	100–200 mg/kg/d	8–12 gm	q 4 hr	Drip over 30 min in 20–30 ml (may increase duration and dilution to decrease discomfort)
Oxacillin	200–400 mg/kg/d	8–12 gm	q 4 hr	"
Penicillin	200,000–400,000 units/kg/d	24 million units	q 2–3 hr	Drip over 30 min or IVP*

*Indications for administration of IV Push:
1. Fluid restriction.
2. Maintain stability of antibiotic.
3. Increase nursing time for nursing duties.
4. Initial medication for infectious disease emergencies.
Definitions:
IVP—5 min.
IV drip—30 min.

Hints:

1. Infants over 4 wk of age suspected of having meningitis or sepsis should be treated initially with ampicillin and chloramphenicol.

2. Enterococcal infections must always be treated with both a penicillin and an aminoglycoside, regardless of reported sensitivities.

3. Klebsiellae are almost never sensitive to ampicillin no matter what the sensitivity testing says. A cephalosporin should be used for *Klebsiella* infections. For serious infections, an aminoglycoside should also be used.

4. Peak levels for aminoglycosides should be obtained 1 half-hour after the end of the 1 half-hour IV administration of the drug (1 hr after IM administration). Trough levels should be obtained just prior to a dose.

DRUG	DESIRED PEAK	DESIRED TROUGH
Gentamicin	4–8 µg/ml	<2 µg/ml
Kanamycin	15–25 µg/ml	<5 µg/ml
Amikacin	"	"
Tobramycin	4–8 µg/ml	<2 µg/ml

Frequent aminoglycoside levels are essential for young infants, seriously ill patients, and patients with impaired renal function.

5. Loading dose for ampicillin 100–200 mg/kg IVP for suspected septicemia or meningitis, i.e., one half of the daily dose.

Guidelines in the Management of Hemophilia

I. HOW TO DECIDE HOW MUCH TO GIVE

Dosage and duration of therapy depend on the type of bleeding seen clinically. Bleeding episodes may roughly be defined as follows:

a. "Open," i.e., from wounds or lacerations of skin and mucous membranes, tooth extractions, or surgery.

b. "Closed"—can be subdivided into:

(i) joint bleeds and nondissecting soft-tissue hematomas, either spontaneous or as a result of injury, and

(ii) dissecting soft-tissue hematomas, some of which may threaten respiration (e.g., visible swelling in the neck, hoarseness, or difficulty swallowing) or peripheral nerve function (e.g., Volkmann's contracture resulting from a circumferential bleed of the forearm).

Expressed in terms of percentage circulating Factor VIII or IX (where normal equals 50–200% and a hemostatic level is roughtly 20%), the following levels are desirable:

a. Open bleeding—achieve a 40% level, then maintain at least 20% until the lesion is adequately healed (e.g., 5–7 days with lacerations or until stitches are out. 10–14 days for surgical procedures).

b. Closed—for joint bleeds a single dose of Factor VIII to achieve a level of 50–60%. Soft-tissue hemorrhage in a critical area warrants a moderate to major replacement dose and hospitalization, with maintenance of a 20–40% level for 48–72 hr.

One must consider rate of disappearance of the plasma factor in planning therapeutic regimens. The in vivo half-life of AHF is 12 hr. The in vivo half-life of Factor IX is 10–84 hr. Therefore, once-a-day replacement is quite feasible for Factor IX-deficient patients. For Factor VIII-deficient patients, one must either boost them every 12 hr, or give 2 times the calculated replacement every 24 hr.

II. WHAT PRODUCTS ARE AVAILABLE?
AND HOW IS THE DOSE CALCULATED?

For Factor VIII-deficient patients.

a. Cryoprecipitate—obtained from blood bank. No crossmatch necessary.

1 pack/10 kg = 20% level

1 pack/5 kg = 40% level

Because of variability of Factor VIII content per pack (roughly 100–150 units), round off to higher number. When smaller patients are treated, always give at least 2 packs.

b. AHF concentrates obtained from pharmacy. Dosage of units of Factor VIII is printed on each vial. (One unit AHF is defined as the activity present in 1 ml of fresh pooled human plasma.)

Calculation: 1 unit of Factor VIII activity/kg body weight raises the Factor VIII level by 2%; e.g., to achieve a 40% level in a 30-kg boy: units Factor VIII needed = 20 x 30 = 600.

For Factor IX-deficient patients:

a. FFP, or recently outdated blood bank plasma (3 wk old) 10 ml/kg. Hypervolemia may complicate therapy.

b. Proplex or Konyne—a stable dried plasma fraction containing Factors II, VII, IX, and X. Each bottle of concentrate contains 500–700 units of Factor IX, and is equivalent to 500–700 ml of plasma.

Calculation: 1 unit of Factor IX activity/kg body weight raises the Factor IX level by 0.5–1.0%.

N.B.: Be sure to administer all factors and concentrates as soon as they are reconstituted, and as rapidly as the patient can tolerate, to ensure peak levels. Factor IX complex and AHF may be given by syringe injection.

III. ADJUVANT THERAPY

1. For dental extractions and for nondental oral bleeds:

a.   Raise level to 20–40% initially.

b.   Administer EACA (Amicar) p.o.—initial dose of 200 mg/kg followed by 100 mg/kg per dose every 4 hr for the first 24 hr. For the next 5–7 days 100 mg/kg per dose every 6 hr is adequate. (Do not exceed a total daily dose of 12 gm in an infant or 24 gm in an older child. (Corrigan: J. Pediatr., *80:*124, 1972.)

c.   Liquid or soft diet.

2. For spontaneous hematuria replacement therapy is *not* indicated. Prednisone 2 mg/kg daily for 3 days has proved effective.

IV. PATIENTS WITH FACTOR VIII
INHIBITORS

Patients with Factor VIII inhibitors who require emergency treatment are best treated with "activated" concentrates. These bypass the inhibitor to promote clotting. One such concentrate is Autoplex; consult the product insert for the correct dosage.

ADVANCED LIFE SUPPORT IN A NUTSHELL

Advanced life support for a patient with cardiac arrest consists of the following elements:

1. Basic life support (A–Airway, B–Breathing, C–Circulation).
2. Use of adjunctive equipment for ventilation and circulation.
3. Cardiac monitoring for dysrhythmia recognition and control.
4. Defibrillation.
5. Establishing and maintaining an intravenous infusion lifeline.
6. Employing definitive therapy, including drug administration
   —to correct acidosis and hypoxemia.
   —to aid in establishing and maintaining effective cardiac rhythm and circulation.
7. Stabilization of the patient's condition.
8. Transportation with continuous monitoring.

Don't forget that it is crucial to maintain uninterrupted basic life support until spontaneous circulation is restored.

Advanced life support can be approached in the following sequence:

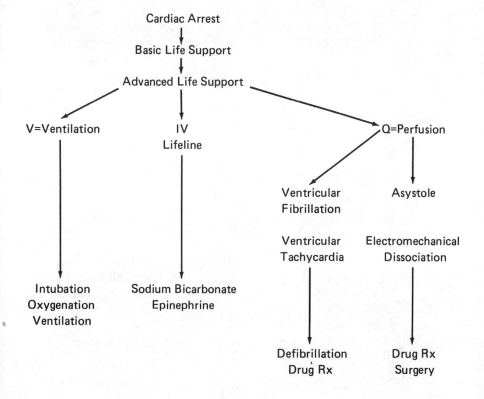

After initiation of basic life support, ventilation (consisting of intubation, oxygenation, and ventilation) and an IV infusion lifeline are established, and sodium bicarbonate and epinephrine are administered. Normal circulation is restored by means of countershock and/or drug therapy, depending on the rhythm disturbance seen with the "quick look" paddles. Keep in mind that by far the most common cause of arrhythmia or bradycardia in pediatric patients is hypoxia.

Objectives of Drug Treatment

1. To correct hypoxia.
2. To correct metabolic acidosis.
3. To increase perfusion pressure during cardiac compression.
4. To stimulate spontaneous or more forceful myocardial contraction.
5. To accelerate cardiac rate.
6. To suppress ventricular ectopic activity.
7. To relieve pain and to treat pulmonary edema.

ESSENTIAL DRUGS	USEFUL DRUGS
Oxygen	Isoproterenol
Sodium bicarbonate	Propranolol
Epinephrine	Procainamide
Atropine	Dopamine
Lidocaine	
Morphine	
Calcium chloride	

Summary of Drug Therapy in Advanced Life Support

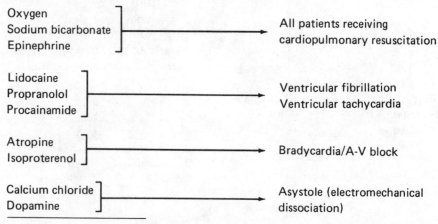

Oxygen
Sodium bicarbonate
Epinephrine
→ All patients receiving cardiopulmonary resuscitation

Lidocaine
Propranolol
Procainamide
→ Ventricular fibrillation
Ventricular tachycardia

Atropine
Isoproterenol
→ Bradycardia/A-V block

Calcium chloride
Dopamine
→ Asystole (electromechanical dissociation)

Reference: Gottlieb, A.J., Zamkoff, K.W., Jastremski, M.S., Scalzo, A., and Imboden, K.J.: The Whole Internist Catalog. Philadelphia, W.B. Saunders Company, 1980, pp. 51–54.

PREDICTION OF OUTCOME FOR PATIENTS IN COMA DUE TO HEAD INJURY

Head injury resulting from accidents constitutes a major source of morbidity and mortality in children. An early prediction of outcome is difficult and cannot be totally accurate. The Glasgow Coma Score provides a rapid and reasonably reliable method of categorizing patients. A high score is prognostic of a good outcome.

GLASGOW COMA SCORE

Eye Opening
- 4 — Spontaneously
- 3 — To voice
- 2 — To pain
- 1 — None

Verbal
- 5 — Oriented
- 4 — Confused
- 3 — Inappropriate
- 2 — Incomprehensible
- 1 — None

Motor
- 6 — Obey command
- 5 — Localize pain
- 4 — Withdraw from pain
- 3 — Abnormal flexion
- 2 — Abnormal extension
- 1 — None

If this scoring system is to be used, two important points must be kept in mind:

1. Major systemic complications, especially shock or hypoxia, must be corrected before a reliable assessment can be made.

2. Some patients, particularly children, make a good recovery in spite of a low score at the time of the original assessment. Vigorous resuscitative and supportive efforts are indicated in all patients.

Reference: Jennett, B., Teasdale, G., Galbraith, S., et al.: J. Neurol. Neurosurg. Psychiatry, *40:*291, 1977.

10
HEART, LUNGS, VESSELS

CONGENITAL HEART DISEASE— THE PRIMARY MANIFESTATION

Different forms of congenital heart disease present in different ways. The primary manifestation may be cyanosis, congestive heart failure, tachycardia or bradycardia, or a heart murmur. Which primary finding suggests which defect? This table should serve as a useful guide.

Marked Cyanosis

Transposition of the great arteries
Pulmonary atresia and stenosis with intact ventricular septum
Tetralogy of Fallot with severe pulmonary stenosis
Complex pulmonary atresias
Tricuspid atresia
Ebstein's malformation of the tricuspid valve

Congestive Heart Failure

Aortic atresia
Coarctation of the aorta
Double outlet right ventricle syndrome
Patent ductus arteriosus
Truncus arteriosus
Ventricular septal defect
Arteriovenous fistulas

Abnormal Heart Rate

Supraventricular tachycardia
Heart block

Heart Murmur

Patent ductus arteriosus
Pulmonary stenosis
Aortic stenosis
Pulmonary artery stenosis
Ventricular septal defect
Arteriovenous fistulas
Atrioventricular valve regurgitations

Reference: Rowe, R., and Mehrizi, A.: The Neonate with Congenital Heart Disease. Philadelphia, W.B. Saunders Company, 1968, p. 105.

*When I first gave my mind to vivisection, as a means of dis-
covering the motions and uses of the heart, and sought to
discover these from actual inspection, and not from the
writings of others, I found the task so truly arduous, so full
of difficulties, that I was almost tempted to think with Fra-
castorius that the motion of the heart was only to be com-
prehended by God.*

William Harvey (1578–1657)
On the Motion of the Heart and
Blood in Animals, Ch. 1

RECURRENCE RISKS FOR CONGENITAL HEART DISEASE

Congenital cardiac lesions are thought to recur in three patterns of
inheritance:
1. As part of a single gene defect syndrome (2 per cent).
2. Chromosomal abnormalities (4 per cent).
3. Multifactorial inheritance (94 per cent).

Some single gene syndromes that often include cardiac defects are
listed in the following table.

*Selected Single Mutant Gene Syndromes with Cardiovascular
Disease Other than Coronary Artery*

AUTOSOMAL DOMINANT	AUTOSOMAL RECESSIVE
Apert	Adrenogenital syndrome
Crouzon	Alkaptonuria
Ehlers-Danlos	Carpenter
Forney	Conradi
Holt-Oram	Cutis laxa
IHSS (not strictly a syndrome)	Ellis-van Creveld
Leopard	Friedreich's ataxia
Marfan	Glycogenosis IIa, IIIa, IV
Myotonic dystrophy	Jervell and Lange-Nielsen
Neurofibromatosis	Laurence-Moon-Biedl
Osteogenesis imperfecta	Mucolipidosis III
Romano-Ward	Mucopolysaccharidosis II, IV, V, VI
Treacher Collins	Osteogenesis imperfecta
Tuberous sclerosis	Refsum
Ullrich-Noonan	Seckel
	Smith-Lemli-Opitz
	Thrombocytopenia with absent radius (TAR)
	Weill-Marchesani

X-LINKED

Incontinentia pigmenti
Mucopolysaccharidosis II
Muscular dystrophy

The recurrence risk for congenital heart disease in families in which one member has one of these syndromes depends on the recurrence risk for the syndrome (generally 25 to 50 per cent) and the frequency with which congenital heart disease is encountered in the syndrome.

The recurrence risk for congenital heart disease due to a chromosomal abnormality depends on the risk of recurrence of the chromosomal defect. A familial tendency for nondisjunction and the presence of a translocation in the chromosomal pattern of one parent may increase the likelihood of recurrence. Some chromosomal defects are associated with particular cardiac abnormalities. The more common chromosomal aberrations and their associated cardiac defects are listed in the following table.

Congenital Heart Disease in Selected Chromosomal Aberrations

POPULATION STUDIED	PERCENTAGE INCIDENCE OF CHD	MOST COMMON LESIONS		
		1	2	3
General population	1	VSD	PDA	ASD
4p—	40	VSD	ASD	PDA
5p—(cri du chat)	25	VSD	PDA	ASD
C mosaic	50	VSD		
13 trisomy	90	VSD	PDA	Dex
13q—	50	VSD		
18 trisomy	90+	VSD	PDA	PS
18q—	50	VSD	AV	ASD
21 trisomy	50	VSD	AV canal	ASD
XO Turner	35	Coarc	AS	ASD
XXXXY	14	PDA	ASD	

VSD = Ventricular septal defect. PDA = Patent ductus arteriosus. ASD = Atrial septal defect. Dex = Dextrocardia. PS = Pulmonic stenosis. AV = Atrioventricular. Coarc = Coarctation of aorta. AS = Aortic stenosis.

The essential components of multifactorial inheritance of congenital heart defects include: (1) a genetic predisposition to cardiovascular maldevelopment, (2) a genetic predisposition to be adversely affected by environmental teratogens, and (3) an environmental insult occurring at a vulnerable period of cardiac development (i.e., very early in pregnancy). Since there is no method of quantitating the presence of these three risks for a given offspring, a few percentages may be kept in mind:

1. In general, the risk of recurrence of congenital heart disease in a given family is 1 to 5 per cent.

2. The more common the heart defect in the affected family member, the more likely that defect is to recur.

3. The risk to subsequent offspring of two parents triples if two existing family members are affected. (For example, the risk of recurrence of a ventriculoseptal defect is about 5 per cent if one previous sibling is affected; however, it increases to approximately 15 per cent if one sibling and one parent or two siblings are affected.)

4. If the majority of family members have some form of congenital cardiac defect, the risk to subsequent offspring approaches 100 per cent. More specifically, if three first-degree family members are affected, the risk in future pregnancies is 60 to 100 per cent.

Reference: Nora, J.J., and Wolf, R.F. Recurrence risks in the family. *In* Kidd, B.S.L., and Rowe, R.D. (eds.): The Child with Congenital Heart Disease after Surgery. Mount Kisco, New York, Futura Publishing Company, 1976, pp. 451–460.

PAROXYSMAL ATRIAL TACHYCARDIA

Paroxysmal atrial tachycardia (PAT) is rare in infancy and childhood, affecting not more than one in every 25,000 children. Studies have revealed patients fall into three groups: (1) patients with the Wolff-Parkinson-White syndrome (WPW); (2) patients whose attacks of PAT begin before 1 year of age; and (3) patients with onset of attacks later in childhood.

In patients with otherwise normal hearts, brief periods of PAT (6 to 24 hours) do not precipitate acute congestive heart failure. The patient who presents in heart failure, therefore, has suffered a prolonged attack of PAT or has an abnormal heart.

Characteristics of these three groups are delineated in the following table.

	PAT PATIENTS WITH ONSET IN INFANCY	PAT PATIENTS WITH ONSET IN CHILDHOOD	PAT PATIENTS WITH WPW (ONSET AT ANY AGE)
Sex predominance	Male	None	None
Likelihood of recurrence	Low	High	High
Presentation at initial attack	Diagnosis frequently made only after patient presents in cardiac failure. Fever may be the presenting feature.	Usually rapid heart rate or palpitations noted by patient or parent. May present with loss of consciousness, vomiting with abdominal pain, or fever.	Characteristics of onset depend upon age of patient and are the same as for patients with PAT without WPW.
Response to treatment	The majority of patients suffer single attacks without recurrences. When attacks recur, they may frequently be treated successfully with digitalis alone or with digitalis and quinidine in combination. Rarely, attacks continue into the second year of life.	Recurrent attacks in this group are short and benign; however, control with digitalis, quinidine, and propranolol is often difficult. Physical means of aborting attacks (eyeball pressure or Valsalva maneuver) may have some success in older children.	Control with digitalis, quinidine, and propranolol is often not completely effective.

Reference: Simcha, A., and Bonham-Carter, R.E.: Lancet, *1*:832, 1971.

10

THE PROLONGED Q-T INTERVAL

What do the deaf child and the child who faints have in common? They should both have an electrocardiogram.

The syndrome of prolonged Q–T interval has been described in patients with congenital deafness and in others with normal hearing. In the latter group the abnormality presents with fainting, atypical seizures, cardiac arrest, or ventricular fibrillation.

Although this disorder is inherited, its inheritance pattern is not known. Some family members of patients with congenital deafness demonstrate the cardiac abnormality but have normal hearing. The true incidence of the syndrome will not be appreciated until appropriate screening becomes more routine.

Episodes of syncope, cardiac arrest, or arrhythmia are typically provoked by stress, exercise, emotional stimulus, or fever. Cardiac catheterization does not demonstrate abnormalities, but it has been reported to incite ventricular fibrillation.

The electrocardiographic abnormality may be intermittent, and adults seem to have less frequent attacks of syncope. Propranolol, the β-adrenergic blocker, has been found to reduce the incidence of attacks, although it does not always correct the electrocardiographic abnormality. Digoxin may shorten the Q–T interval, but it does not prevent syncope. Adrenergic drugs tend to induce ventricular fibrillation. Quinidine, procainamide, and the phenothiazines further prolong the Q–T interval. Blockade of the left stellate ganglion and ganglionectomy have reportedly been successful in preventing both the attacks and the electrocardiographic abnormality.

Recommendations

1. An electrocardiogram should be performed in all children with syncope or atypical seizures.

2. If a child is shown to have prolongation of the Q–T interval, the child's entire family should be screened with an electrocardiogram and audiogram.

3. Electrocardiographic screening should be undertaken for all children with congenital deafness and their family members — whether the latter are deaf or not.

4. The families of children who die unexpectedly without apparent cause should have electrocardiographic screening.

5. When the prolonged Q–T interval is demonstrated, even in asymptomatic children, prophylactic treatment with propranolol should be instituted at least until adulthood. Remember: the first episode of syncope may end in death.

Reference: Frank, J.P., and Friedberg, D.Z.: Am. J. Dis. Child., *130*:320, 1976. Furberg, C., and Hörnell, H.: Acta Paediatr. Scand., *64*:777, 1975.

THE SICK SINUS SYNDROME

If the sinus node fails to depolarize, a patient experiences cardiac arrest or another pacemaker takes over — usually the atrioventricular node. Patients who suffer from chronic or intermittent dysfunction of the sinus node are said to have the sick sinus syndrome. The secondary pacemaker may produce bradycardia or tachycardia. The symptomatic patient may have syncope, dizzy spells, convulsions, or sudden death. Many of the patients described with this syndrome have undergone cardiac surgery or have congenital heart defects. In some patients the dysfunction has been secondary to myocarditis. In others there has been no demonstrable cardiac lesion. In the latter patients there has been no evidence of a similar condition in family members.

Drug therapy in the sick sinus syndrome is not helpful. Treatment — and the only insurance against sudden death — consists of the insertion of a cardiac pacemaker.

All patients with attacks of syncope, dizziness, or tachycardia should have measurement of their resting pulse rate and an electrocardiogram performed. Electrocardiographic recordings should be made for at least 1 minute and should be repeated at intervals. Recordings should also be made after exercise, especially if the pulse rate at rest is below 60 beats per minute. The sick sinus syndrome should be suspected if one of the following conditions exists:

1. Low voltage, broad P waves, which may be bifid.
2. P waves which alter their shape and direction during the recording.
3. Periods of sinus arrest often followed by nodal escape beats.
4. Failure to increase heart rate more than 30 per cent after exercise on a treadmill at 2 miles per hour for 2 minutes.
5. Onset of an abnormal rhythm which may be slow after exercise.
6. Failure to increase the heart rate by more than 30 per cent after administration of atropine, 0.01 mg per kg intravenously.

This is another one of those diagnoses that will only be found if we look for it expectantly.

References: Radford, D.J., and Izukawa, T.: Arch. Dis. Child., *50*:879, 1975. Scott, O., Macartney, F.J., and Deverall, P.B.: Arch. Dis. Child., *51*:100. 1976.

MITRAL VALVE PROLAPSE

Incidence   Occurs predominantly in females in the younger population. One survey indicates a 6.3 per cent incidence of mitral valve prolapse in 1169 healthy young women. An association with stroke has been made.

Pathophysiology	Posterior protrusion of valve leaflets beyond the mitral ring during ventricular systole; often associated with mitral insufficiency. Redundancy of the posterior or both valve leaflets is associated with dilatation of the annulus and lengthening of the chordae.
Etiology	The various hypotheses include: 1. Myxomatous degeneration of the valve. 2. Segmental cardiomyopathy of the left ventricle with secondary valvular changes.
Association	1. Congenital heart disease (especially secundum atrial defect). 2. Marfan's syndrome. 3. Collagen-vascular disorders. 4. Familial occurrence. 5. Thoracic deformities (pectus excavatum, straight back syndrome, scoliosis). 6. Wolff-Parkinson-White syndrome.
Presentation	1. Majority asymptomatic (see incidence). 2. Palpitations; fatigability; shortness of breath; atypical chest pain. 3. Symptoms seen in tall, slender females and in patients with developmental thoracic deformities.
Physical Exam	Highly variable, even in the same patient. Apical midsystolic click followed by a late systolic murmur. Maneuvers that decrease left ventricular chamber size, and consequently increase mitral leaflet malposition, increase the intensity of the murmur (and vice versa).

When patient is sitting or standing, murmur is prolonged and click moves closer to S_1.

When patient is squatting, murmur becomes shorter and click moves closer to S_2.

Holosystolic murmur of mitral insufficiency: "Honk" or "whoop" may be heard because of resonation of leaflets and chordae.

X-ray	Cardiac fluoroscopy normal except in the presence of insufficiency, congenital heart disease, or thoracic abnormalities.

ECG Abnormalities in about one third of patients unless overt mitral insufficiency is present:

1. T-wave inversion in II, III, AVF.
2. Supraventricular tachycardia.
3. Ventricular premature beats.

Abnormalities may be manifest only on exercise testing.

Echo/Phono Best test for documentation. A negative echostudy does *not* rule out mitral valve prolapse. Echocardiographic findings include:

1. Late systolic dip of the posterior or both valve leaflets occurring with the click.
2. Gradual "hammocking" of the mitral leaflets through systole.

Natural History Probably benign in most asymptomatic patients. There is as yet little evidence to suggest the progressive development of mitral insufficiency. Sudden death may take place, presumably secondary to ventricular arrhythmias. Bacterial endocarditis may occur. A typical chest pain that is non-ischemic in origin and refractory to therapy may be troublesome.

10

Management Reassurance for the asymptomatic patient without ECG abnormalities on rest and exercise. Prophylactic treatment of arrhythmias. Try propranolol for chest pain. Specific therapy of mitral insufficiency when present. Prophylactic antibiotics should be used along with dental or "dirty" surgical procedures.

Reference: Procacci, P.M., Savran, S.V., Schreiter, S.L., and Bryson, A.L.: N. Engl. J. Med., *249:*1086, 1976. Devereux, R.B., Perloff, J.K., Reichek, N., and Josephson, M.D.: Circulation, *54:*3, 1976.

EXTRACARDIAC MANIFESTATIONS OF BACTERIAL ENDOCARDITIS

The patient with bacterial endocarditis presents both a diagnostic and a therapeutic challenge. The myriad manifestations of the disease result from the hemodynamic, embolic, and immunologic sequelae of the endovascular infection.

The following review of the more common extracardiac manifestations may serve as an aid in diagnosis and management of this disease.

MANIFESTATION	COMMENT

I. Renal
1. Microscopic hematuria and proteinuria
2. Occasionally azotemia
3. Abnormalities usually resolve with effective antimicrobial therapy
	1. Biopsy
	  a. Focal glomerulonephritis *or*
	  b. Diffuse proliferative glomerulonephritis

II. Neurologic
1. Major neurologic complications are:
  a. Cerebral infarction in region of middle cerebral arteries secondary to emboli (most common neurologic complication)
  b. Meningeal signs and symptoms
  c. Seizures
  d. Intracranial hemorrhage
  e. Large macroscopic brain abscesses are uncommon
  f. Microscopic brain abscesses are common and reflect multiple microemboli
	1. Neurologic complications occur in 25–40% of patients with bacterial endocarditis
	2. The mortality of patients with neurologic complications is >50%
	3. Embolic phenomenon are usually seen in endocarditis due to *S. aureus, Pneumococcus, Enterobacteriaceae,* and anaerobic streptococci
	4. *Mitral* valve endocarditis produces major cerebral emboli more frequently than *aortic* valve endocarditis
	5. Mycotic aneurysms occur more frequently in the *early* course of *acute* endocarditis than *late* in the course of *subacute* endocarditis
	6. CSF exam tends to reflect the nature of the infecting organisms; i.e., virulent organisms are more likely to produce meningitis with a purulent CSF than are less virulent organisms, which are likely to produce a sterile "aseptic" CSF

III. Musculoskeletal

1. Arthralgia—usually in shoulder, knee, hip
2. True synovitis
   a. Ankle, knee, wrist most frequent
   b. Usually sterile
   c. Biopsy shows acute inflammatory changes
3. Low back pain
   a. Often severe
   b. Often demonstrates spinal tenderness and decreased range of motion
   c. X-rays usually normal
   d. Usually not secondary to disc space infection
4. Myalgias—often localized to thighs and calves
5. Miscellaneous
   a. Clubbing of the digits
   b. Hypertrophic osteo-arthropathy
   c. Avascular necrosis of hip

1. Musculoskeletal findings are seen in approximately 44% of patients with bacterial endocarditis

IV. Skin

1. Petechiae
2. Osler's nodes
3. Janeway lesions
4. Periungual erythema
5. Subungual "splinter" hemorrhages

V. Hematologic

1. Anemia
2. Thrombocytopenia (in the absence of disseminated intravascular coagulation)
3. Monocytosis
4. Splenomegaly
5. Plasmacytosis of bone marrow
6. Disseminated intravascular coagulation

10

Continued

MANIFESTATION	COMMENT
VI. Serologic	
1. Elevated ESR	1. Titers of circulating immune
2. Elevated serum gamma	complexes highest in patients with:
globulins	a. Right-sided endocarditis
3. Positive rheumatoid factor	b. Extravascular manifestations
4. Positive antinuclear	c. Signs of infection for more
antibody	than 4 weeks
5. Circulating immune	
complexes	
6. Presence in serum of	
cryoglobulins	
7. Low serum complement	

References: Pruitt, A.A., Rubin, R.H., Karchmer, A.W., and Duncan, G.W.: Medicine, *57:*329, 1978. Churchill, M.A., Geraci, J.E., and Hunder, G.G.: Ann. Intern. Med., *87:*754, 1977. Bajer, A.S., Theofilopoulos, A.N., Eisenberg, R., et al.: N. Engl. J. Med., *295:*1500, 1976.

EVALUATION OF HYPERTENSION

The conventional wisdom is that most hypertension detected in infants, children, and adolescents is secondary to a definable disease. Recently, it has been suggested that essential hypertension also manifests itself in late childhood and early adolescence and may be responsible for as much as 30 per cent of all observed elevations in blood pressure.

When confronted with a patient with hypertension, one must determine the following:

1. Is it transient or persistent?
2. Is it secondary to another process?

It is unfortunate that most pediatric patients do not have their blood pressure recorded. A survey revealed that in only 5 per cent of all pediatric out-patient visits was the blood pressure recorded, and in only 62 per cent of hospital admissions was the blood pressure measured. In patients less than 1 year of age, blood pressure was recorded in 0.4 per cent of out-patients and 56 per cent of in-patients.

A complete physical examination must include a blood pressure measurement. The blood pressure should be measured in all acutely ill patients, particularly those with complaints referable to the heart, kidneys, or central nervous system.

The Normal Blood Pressure

The normal systolic and diastolic blood pressures to be expected in children at various ages are shown in Figures 10-1 and 10-2.

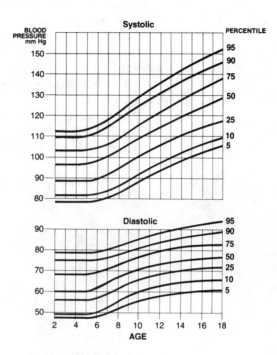

FIG. 10-1

Percentile for blood pressure measurement in boys (right arm, seated).

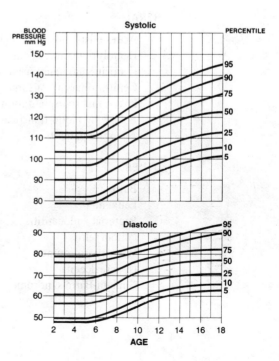

FIG. 10-2

Percentile for blood pressure measurement in girls (right arm, seated).

The following guidelines should be employed when obtaining a conventional office blood pressure.

1. The patient should be supine.
2. The cuff should be at least 20 per cent wider than the diameter of the arm and cover approximately two-thirds to three-quarters of the arm as measured from elbow to axilla.
3. The examiner should be at eye level with the manometer.
4. The meniscus of the manometer should be checked weekly for zero calibration.
5. While measuring, the rate of fall should be approximately 2 to 3 mm Hg per heart beat.
6. Readings should be made to the nearest 2 mm Hg.

Guidelines for the 95th percentile of acceptable blood pressure are:

AGE (years)	SYSTOLIC (mm Hg)	DIASTOLIC (mm Hg)
0–3	110	65
3–6	120	70
6–11	125	78
11–15	140	80

Conditions Associated with Acute Transient Hypertension or Intermittent Hypertension

RENAL

Acute poststreptococcal glomerulonephritis
Hemolytic-uremic syndrome
Henoch-Schönlein purpura with nephritis
Genitourinary tract surgery
Post–renal transplantation
Following blood transfusion in patients with azotemia
Anephric patients

OTHER

Burns
Leukemia
Bacterial endocarditis
Poliomyelitis
Mercury poisoning
Hypercalcemia
Guillain-Barré syndrome

Stevens-Johnson syndrome
Hypernatremia
Familial dysautonomia
Increased intracranial pressure
Corticosteroid therapy
Amphetamines

Potentially Curable Forms of Hypertension

RENAL

Unilateral hydronephrosis
Unilateral pyelonephritis
Unilateral dysplastic kidney
Traumatic damage
Tumors
Unilateral multicystic kidney
Unilateral ureteral occlusion
Ask-Upmark kidney (segmental dysplasia of small renal arteries)

VASCULAR

Coarctation of the aorta
Renal artery abnormalities
  Stenosis
  Arteritis
  Fibromuscular dysplasia
  Neurofibromatosis
  Fistula
  Aneurysm
Renal artery thrombosis

ADRENAL

Neuroblastoma
Pheochromocytoma
Adrenogenital syndrome
Cushing's disease
Primary aldosteronism
  Adenoma
  Hyperplasia

OTHER

Vascular or renal parenchymal abnormalities after irradiation
Ingestion of excessive amounts of licorice
Administration of glucocorticoids

Incurable, but Therapeutically Controllable, Forms of Chronic Hypertension

RENAL

Chronic glomerulonephritis
Chronic bilateral pyelonephritis
Congenital dysplastic kidneys (bilateral)
Polycystic kidneys
Medullary cystic disease
Post–renal transplantation

VASCULAR

Surgically irremediable main renal artery abnormalities
Surgically irremediable coarctation of the aorta
Generalized hypoplasia of the aorta

MISCELLANEOUS

Essential hypertension
Lead nephropathy (late)
Radiation nephritis

The Diagnostic Evaluation

ACUTE OR CHRONIC? FAMILIAL OR ISOLATED?

Careful physical examination (lupus? Cushing's syndrome? neurofibromatosis? adrenogenital syndrome? abdominal mass?)
Blood pressure in all four extremities
Blood pressure measurements in parents and siblings
Examination of the ocular fundus
Examination of the heart
Chest roentgenogram for cardiac size
Electrocardiogram

RENAL PARENCHYMAL?

Urinalysis
Blood urea nitrogen
Creatinine

If renal parenchymal disease is suspected, then a judgment must be made as to whether it is acute or chronic. Urine culture, measurements of serum complement components, and intravenous pyelogram are useful in reaching this decision. Renal biopsy may be required to establish a diagnosis.

NONRENAL PARENCHYMAL?

Vascular abnormality
 Renal flow study: renal scan and arteriography
Endocrine abnormality
 Aldosteronism (serum electrolytes–hypokalemia, plasma renins)
 Neuroblastoma (catecholamines)
 Cushing's syndrome (plasma cortisol)
 High renin essential hypertension (plasma renin)

The physician should proceed with the premise that almost all hypertension in children under 6 years of age has an identifiable cause, and that 60 to 80 per cent of hypertension in children 6 to 12 years of age is secondary to a diagnosable disease.

References: Loggie, J.M.H., and McEnery, P.T.: *In* Rubin, M.I. (Ed.): Pediatric Nephrology. Baltimore, Williams & Wilkins Company, 1976, p. 417. Pazdrai, P.T., Lieberman, H.M., Pazdrai, W.E., et al.: J.A.M.A., *235*:2320, 1976. Lieberman, E., and Holliday, M.A.: Pediatric Portfolio, Vol. II, Number 2, 1972.

ASTHMA IN CHILDHOOD—
CHARACTERISTICS AND PROGNOSIS

What is the natural history and the clinical and physiologic manifestations of asthma in children? A review of 315 children who were all evaluated at age 14 years provides many insights. The children were classified by history as follows:

CLASS	DEFINITION
A	No more than five episodes of wheezing up to 14 years of age.
B	More than five episodes of wheezing but none within 12 months of their 14th birthday.
C	Continuing history of episodic asthma with attacks within 12 months of the 14th birthday.
D	History of very frequent or chronic unremitting asthma having either periods of severe or prolonged asthma during the 13th year of life with remissions of less than one month or more than 10 attacks within three months of 14th birthday.

10

The following table describes the characteristics of these four groups of patients. From this table it can be seen that the characteristics of severe persistent asthma include onset usually in the first three years of life, a high frequency of attacks within the initial year, clinical and physiologic evidence of persisting airway obstruction and pulmonary hyperinflation, chest deformity, and impairment of growth. In contrast, mild asthma usually begins later in childhood, is episodic, and is not associated with evidence of airway obstruction between attacks. Most of the patients with mild asthma will have no further difficulty after age 10 years.

Asthma — Prognosis and Characteristics

CLASS	FREQUENCY (%)	USUAL AGE OF ONSET	AGE AT REMISSION	SEX PREVALENCE	PHYSICAL CHARACTERISTICS AT AGE 14	ASSOCIATED ALLERGIES (ANYTIME BEFORE AGE 14)		
						Hay Fever (%)	Eczema (%)	Urticaria (%)
A	20	After 3	8	None	Normal	44	14	55
B	28	2 to 3	5 to 14	60% males 40% females	Normal	55	22	54
C	34	2 to 3	After 10	68% males 32% females	7% Pigeon chest 15% Barrel chest Decreased weight 10% pulmonary hyperinflation by x-ray	72	56	57
D	18	Before 2 (28% before 6 months)	After 10	79% males 21% females	25% Pigeon chest 48% Barrel chest Decreased weight and height 27% pulmonary hyperinflation by x-ray	80	67	57
					Controls	18	11	30

Reference: McNicol, K.N., and Williams, H.B.: Br. Med. J., 4:7, 1973.

CLASS	POSITIVE SKIN TESTS AT AGE 14 YEARS (%)	BLOOD EOSINOPHIL COUNT (PER mm³)	PROPORTION OF EOSINOPHILS IN NASAL SMEAR (% eosinophils – % patients)		MEAN SERUM IgE AT AGE 14 (ng/ml)
A	43	293 ± 271 ($2\% > 1000/mm^3$)	$> 5 - 9$	$>20 - 3$	607 ± 448
B	45	300 ± 290 ($8\% > 1000/mm^3$)	$> 5 - 11$	$>20 - 1$	607 ± 448
C	80	554 ± 369 ($18\% > 1000/mm^3$)	$> 5 - 23$	$>20 - 3$	1005 ± 508
D	81	657 ± 297 ($27\% > 1000/mm^3$)	$> 5 - 24$	$>20 - 7$	2163 ± 1800
	Control: 10	Control: 213 ± 250 ($0\% > 1000/mm^3$)	Control: $> 5 - 7$	$>20 - 1$	Control: 79 ± 156

10

THE TWENTY-NINE FACES OF CYSTIC FIBROSIS

Most pediatricians now appreciate the fact that juvenile rheumatoid arthritis may present in a variety of ways; this fact has been captured by the phrase, "the three faces of juvenile rheumatoid arthritis." Cystic fibrosis is a far more prodigious imitator. Are you aware of "the 29 faces of cystic fibrosis"?

Listed below are the 29 ways in which cystic fibrosis may initially manifest itself. Be suspicious and perform a sweat test when these problems are encountered without a suitable alternative explanation.

Meconium ileus and meconium peritonitis
Pancreatic insufficiency and growth failure
Recurrent pulmonary infections
Intestinal impaction and obstruction (may produce intussusception)
Rectal prolapse
Prolonged neonatal hyperbilirubinemia
Cirrhosis of the liver
Portal hypertension
Glucose intolerance
Diabetes
Acute and recurrent pancreatitis
Vitamin K deficiency with bleeding
Vitamin A deficiency
Vitamin E deficiency, muscle weakness, and creatinuria
Night cramps
Hypoproteinemia in infancy with edema and anemia (seen usually in
   infants fed soybean formulas or human milk)
Lactase deficiency
Duodenal ulcer
Cholelithiasis and cholecystitis
Chronic obstructive airway disease
Cor pulmonale
Recurrent episodes of asthma
Hypertrophic pulmonary osteoarthropathy
Nasal polyps
Optic neuritis
Salty taste of infant noted by mother
Hyponatremic dehydration in warm weather
Heat stroke
Infertility in males

THE FALSE-POSITIVE SWEAT TEST

The most common cause of a false-positive sweat test is laboratory error. Careful collection and analysis must be employed to achieve reliable results. The following points should be kept in mind:

1. At least 100 mg of sweat must be collected, and sweat volumes should be reported along with electrolyte concentrations.
2. The most reliable method of sweat collection is the pilocarpine iontophoresis method of Gibson and Cooke.
3. Electroconductivity methods of electrolyte composition are unreliable. Sodium and chloride determinations should be made by quantitative methods.
4. Normal adolescents and adults may have somewhat higher sweat chloride values than children. The upper limit of normal for a child is usually 60 mEq/L, but an adult with a sweat chloride of 60 to 80 mEq/L may be normal, and the test should be repeated when such results are obtained.

When the test has been carefully performed, other causes of elevated sweat chloride must be considered before making a diagnosis. These other causes include:

Adrenal insufficiency, untreated
Ectodermal dysplasia
Hereditary nephrogenic diabetes insipidus
Glucose-6-phosphatase deficiency
Pupillatonia, hyporeflexia, and segmental hypohydrosis with autonomic dysfunction
Hypothyroidism
Mucopolysaccharidoses
Malnutrition
Fucosidosis

False-negative sweat chloride results may be caused by edema.

A diagnosis of cystic fibrosis should not be made on the basis of a positive sweat test alone. At least one of the following three criteria must also be present:

1. Documented family history of cystic fibrosis
2. Chronic pulmonary disease
3. Pancreatic insufficiency

Reference: Wood, R. E., Boat, T. F., and Doershuk, C. F.: Am. J. Respir. Dis., *113:*833, 1976.

CLINICAL ASSESSMENT OF PATIENTS WITH CROUP

Objective evaluation of the child with croup is often difficult. The scoring system below provides a method of determining the severity of respiratory distress without the need for arterial blood gas determinations.

CLINICAL CROUP SCORE

	0	1	2
Inspiratory breath sounds	Normal	Harsh with rhonchi	Delayed
Stridor	None	Inspiratory	Inspiratory and expiratory
Cough	None	Hoarse cry	Bark
Retractions and flaring	None	Flaring and suprasternal retractions	As under 1, plus subcostal and intercostal retractions
Cyanosis	None	In air	In 40% O_2

A score of 4 or more indicates moderately severe airway obstruction.

A score of 7 or more, particularly when associated with $Pa_{CO_2} \geqslant 45$ torr and $Pa_{O_2} \leqslant 70$ torr (in room air) indicates impending respiratory failure. Consideration should be given to placing an artificial tracheal airway.

Reference: Downes, J.J., and Raphaely, R.C.: Anesthesiology, *43:*238, 1975.

> *Adam's apple* — The prominence of the thyroid cartilage in the front of the neck was attributed to a piece of the forbidden fruit that became stuck in Adam's throat.

STUMPED BY STRIDOR?

Stridor is always pathological. Think in anatomic terms and you will usually find the cause.

Stridor at the Epiglottis

Congenital anomalies
  Aryepiglottic cyst
  Dermoid cyst
  Thyroglossal duct cyst
  Lingual thyroid
  Flabby epiglottis

Inflammatory disease
  Epiglottitis: bacterial origin
              allergic origin

Stridor at the Larynx and Subglottic Region

Congenital anomalies
  Hemangioma or lymphangioma
  Unilateral or bilateral vocal cord paralysis
  Laryngeal and/or subglottic stenosis
  Laryngomalacia
  Laryngeal cyst
  Papilloma

Trauma
  Birth injury
  Postlaryngoscopy
  Postlaryngeal catheterization

Inflammatory disease
  Laryngitis
  Laryngeal abscess
  Subglottic edema (of allergic origin)

Foreign body
  Radiopaque or radiolucent

Metabolic disorders
  Laryngismus stridulus (rickets)

Stridor from the Trachea

Congenital anomalies
    Hemangioma or lymphangioma
    Tracheomalacia
    Cartilage ring abnormalities ("segmental malacia")

Foreign body
    Radiopaque or radiolucent

Postoperative
    After tracheal intubation
    Stricture after tracheostomy
    Narrowing at the level of tracheoesophageal fistula

Stridor from Causes Originating Outside the Respiratory Tract

Congenital anomalies
    Vascular ring or anomalous innominate artery
    Esophageal atresia
    Tracheoesophageal fistula
    Aberrant or ectopic thyroid tissue
    Congenital goiter
    Carcinoma of thyroid

Inflammatory origin
    Retropharyngeal abscess
    Retroesophageal abscess

Foreign body
    Within the esophagus

Postoperative
    After tracheoesophageal fistula closure
    After mid-mediastinal surgery

Reference: Grünebaum, M.: Clin. Radiol., *24*:485, 1973.

ASTHMA OR BRONCHIOLITIS

Given a first attack of wheezing associated with hyperinflated lungs in an infant, one is hard pressed to determine if this represents the initial attack of asthma or, instead, represents an attack of bronchiolitis as a result of a lower respiratory tract infection of viral etiology.

The table below provides some clues for distinguishing the two conditions.

Clinical Features

	BRONCHIOLITIS	ASTHMA
Occurrence	Within the first 2 years, usually within the first 6 months	Any age
Frequency of attacks	Usually 1, occasionally 2 or 3	Three or more episodes
Season	Winter, spring	Anytime
Etiology	Associated with RSV epidemics and other respiratory viral infections	Allergy, infections, exercise, aspirin, pollutants
Signs	1. Fine rales predominate 2. Expiration = inspiration 3. Shallow, rapid respirations	1. Wheezing predominant 2. Expiration prolonged 3. Tachypnea and hyperpnea
X-ray	Hyperinflation ± scattered infiltrates	Hyperinflation ± atelectasis
Response to sympathomimetics	Generally none	Generally some reversal of bronchospasm
Prognosis	Excellent	Variable, may become chronic

Perhaps of even greater value in determining if the patient has asthma or will subsequently develop asthma are the following:

Prognostic Indicators of Future Asthma in Bronchiolitis

1. Family history of allergy
2. Nasal eosinophilia
3. Signs of atopic diathesis (eczema)
4. Sympathomimetic reversal of symptoms
5. Elevated total serum IgE

Reference: Dunsky, E.: Pediatr. Ann., 6:447, 1978.

PLEURAL EFFUSIONS: EXUDATES OR TRANSUDATES?

Pleural effusions are classically divided into "transudates" or "exudates." A transudate occurs when the mechanical factors influencing the formation or reabsorption of pleural fluid are altered. Decreased plasma oncotic pressure, and elevated systemic or pulmonary hydrostatic pressure are alterations that commonly produce transudates. In contrast, an exudate results from inflammation or other diseases of the pleural surface. Common conditions producing an exudate include: pneumonia, tuberculosis, pancreatitis, pulmonary infarction, and systemic lupus erythematosus.

Reliance on a single test to distinguish an exudate from a transudate will frequently be misleading. In the past, the measurement of pleural fluid protein, or specific gravity, or cell count has been employed as a diagnostic aid. Any single test will give unacceptably high "false positive" or "false negative" results.

The use of the following three tests will enable you to correctly classify virtually all pleural effusions:

1. $\dfrac{\text{Pleural fluid protein}}{\text{Serum protein}}$ $\geqslant 0.5$ (suggests exudate)

2. Pleural fluid LDH $\geqslant 200$ IU (suggests exudate)

3. $\dfrac{\text{Pleural fluid LDH}}{\text{Serum LDH}}$ $\geqslant 0.6$ (suggests exudate)

The presence of two of these criteria strongly suggests a diagnosis of exudate — the presence of all three virtually assures it.

Some other helpful facts include:

About 80 per cent of transudates will have a white cell count of less than $1000/\text{mm}^3$, while 80 per cent of exudates will have white cell counts above $1000/\text{mm}^3$.

Pancreatitis often produces a left-sided pleural effusion.

If congestive heart failure is associated with a unilateral effusion, it is usually right-sided.

Reference: Light, R. W., MacGregor, M. I., Luchsinger, P. C., and Ball, W. C., Jr.: Ann. Int. Med., 77:507, 1972.

11
GASTRO-INTESTINAL

DIARRHEA—CLUES TO THE DIAGNOSIS

Certain features of the patient's history in conjunction with physical findings and the appearance of the stool will allow you to make the correct etiologic diagnosis in approximately 75 per cent of all patients you see with diarrhea. The important clinical features of acute diarrheal disease that are useful in differential diagnosis are described on the next page.

Reference: Nelson, J., and Haltalin, K.: J. Pediatr., *78*:519, 1971.

Diaper—From the old French. *Diaspre* means ornamental cloth. The word originally came from the Greek *dia*, meaning through, and the Byzantine *aspros*, meaning white. The word aspros appears in the Greek aspropatos, which means "bottoms up" and suggests the transparent bottom of the bottle as the last of the wine is drunk. Bottoms up is, of course, applicable to the baby as the diaper is being applied.

11

Clinical Features of Acute Diarrheal Disease Useful in Differential Diagnosis

CLINICAL FEATURES	SHIGELLA	ENTEROPATHOGENIC E. COLI	SALMONELLA (EXCLUDING TYPHOID FEVER)	NONBACTERIAL
Age	6 months to 5 years (rare in neonate)	Less than 2 years	Any age	Any age
Diarrhea in household	Common (>50%)	No	Variable	Variable
Onset	Abrupt	Gradual	Variable	Abrupt
Vomiting as a prominent symptom	Absent	Uncommon	Common	Common
Fever (over 102° F)	Common	Absent	Variable	Uncommon
Respiratory symptoms	Common (bronchitis)	Absent	Uncommon (except in septicemia form)	Common (upper respiratory)
Convulsion	Common	Rare	Rare	Rare
Anal sphincter	Lax tone (rarely, rectal prolapse)	Normal	Normal	Normal
Stools: Consistency	Watery	Loose, slimy	Loose, slimy	Loose
Odor	Relatively odorless	Foul	Foul (rotten egg)	Unpleasant
Blood	Common	Rare	Rare	Rare
Color	Yellow-green (almost colorless in severe cases)	Green	Green	Variable
Mucus	Present	Variable	Variable	Absent
Time after onset when seen by physician	Early	Several days	Several days	Early
Early course, untreated	Slight or no improvement	Persistent or relapsing	Persistent	Daily improvement

THE PATIENT WITH CHRONIC DIARRHEA

The infant or child with chronic diarrhea always poses a diagnostic and therapeutic challenge. In such patients in whom a number of diagnostic possibilities exist, an orderly and relatively simple and inexpensive approach to investigation should be pursued. One such approach, employing three stages of diagnostic procedures, is outlined below.

STAGE 1

DIAGNOSTIC TEST	DIAGNOSTIC INFORMATION
Examination of the stool	A mucoid stool with blood suggests infection.
	A mucoid stool without blood suggests an irritable colon.
	White flecks and beanlike curds are seen in protein allergies.
	Soufflelike stools, with the smell of vinegar, suggest disaccharide intolerance.
	Oil droplets in the stool suggest steatorrhea.
Test for reducing substances	Positive test suggests disaccharide intolerance.
pH	Stool pH below 6.0 suggests disaccharide intolerance.
Stool trypsin	If no digestion of gelatin in dilution of 1:100, it suggests pancreatic insufficiency.
Stool supernatant tested for precipitins to milk, soy, and gluten	Protein intolerance.
Stool for ova and parasites	Parasitic infection.
Smear of stool for leukocytes	If leukocytes present, it suggests presence of bacterial infection or ulcerative colitis.
Stool culture	
Sweat test	Cystic fibrosis.
Complete blood count	Neutropenia suggests pancreatic insufficiency.
	Macrocytic anemia suggests small bowel disease with folic acid deficiency.
	Hypochromic anemia suggests iron deficiency with gastrointestinal bleeding as a result of protein allergy or ulcerative colitis.
Serum carotene	If low, suggests presence of fat malabsorption.
Serum folate	If low, suggests presence of small bowel disease.

If No Diagnosis Is Established or Tests Suggest Presence of Malabsorption, then Proceed to Stage 2 Tests

STAGE 2

DIAGNOSTIC TEST	DIAGNOSTIC INFORMATION
72-hour stool collection for quantitative fat determination	Steatorrhea documents the presence of malabsorption. Common causes include cystic fibrosis, celiac syndrome, and inflammatory disease of the small bowel.
Disaccharide tolerance test. Perform in patients with acid stools or patients with reducing substance in stool	Administer 2 gm/kg of disaccharide — start with lactose. Should produce a rise in blood glucose of at least 20 mg/dl in 20 to 60 minutes. Lack of appropriate response indicates disaccharidase deficiency.
Xylose tolerance test. Administer 0.5 gm/kg after a 4-hour fast. Collect all urine for 5 hours	Infants 0 to 6 months of age should excrete 8 to 16 per cent of dose; infants and children over 6 months of age should excrete 20 to 25 per cent of dose. Impaired absorption indicates impaired small bowel function. Falsely low values seen with gastric retention, impaired renal function, or inadequate hydration.
Radiologic examination of small and large bowel. Begin with barium enema	Look for malrotation, Hirschsprung's disease, colitis, chronic granulomatous disease, small bowel pattern of malabsorption.
Sigmoidoscopy. Consider in patients with diarrhea accompanied by occult or gross gastrointestinal bleeding	Ulcerative colitis. Chronic granulomatous disease.

If No Diagnosis Has Been Established or Definitive Proof Is Required, then Proceed to Stage 3 Tests

These include:

Small bowel biopsy
Duodenal intubation for collection of pancreatic enzymes and
    bile acids, and for culture of small bowel flora
Urine collection for catecholamines, amino acids, and keto acids

Reference: Gryboski, J.: Gastrointestinal Problems in the Infant. Philadelphia, W.B. Saunders Company, 1975, p. 676.

COMMON CAUSES OF CHRONIC DIARRHEA

Chronic diarrhea, like every other illness, must begin sometime. The age of onset should provide a valuable clue to the cause of diarrhea, as outlined below.

DURING THE FIRST 4 MONTHS OF LIFE (IN DECREASING ORDER):

1. Cow and soy protein-induced mucosal injury
2. Malabsorption following infectious insult
3. Cystic fibrosis
4. Short bowel syndrome
   a. Resection-NEC atresia
   b. Congenital short bowel
5. Congenital monosaccharide transport defects
6. Congenital disaccharidase deficiency

FROM 4 MONTHS TO 3 YEARS OF AGE:

1. Chronic nonspecific diarrhea
   a. Postinfectious
   b. Postantibiotic
   c. Irritable bowel
   d. Psychosocial
2. Milk and/or protein sensitivity
3. Cystic fibrosis
4. Giardiasis
5. Celiac sprue
6. Sucrase-isomaltase deficiency

FROM 3 YEARS OF AGE UNTIL THE END OF CHILDHOOD:

1. Giardiasis
2. Celiac disease
3. Inflammatory bowel disease
4. Developmental disaccharidase-base deficiency
5. Irritable bowel syndrome

Reference: Ament, M.E., and Barclay, G.: Continuing Education, *14:*26, 1981.

IRRITABLE COLON SYNDROME OF CHILDHOOD

The infant or young child with persistent or recurrent diarrhea who has adequate weight gain may have the irritable colon syndrome. The irritable colon syndrome is characterized by the following facts:

Onset is usually between 6 and 20 months of age, but diarrhea may begin at an earlier age.

Bowel movements occur usually in the early hours of the day. There are usually no more than three or four bowel movements per day.

The first stool of the day may be large and sometimes totally or partially formed, but subsequent stools are smaller, looser, and contain more vegetable fibers and mucus. A small amount of blood may be present.

Malabsorption is not an etiologic factor. Starch granules may be present in the stool, but these are a result of premature evacuation of the colon.

The condition is not influenced by diet.

The diarrhea is not caused by infection, but exacerbations do seem to be associated with respiratory infections and teething.

Affected children often have a history of constipation prior to the onset of diarrhea, and many suffered from infantile colic. Following clearance of diarrhea, many affected children develop constipation.

There is frequently a family history of functional bowel complaints.

Clearance of diarrhea is gradual and occurs in 90 per cent of cases by 36 to 39 months of age.

Etiology is unknown, but hypotheses include a psychosomatic origin and hereditary predisposition.

Treatment consists of maintaining a normal diet with elimination of chilled liquids (these seem to promote colonic motility). Diodoquin may be helpful for some patients but should be used for very limited periods of time because it may produce optic atrophy.

Infection may be ruled out by examination of the stool for leukocytes. Malabsorption must be considered in the child who fails to gain weight.

Reference: Davidson, M., and Wasserman, R.: J. Pediatr., *69*:1027, 1966.

THE DIAGNOSIS OF REGIONAL ENTERITIS (CROHN'S DISEASE)

The diagnosis of regional enteritis is often unnecessarily delayed. The physician is frequently misled by the nongastrointestinal manifestations of the disease. In over one-third of patients, an initial diagnosis of an infection or collagen vascular disease is incorrectly made. In another one-third of patients, the initial diagnosis is appendicitis or other gastrointestinal disease. The average delay in correct diagnosis may be one full year.

The table below illustrates the more common clinical manifestations of regional enteritis in children and young adolescents.

CLINICAL MANIFESTATIONS	PER CENT OF PATIENTS
Abdominal pain	86
Fever	83
Weight loss	80
Diarrhea	72
Growth retardation	30
Joint symptoms (polyarthritis and arthralgia)	25
Anorectal disease	24
Gastrointestinal bleeding	14
Nonspecific rash or erythema nodosum	10
NONSPECIFIC LABORATORY ABNORMALITIES	
Increased erythrocyte sedimentation rate	84
White cell count over 10,000/mm^3	70
Decreased serum albumin	64
Hypochromic, microcytic anemia	50
Stools positive for occult blood	36

Regional enteritis should be considered in the differential diagnosis of all children with prolonged fever and arthralgia even in the absence of gastrointestinal symptoms. On some occasions, the nongastrointestinal manifestations of the disease may precede the radiographic evidence of disease in the bowel by as much as 2 years.

Reference: Burbige, E.J., Huang, S.S., and Bayless, T.M.: Pediatrics, 55:866, 1975.

IS IT ULCERATIVE COLITIS OR REGIONAL ENTERITIS?

Are you a lumper or a splitter? If you are a lumper you will classify all inflammatory bowel disease simply as "inflammatory bowel disease." As a splitter you would agree that, more often than not, there are enough distinguishing characteristics to permit the differentiation of ulcerative colitis from regional enteritis (Crohn's disease). See the table below for a comparison of the features of ulcerative colitis and Crohn's disease.

Clinical, Pathologic, and Radiographic Features

FEATURES	ULCERATIVE COLITIS	CROHN'S DISEASE
Diarrhea	Severe	Moderate or absent
Rectal bleeding	Common	Rare
Abdominal pain	Frequent	Common
Weight loss	Moderate	Severe
Growth retardation	Mild	Severe
Extraintestinal manifestations	Common	Common
Percentage with bowel involvement		
Anus	15	85
Rectum	95	50
Colon	100	50
Ileum	0 (except for backwash ileitis)	80
Distribution of lesions	Continuous	Skip areas
Pathologic features	Diffuse mucosal disease	Granulomas, focal disease
Radiographic features	Loss of haustra	Thumbprinting
	Superficial ulcers	Skip areas
	No skip areas	String sign
Cancer risk	High	Less than with ulcerative colitis but still increased

Reference: Graef, J.W., and Cone, T.E.: *In* Manual of Pediatric Therapeutics. Boston, Little, Brown & Company, 1980, p. 267.

CELIAC DISEASE, CYSTIC FIBROSIS, OR GASTROINTESTINAL ALLERGY

	CELIAC DISEASE	CYSTIC FIBROSIS	GASTROINTESTINAL ALLERGY
Family history	Occasionally +	Often +	Often +
Onset	Usually 8 months to 2 years	<6 months	1 to 6 months
Respiratory symptoms	—	95% by 1 year	Asthma, bronchitis 4 years or so
Appetite	Poor	Excessive	Normal
Stools	Bulky, foul, liquid	Greasy, bulky	Soft to watery, mucoid
Blood in stools	—	—	+
Growth	Normal to 8 to 10 months	Retarded	Variable
Sweating	—	+	—
Vitamin deficiencies	Unusual	Sometimes	Sometimes
Calcium deficiency	+	Rare	Sometimes

> *Celiac*—From the Greek word *koilia*, which means belly. The name celiac disease is derived from the enlarged belly these children normally demonstrate.

11

	CELIAC DISEASE	CYSTIC FIBROSIS	GASTROINTESTINAL ALLERGY
Glucose tolerance	Flat	Normal to ↑	Normal
Vitamin A	Low normal	Below normal 80%	Variable
Proteins	May be low	Often low	Often low
Carotene	Very low	Very low	Usually normal
Finger clubbing	+	+	—

Reference: Gryboski, J.: Gastrointestinal Problems in the Infant. Philadelphia, W.B. Saunders Company, 1975, p. 653.

MALABSORPTION SYNDROMES — DIAGNOSIS BY AGE

One of the simplest clues to the etiology of a malabsorption state is the age of onset. This, together with a careful history and stool examination should put one well on the way to a specific diagnosis. The likely age of onset of the malabsorption syndromes are listed below: syndromes are listed below:

Malabsorption Syndromes which may Present at Different Ages

NEONATAL PERIOD	1 MONTH TO 2 YEARS	2 YEARS TO PUBERTY
Congenital lactase deficiency	Sucrase-isomaltase deficiency	Secondary disaccharidase deficiency
Secondary disaccharidase deficiency	Secondary disaccharidase deficiency	Celiac sprue
Congenital glucose-galactose malabsorption	Secondary monosaccharide malabsorption	Tropical sprue
Secondary monosaccharide malabsorption	Enterokinase deficiency	Parasites
Congenital chloridorrhea	Cow's milk protein sensitivity	Stasis syndrome
Enterokinase deficiency	Soy protein sensitivity	Primary immune defects
Cow's milk protein intolerance	Primary immune defects — Wiskott-Aldrich syndrome; Thymic aplasia with agammaglobulinemia	
Soy protein intolerance	Cystic fibrosis	
Primary immune defects — Wiskott-Aldrich syndrome	Neonatal hepatitis — biliary atresia — choledochal cyst	
Cystic fibrosis	Parasites	
Short bowel syndrome	Pancreatic insufficiency with bone marrow failure	
Neonatal hepatitis — biliary atresia	Celiac sprue	
Primary hypomagnesemia	Abetalipoproteinemia	
	Intestinal lymphangiectasia	
	Whipple's disease	
	Wolman's disease	
	Amino acid malabsorption	
	Vitamin B_{12} malabsorption syndromes	
	Congenital malabsorption of folic acid	
	Stasis syndrome	

Reference: Ament, M. E.: J. Pediatr., *81:*685, 1972.

THE FLOATING STOOL

The myth of the floating stool has been exploded in recent literature. Here is poetic testimony to the fact that it's the air in stool that causes it to float, not the fat.

> While safe's the stool that comes a sinker
> The floater's apt to be a stinker
>
> So it's not the fat but, rather, flatus
> Imparts the elevated status.

References: Levitt, M.D., and Duane, W.C.: N. Engl. J. Med., *286:*973, 1972. Teller, J.D.: N. Engl. J. Med., *287:*52, 1972.

The jejunum is more exempt from morbid conditions than any other portion of the alimentary canal.

Sir William Withey Gull *(1816–1890)*
St. Bartholomew's Hospital Reports,
52:45, 1916.

11

SHWACHMAN'S SYNDROME — PANCREATIC INSUFFICIENCY/ NEUTROPENIA

Shwachman's syndrome is a rare disorder that is now known to be a multiorgan disease. The first case descriptions emphasized the pancreatic insufficiency and neutropenia, but the last 20 years have afforded proof of the diverse presentation that may occur in association with Shwachman's syndrome. The table lists the variety of features of this disorder. It has been speculated that the basic defect in Shwachman's syndrome may lie in the function of the microtubular and microfilament elements of many different cell types in the body. Too little is known about the mechanisms of such dysfunctions to enable one to be specific, but such defects could easily explain the abnormal appearance of chondrocytes, impaired granulocytic function, bone marrow dysfunction, and pancreatic and liver disease.

Features Associated with Shwachman's Syndrome

Exocrine pancreatic insufficiency
  Steatorrhea
Growth retardation
Skeletal abnormalities
  Metaphyseal dyschondroplasia, delayed maturation, rib abnormalities, long bone
  tubulation, clinodactyly
Narrow thorax
Hematologic abnormalities
  Bone marrow hypoplasia, neutropenia, thrombocytopenia, raised HbF,
  lymphoproliferative and myeloproliferative neoplasia
Recurrent infections
Defective neutrophil mobility
Neonatal problems
  Poor feeding, respiratory distress
Psychomotor retardation
Hypotonia
Hepatomegaly
  Raised SGOT and SGPT
Renal tubular dysfunction
Ichthyosis
Dental abnormalities
Delayed puberty
Diabetes mellitus
Dysmorphic features
Endocardial fibrosis
Hirschsprung's disease

Reference: Shwachman, H., Diamond, L.K., Oski, F.A., and Khow, K.T.: J. Pediatr., *65:*645, 1964. Aggett, P.J., Cavanagh, N.P.C., Matthew, D.J., Pincott, J.R., Sutcliffe, J., and Harries, J.T.: Arch. Dis. Child., *55:*331, 1980.

GASTROINTESTINAL HEMORRHAGE

Gastrointestinal hemorrhage in infants and children has many causes. Some forms of bleeding can present an immediate threat to life. Management includes prompt diagnosis. It is important to be aware of the more common causes of gastrointestinal bleeding and the fact that the relative frequency of different lesions changes with the age of the patient.

Lesions Producing Gastrointestinal Hemorrhage

	RELATIVE FREQUENCY (%)	
	Under 1 Year of Age	Over 1 Year of Age
Anal fissure	43.0	12.5
Duodenal ulcers	6.0	6.0
Duplication of colon	0.7	0.0
Esophageal varices	0.0	10.5
Gastric ulcers	5.6	8.0
Gangrenous bowel	9.0	0.0
Hemorrhoids	0.0	0.8
Intussusception	31.9	9.0
Meckel's diverticulum	3.8	1.2
Polyps	0.0	50.0
Ulcerative colitis	0.0	2.0

11

Reference: Spencer, R.: Surgery, 55:718, 1964.

THE BLACK STOOL

When you test a black stool for occult blood and it proves to be negative, do not be frustrated — get more history. Other causes of a black stool include:

Ingestion of iron preparations
Ingestion of bismuth (Pepto-Bismol)
Ingestion of lead
Eating licorice
Eating charcoal, coal, or dirt

If the patient is taking large quantities of ascorbic acid, you may get a false-negative test for occult blood even with significant bleeding. The vitamin C interferes with the color change normally produced by the peroxidase activity of the heme.

Reference: Jaffe, R.M.: Ann. Intern. Med., *83*:824, 1975.

"A baby is God's opinion that the world should go on."

Carl Sandburg

THE USE OF ALGORITHMS FOR THE DIAGNOSIS OF JAUNDICE IN CHILDHOOD

Jaundice in the neonatal period has multiple causes that are unique to that period of life (see pages 113 to 118). The algorithms on the following pages are designed to provide a diagnostic guide to the evaluation of jaundice when it presents in late infancy and childhood.

Some points that should prove useful in employing these algorithms include the following:

1. Begin the differential diagnosis of jaundice with an examination of the urine. A positive urine test for bilirubin indicates the retention of conjugated bilirubin in the serum. The urine tests are positive in approximately 70 per cent of patients with conjugated bilirubin levels in the range of 1 to 2 mg/100 ml and in virtually all patients with serum conjugated bilirubin levels in excess of 2 mg/100 ml. The Ictotest (Ames Laboratories) is negative in patients with unconjugated hyperbilirubinemia.

2. Confirm the urinary findings with a measurement of the serum fractions of both conjugated and unconjugated bilirubin. The upper limit of normal for total bilirubin is 1.0 mg/100 ml with a conjugated (direct reacting fraction) of less than 0.2 mg/100 ml.

3. In pure unconjugated hyperbilirubinemia, at least 85 per cent of the total bilirubin should be of the unconjugated form. In conjugated hyperbilirubinemia, there is at least 30 per cent, and usually close to 50 per cent, of the total bilirubin in the direct or conjugated form.

4. Obstructive jaundice and acute hepatocellular disease tend to give values greater than 50 per cent direct reacting bilirubin, while in chronic liver disease the conjugated fraction is usually in the 30 to 50 per cent range.

5. Patients with 15 to 30 per cent conjugated bilirubin generally have hepatocellular or cholestatic jaundice complicated by hemolysis.

6. Unconjugated hyperbilirubinemia can be arbitrarily separated into patients with indirect bilirubin levels of above and below 6.0 mg/100 ml. This is not a precise distinction. Some patients with Gilbert's syndrome may have unconjugated bilirubin levels as high as 8.0 mg/100 ml, while patients with Arias Type II syndrome may have values as low as 3.0 mg/100 ml.

7. Gilbert's syndrome has multiple causes. The unconjugated hyperbilirubinemia is always in excess of that which would be expected for the red cell life span.

8. In both Gilbert's syndrome and Arias Type II conjugation defect, there is impaired conjugation of bilirubin with glucuronic acid. The Type I defect (Crigler-Najjar syndrome) presents no diagnostic difficulty because in this syndrome the unconjugated hyperbilirubinemia first develops in the neonatal period and the conjugation defect is complete.

9. Cholestatic jaundice can usually be distinguished from hepatocellular jaundice by the measurement of alkaline phosphatase. Approximately 90 per cent of patients with cholestasis will have alkaline phosphatase values that are more than three times normal, while 90 per cent of patients with hepatocellular jaundice will have elevations of alkaline phosphatase that do not exceed three times normal. Patients with drug-induced cholestasis tend to have values one to three times normal.

10. Although the diagnosis of Dubin-Johnson syndrome can be confirmed by liver biopsy that demonstrates the characteristic finding of brown to black centrilobular granular pigment, this is seldom necessary. Sulfobromophthalein (BSP) kinetic studies will identify the minuscule transfer maximum for BSP into bile. In addition, analysis of the isomers of coproporphyrin in the urine will show the characteristic increases in the total quantity of the isomer 1 and in the ratio of isomer 1 to isomer 3.

Reference: Ostrow, J.D.: J.A.M.A., *234*:522, 1975.

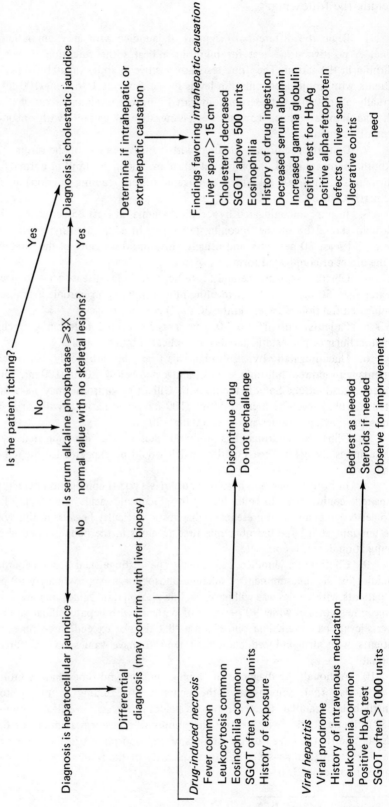

Diagnosis of Unconjugated Hyperbilirubinemia

Is the patient itching?

No → Is serum alkaline phosphatase ≥3X normal value with no skeletal lesions?

Yes → Diagnosis is cholestatic jaundice

No → Diagnosis is hepatocellular jaundice

Yes → Diagnosis is cholestatic jaundice

Diagnosis is hepatocellular jaundice → Differential diagnosis (may confirm with liver biopsy)

Drug-induced necrosis
Fever common
Leukocytosis common
Eosinophilia common
SGOT often >1000 units
History of exposure

→ Discontinue drug
Do not rechallenge

Viral hepatitis
Viral prodrome
History of intravenous medication
Leukopenia common
Positive HbAg test
SGOT often >1000 units

→ Bedrest as needed
Steroids if needed
Observe for improvement

Diagnosis is cholestatic jaundice → Determine if intrahepatic or extrahepatic causation

Findings favoring *intrahepatic causation*
Liver span >15 cm
Cholesterol decreased
SGOT above 500 units
Eosinophilia
History of drug ingestion
Decreased serum albumin
Increased gamma globulin
Positive test for HbAg
Positive alpha-fetoprotein
Defects on liver scan
Ulcerative colitis

need

Liver biopsy or mini-laparotomy

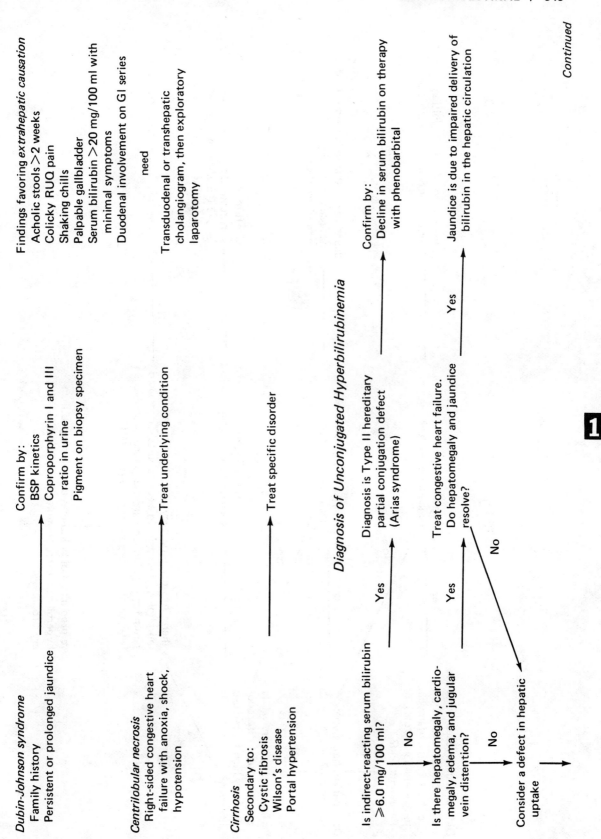

Dubin-Johnson syndrome
Family history
Persistent or prolonged jaundice

Confirm by:
BSP kinetics
Coproporphyrin I and III
ratio in urine
Pigment on biopsy specimen

Centrilobular necrosis
Right-sided congestive heart
failure with anoxia, shock,
hypotension

→ Treat underlying condition

Cirrhosis
Secondary to:
Cystic fibrosis
Wilson's disease
Portal hypertension

→ Treat specific disorder

Findings favoring *extrahepatic causation*
Acholic stools >2 weeks
Colicky RUQ pain
Shaking chills
Palpable gallbladder
Serum bilirubin >20 mg/100 ml with
minimal symptoms
Duodenal involvement on GI series

need

Transduodenal or transhepatic
cholangiogram, then exploratory
laparotomy

Diagnosis of Unconjugated Hyperbilirubinemia

Is indirect-reacting serum bilirubin
≥6.0 mg/100 ml?

Yes → Diagnosis is Type II hereditary
partial conjugation defect
(Arias syndrome)

No

Is there hepatomegaly, cardio-
megaly, edema, and jugular
vein distention?

Yes → Treat congestive heart failure.
Do hepatomegaly and jaundice
resolve?

No

Consider a defect in hepatic
uptake →

Yes → Jaundice is due to impaired delivery of
bilirubin in the hepatic circulation

No

Confirm by:
Decline in serum bilirubin on therapy
with phenobarbital

Continued

11

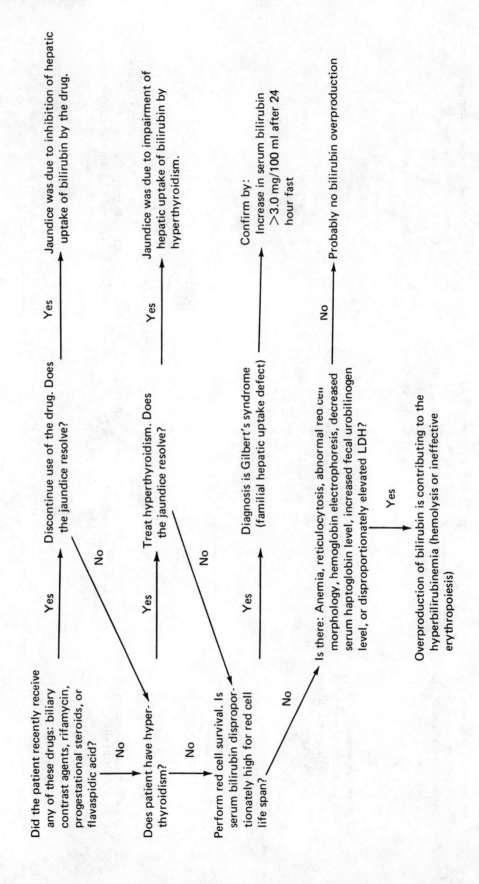

Did the patient recently receive any of these drugs: biliary contrast agents, rifamycin, progestational steroids, or flavaspidic acid?

Yes → Discontinue use of the drug. Does the jaundice resolve?

Yes → Jaundice was due to inhibition of hepatic uptake of bilirubin by the drug.

No

Does patient have hyper-thyroidism?

Yes → Treat hyperthyroidism. Does the jaundice resolve?

Yes → Jaundice was due to impairment of hepatic uptake of bilirubin by hyperthyroidism.

No

Perform red cell survival. Is serum bilirubin disproportionately high for red cell life span?

Yes → Diagnosis is Gilbert's syndrome (familial hepatic uptake defect)

No

Is there: Anemia, reticulocytosis, abnormal red cell morphology, hemoglobin electrophoresis, decreased serum haptoglobin level, increased fecal urobilinogen level, or disproportionately elevated LDH?

Yes → Overproduction of bilirubin is contributing to the hyperbilirubinemia (hemolysis or ineffective erythropoiesis)

Confirm by:
Increase in serum bilirubin >3.0 mg/100 ml after 24 hour fast

No → Probably no bilirubin overproduction

> *Abdomen* — Known to children as "tummy" and to unsophisticated adults as "belly," this term probably derives from two Latin words: *abdere,* to hide, and *omen,* augury. The abdomen is thus visualized as a container hiding the viscera from which ancient augurs used to foretell future events.

INADEQUATE HEPATIC METABOLISM OF BILIRUBIN

The uptake, conjugation, and excretion of bilirubin by the liver require a variety of enzymes. The absence of any of these enzymes may produce jaundice. The table below lists the clinical features of syndromes caused by deficiencies in hepatic metabolism. Of the five syndromes described in the table, only Gilbert's syndrome is seen frequently.

11

Syndromes of Deficient Hepatic Metabolism

	GILBERT'S SYNDROME	DUBIN-JOHNSON SYNDROME	ROTOR'S SYNDROME	CRIGLER-NAJJAR TYPE I	CRIGLER-NAJJAR TYPE II
SGOT, Alk phos, PT/PTT, alb	Normal	Normal	Normal	Normal	Normal
BSP	Normal	Abnormal retention; mostly unconjugated (10–20% retention)	Abnormal retention; mostly conjugated	Normal <7%	Normal <7%
Oral cholecystogram	Normal	Not visualized or very faint visualization	Normal	Normal	Normal
Liver biopsy	Normal	Black or deep blue or green grossly, pigment in liver by histology	Normal	Normal; bile stasis in hepatic canaliculi	Normal
Bilirubin	Unconjugated; about 3 mg/100 ml may fluctuate	Usually below 6 mg/100 ml (0–19); 60% direct	Conjugated (mostly) or 50% & 50%	13–48 mg/100 ml unconjugated	6–22 mg/100 ml unconjugated
Complaint	Anorexia, malaise, abdominal pain	Vague abdominal pain	----	Kernicterus in neonatal age	May remain asymptomatic age 2 - 40 years
Prognosis	Good	Good	Good	Poor	Generally good
Inheritance	Autosomal dominant	Autosomal dominant	Autosomal dominant	Autosomal recessive	? Autosomal dominant
Test	1. Bilirubin clearance 2. Starvation → Indirect bilirubin elevation	Physical exercise, alcohol, surgery, infection, pregnancy, → bilirubin elevation	Infection, emotion, fatigue	Deficiency of Glucuronyl transferase	Glucuronyl transferase deficiency
Rx	Phenobarbital	----	----	----	Phenobarbital

ACUTE PANCREATITIS IN CHILDREN

Pancreatitis is an acknowledged but infrequently recognized cause of abdominal pain in children. The diagnosis is sometimes difficult. The following clinical description may help.

Etiology

Drugs/toxins

    Thiazides   Salicylazosulfapyridine
    Steroids   Chlorthalidone
    Azathioprine   Furosemide
    Alcohol   *L*-asparaginase
    Tetracycline   Oral contraceptives

Trauma/surgery

Biliary tract disease
    Choledochal cyst
    Stricture of the common bile duct
    Congenital stenosis of the ampulla of Vater
    Anomalous insertion of the common bile duct
    Cholelithiasis/cholecystitis

Infection
    Mumps (even in the absence of parotitis)
    Hepatitis B virus
    Coxsackie B5
    Epstein-Barr virus
    Mycoplasma
    Influenza B

Diabetes mellitus (ketoacidosis)

Perforated duodenal ulcer

Miscellaneous
    Hyperparathyroidism   Acute porphyria
    Septic shock   Kwashiorkor
    Cystic fibrosis   Hyperlipoproteinemia I and V
    Pregnancy   Scorpion bites

Idiopathic

11

Signs and Symptoms

1. *Abdominal pain.* Children may not localize the pain very well. It is usually noted to be in the upper quadrants or the periumbilical area. The pain is usually constant, but it may be intermittent, and it may be made worse by eating. The knee-chest position will usually relieve the pain.

2. *Vomiting.* Vomiting is aggravated by eating or drinking. It does not relieve the pain.

3. *Abdominal tenderness.* Tenderness may be accompanied by guarding and rebound. Maximal tenderness is usually in the midepigastric region. Bowel sounds may be normal, hypoactive, or absent.

4. *Fever.*

5. *Upper gastrointestinal hemorrhage.* The hemorrhage is thought to result from stress and may originate in the stomach, duodenum, or be caused by penetration of an ulcer into the head of the pancreas.

Laboratory Evaluation

1. *Elevated bilirubin.* This may be due to a stone in the common duct or to edema in the head of the pancreas.

2. *X-ray changes.* X-rays may document pleural effusion (most commonly on the left side) and/or ascites. There may also be a dilated segment of small bowel adjacent to the inflamed pancreas (sentinel loop). Isolated gaseous distention of the ascending colon and hepatic flexure may be present (colon cutoff sign).

3. *Hyperglycemia.* Diabetes mellitus may or may not follow pancreatitis.

4. *Hypocalcemia.*

5. *Elevated serum amylase.* The serum amylase usually begins to rise within hours of the onset of symptoms. It usually peaks within the first 24 hours of illness and returns to normal within 48 to 72 hours. Daily amylase determinations are helpful in following patients. If the amylase remains elevated for over two weeks, a pseudocyst should be suspected. Amylase values may be normal in patients with acute hemorrhagic pancreatitis.

6. *Elevated serum lipase.* These values tend to follow those of the serum amylase.

7. *Elevated urinary diastase.* Timed urine collections are necessary for this determination.

8. *Amylase clearance test.* Amylase clearance may be elevated in patients with severe burns or diabetic ketoacidosis, as well as in those with pancreatitis. It is calculated from the following formula:

$$\frac{Cam \text{ (clearance of amylase)}}{Ccr \text{ (clearance of creatinine)}} = \frac{Amylase \text{ (urine)}}{Amylase \text{ (serum)}} \times \frac{Creatinine \text{ (serum)}}{Creatinine \text{ (urine)}} \times 100$$

Treatment

1. *Relief of pain.* This is best accomplished with meperidine given every three hours. Its effect may be potentiated by promethazine.

2. *Reduction of exocrine pancreatic secretion.* The patient should fast, and intravenous fluids should be supplied. If intravenous fluids are required for more than five days, parenteral alimentation should be initiated. A nasogastric tube should be placed if the patient is nauseated or vomiting, or has an ileus.

When oral feedings are initiated, they should consist of carbohydrates alone initially, because they cause the least stimulation to the pancreas.

Feedings should be restarted when abdominal tenderness has disappeared, any ileus has resolved, and urinary diastase or amylase clearance has become normal.

3. *Treatment of shock and electrolyte abnormalities.*

Although anticholinergic drugs and antibiotics have been used in the treatment of pancreatitis, their use has not improved the prognosis. Mortality may range from about 20 per cent with acute interstitial pancreatitis to about 80 per cent with hemorrhagic pancreatitis.

Reference: Jordan, S.C., and Ament, M.E.: J. Pediatr., *91*:211, 1977.

Omentum — Probably derived from the Latin *omen,* this term for the covering of the abdominal contents reflects the ancient practice of foretelling the future by inspecting animal viscera.

11

12
GENITOURINARY

DEVELOPMENT OF RENAL FUNCTION

In the evaluation of the newborn or young infant for possible renal disease, one must be aware of the normal kidney function during this early period of life in order to appropriately interpret the laboratory values. The following table should prove useful.

Functional Development of the Kidney

	PREMATURE INFANT	FULL-TERM NEONATE	ADULT	AGE OF MATURATION (IN MONTHS)
Glomerular filtration rate (ml/min/1.73 m^2)	30–50	40–60	120	12–24
Renal plasma flow (ml/min/1.73 m^2)		120–150	630	3–6
Filtration fraction (per cent)		30–40	20	6–36
Tm PAH (mg/min/1.73 m^2)		12–30	75	12–24
Tm glucose (mg/min/1.73 m^2)		35–100	300	12–24
Urea clearance (ml/min/1.73 m^2)	15–30	20–50	75	12–24
Extreme dilution of urine (mOsm/liter)	50	50	50	
Maximal concentration of urine (mOsm/liter)	400–600	400–600	1400	3
Maximal U/P osmolar ratio	2.5		4	3
Ammoniogenesis	Lowered	Normal		
Lowering of urinary pH	Normal	Normal		
Hydrogen ion excretion	Lowered	Normal or lowered		

Tm, Maximal tubular reabsorption; PAH, para-aminohippurate; U/P, urine/plasma.

Reference: Royer, P., Habib, R., Mathieu, H., and Broyer, M.: *In* Pediatric Nephrology. Philadelphia, W.B. Saunders Company, 1974, p. 118.

12

THE CHILD WITH EXCESSIVE URINATION

The concern of parents about urinary frequency or excessive urine volume in their child should be approached in a systematic manner. After a thorough history and physical examination, the next step should be a comparison of the number of the child's voids per 24 hours with the normal values.

AGE	NORMAL NUMBER OF VOIDS PER 24 HOURS
3–6 months	20
6–12 months	16
1–2 years	12
2–3 years	10
3–4 years	9
12 years–adulthood	4–6

This step alone may be sufficient to allay parental and physician concern.

If, however, the number of voids is above normal or if the initial concern was excessive urine volume, then a urinalysis and 24-hour urine volume will further clarify the situation, as illustrated in the accompanying algorithm.

References: Hollerman, C.E., Jose, P., and Calcagno, P.L.: *In* Neonatology, Pathophysiology and Management of the Newborn. Philadelphia, J.B. Lippincott Company, 1975, p. 487. Illingworth, R.S.: *In* Common Symptoms of Disease in Childhood. 5th Ed. Oxford, Blackwell Scientific Publications, 1975, p. 299.

An Approach to Polyuria and/or Frequency

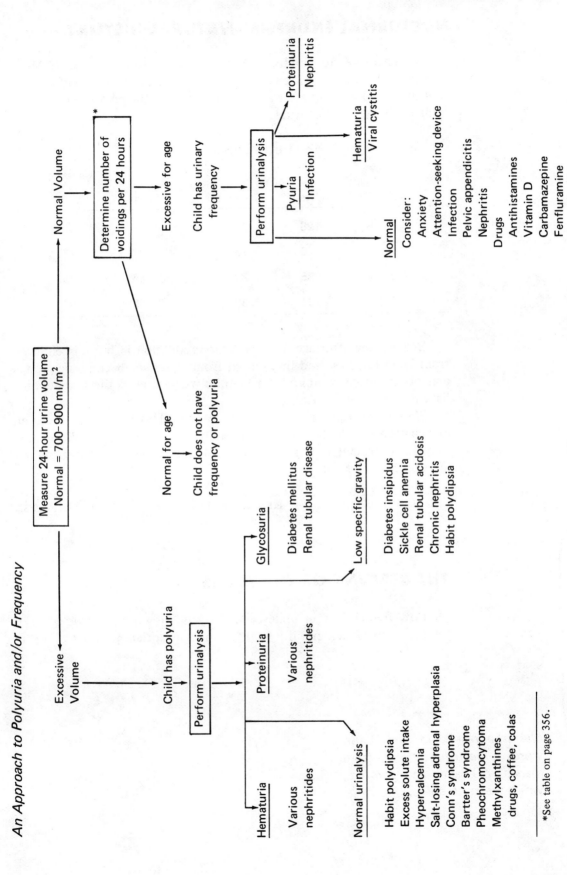

Measure 24-hour urine volume
Normal = 700–900 ml/m²

Normal Volume

Determine number of
voidings per 24 hours *

Excessive for age

Child has urinary
frequency

Perform urinalysis

Proteinuria
Nephritis

Hematuria
Viral cystitis

Pyuria
Infection

Normal
Consider:
Anxiety
Attention-seeking device
Infection
Pelvic appendicitis
Nephritis
Drugs
Antihistamines
Vitamin D
Carbamazepine
Fenfluramine

Normal for age

Child does not have
frequency or polyuria

Excessive
Volume

Child has polyuria

Perform urinalysis

Glycosuria

Diabetes mellitus
Renal tubular disease

Low specific gravity

Diabetes insipidus
Sickle cell anemia
Renal tubular acidosis
Chronic nephritis
Habit polydipsia

Proteinuria

Various
nephritides

Hematuria

Various
nephritides

Normal urinalysis

Habit polydipsia
Excess solute intake
Hypercalcemia
Salt-losing adrenal hyperplasia
Conn's syndrome
Bartter's syndrome
Pheochromocytoma
Methylxanthines
drugs, coffee, colas

*See table on page 356.

12

NOCTURNAL ENURESIS—NATURAL HISTORY

At what age do children normally stop wetting their bed? Most parents, as well as physicians, have unrealistic expectations and assume that most bed-wetting after age 4 years suggests the presence of under-lying renal disease. Not true!

Age by which bed-wetting stopped:

AGE	BOYS		GIRLS	
	White (%)	Black (%)	White (%)	Black (%)
<2	28	37	37	35
2–3	70	73	80	77
4–5	85	83	89	90
6–7	91	89	92	92

Bed-wetting after age 4 years is more common in boys, in children from large families, and in children from lower socioeconomic groups and occurs more commonly in families where one of the parents may have been a bed-wetter.

When bed-wetting recurs after a period of dryness, then an explanation should be sought. The polyuria of diabetes mellitus may frequently present in this way. Also rule out urinary tract disease and diabetes insipidus.

Reference: Dodge, W.F., West, E.F., Bridgforth, E.B., et al.: Am. J. Dis. Child., *120*:32, 1970.

THE DESCENT OF THE TESTIS

How frequent is an undescended testis? How long should it take for the testis to descend if it is not in the appropriate position at birth?

Masturbation—From the Latin word *manustupratio*; from *manus*, or hand, and *stuprare*, which means to defile.

Here are some guidelines.

1. A testis 4 cm below the pubic crest in a term infant may be considered descended. In the infant weighing less than 2500 grams, a distance of 2.5 cm below the pubic crest may be used as a criterion for descent.

2. In approximately 97 per cent of term infants, the testes are in the correct position. In males who weigh less than 2500 grams at birth, the incidence of descended testes is 79 per cent.

3. In the term infant, the testis, if it is to descend, will have done so by 6 weeks of age. In the premature infant, this descent should be completed at the same gestational age – approximately 46 weeks.

4. The ultimate incidence of undescended testis in term infants is approximately 0.8 per cent or about 1 per 1000.

5. The testis that has not completely descended by 6 weeks of age in the term infant will always remain higher than its mate and will always remain smaller. There is no justification for deferring surgery beyond 4 years of age in the expectation that descent will eventually occur.

6. Ten per cent of patients with cryptorchidism have upper urinary tract abnormalities, such as duplication, hydroureter, hydronephrosis, horseshoe kidney, and hypoplastic kidney. The anomalies are more common when associated with unilateral cryptorchidism.

References: Grossman, H., and Ririe, D.G.: Am. J. Roentgenol., *103*:210, 1968. Scorer, C.G.: Arch. Dis. Child., *39*:605, 1974.

RENAL SCANNING

There are a number of situations in which radionuclide imaging of the urinary tract can provide useful information which is either not available from excretory urography (IVP) or which supplements the information provided by IVP. Radiation exposure during a renal scan is significantly less than during IVP. A variety of radionuclides are available for use. Their selection is determined by the renal function to be evaluated, i.e., glomerular filtration rate, tubular secretion, or tubular reabsorption.

12

Indications for renal scanning include:

INDICATION	COMMENT ON SCAN
Contrast media sensitivity	No adverse reactions to radionuclides used in renal scanning reported
Uremia	May be used even in severe uremia (BUN ≥100)
Trauma	Provides additional and supplementary information to IVP
In preparation for radiotherapy port placement or for renal biopsy	Significantly less radiation than fluoroscopy
Congenital anomalies	Complements IVP
Pyelonephritis	IVP often normal in acute situation; cortical scan may be useful in diagnosis and follow-up; especially useful in chronic pyelonephritis
Transplant evaluation	Baseline study crucial for follow-up; very sensitive in detecting early rejection
Quantitative or differential renal function studies	May replace ureteral catheterization, which is a difficult procedure
Obstructive disease	Superior to IVP in situations of poor renal concentrating ability. Can illustrate intact cortical tissue in patients with major hydronephrosis
Azotemia in the newborn	Because of decreased concentrating ability, the IVP may not be helpful in the neonate
Bladder abnormalities (including reflux and residual volume)	Equal to or superior to IVP; 100 to 1000 times less gonadal radiation exposure

Reference: Handmaker, H., and Lowenstein, J.M.: Curr. Probl. Pediatr., 6:29, 1975.

RENAL STONES

Kidney stones are responsible for both urinary tract infections and progressive renal failure in infants and children. Kidney stones are far more common than is generally appreciated and have been found in 1 per cent of autopsies in infants and children.

Approximately 30 per cent of all recognized cases occur in children before the age of 2 years, and over one-half occur before the age of 4. Stones may be found in neonates.

In young infants the stones tend to be bilateral, while they are unilateral in about 90 per cent of older children. Boys are affected in 80 to 85 per cent of cases under 2 years of age; 60 to 65 per cent of patients 4 to 10 years of age are male; and 55 per cent of adult patients with stones are male.

Stones may produce pyuria, hematuria, abdominal distention, vomiting, disturbances of micturition, urinary retention, and even anuria.

In approximately 50 per cent of patients, a cause for the stone can be determined. About 25 per cent of stones are associated with malformations of the urinary tract, and 25 per cent are a result of a metabolic disorder.

The evaluation of patients with renal stones should include the following:

1. Plain film of the abdomen.
2. Intravenous urography.
3. Measurement of both urine and plasma concentration of: calcium, magnesium, oxalic acid, and uric acid.
4. Chemical analysis of the stone.
5. Urinary amino acid chromatogram (if other chemical analyses have been nondiagnostic).

Some characteristics of the various disorders associated with stone formation are described in the accompanying table.

Diagnostic Features of Renal Stone Diseases in Infants and Children

ETIOLOGY	X-RAY FILM APPEARANCE	DIAGNOSTIC FEATURES
Urinary tract malformations	Radiopaque	Obstruction at ureteropelvic junction most common abnormality. Frequently associated with infections. Stones usually composed of calcium phosphate and magnesium ammonium phosphate.
Metabolic Disorders		
Calcium stones	Radiopaque	Responsible for approximately one-half of stones of metabolic origin. Hypercalciuria present. Usually single stones. May be associated with nephrocalcinosis.
Cystine stones	Radiopaque	Account for 1 to 5 per cent of stones. Most common stone formed in renal tubular disorders (cystinuria and hypercystinuria). Calculi are generally large, multiple, and molded to the outline of the calyces and pelvis. Stones are soft, yellow, and waxy. Urinary cystine concentration increased.
Uric acid stones	Slightly radiopaque	Less common in children than adults. Most commonly associated with hyperuricemia due to a variety of causes. Hereditary form exists without either hyperuricemia or hyperuricosuria.

Continued

ETIOLOGY	X-RAY FILM APPEARANCE	DIAGNOSTIC FEATURES
Oxalic stones	Radiopaque	Stones are large and regular in outline, and bristle with tiny spikes. Often produce hematuria. May be associated with primary hyperoxaluria or oxalosis. Oxaluria seen in glycinuria and hypercalciurias. Oxaluria may be caused by large consumption of vitamin C.
Xanthine stones	Radiolucent	Rare disorder. Stones are yellowish-brown and friable. Urine xanthine concentration increased. May be associated with xanthine oxidase deficiency. In this disorder, blood and urine uric acids are low.
Syndrome of lithiasis, psychomotor retardation, and hip malfunction	Radiopaque	Stones of calcium phosphate. Stones numerous and bilateral. Retardation of both growth and psychomotor development. Hip disorder simulates osteochondritis. No biochemical or histologic renal disease. Prognosis excellent for mental, renal, and hip function. Etiology unknown.
Unknown origin	Radiopaque	Stones of calcium phosphate or magnesium ammonium phosphate. Prognosis good if no serious renal damage. Usually do not recur.

Reference: Royer, P., Habib, R., Mathieu, H., and Broyer, M.: Pediatric Nephrology. Philadelphia, W.B. Saunders Company, 1974, p. 193.

DANGERS OF THE DIPSTICK

The urine dipstick is an extremely quick and convenient method of screening for pH, protein, glucose, hemoglobin, ketones, bilirubin, and urobilinogen. The dipstick is a screening test, however, and its limitations must be kept in mind. The situations in which false positive and false negative results may be obtained are listed below:

pH. This determination is not altered except when the pH of the urine is actually altered by drugs.

Protein. A highly alkaline urine may cause a false positive dipstick for protein. The skin disinfectant benzalkonium chloride contains quarternary ammonium salts and may cause a false positive test for this reason.

The alternate test used for detecting protein other than albumin involves denaturing the protein with heat or sulfosalicylic acid to produce turbidity. A false positive result in this alternate test may be produced by:

Buniodyl
Chlorpromazine
Promazine
Carinamide
Cephaloridine
Cephalothin
Radiographic agents such as iopanoic acid, iodopyracet, and iophenoxic acid
Sulfamethoxazole
Thymol
Tolbutamide

Glucose. The dipstick technique for glucose may be falsely positive in the presence of bleach in the collecting vessel and vaginal powders containing glucose.

Ascorbic acid may produce a false negative result by retarding color development.

The Clinitest method may be used to quantitate the urinary glucose; however, other reducing agents may produce a false positive result. These include:

Sugars galactose, lactose, levulose, maltose, or pentose
Homogentisic acid
Glucuronic acid
Bleach

Drugs that produce a false positive Clinitest result include:

Acetanalide
p-aminosalicylic acid
Antipyrine
Cephaloridine
Cephalithin
Chloramphenicol
Chlortetracycline
Cinchophen
Diatrizoate
Isoniazid
Levodopa
Nalidixic acid
Oxytetracycline
Tetracycline

Hemoglobin. A false positive test may be produced by myoglobin or the presence of oxidizing agents such as ascorbic acid.

Ketones. Aspirin may cause ketonemia in children, but the presence of aspirin in a ketonuric urine may produce a false negative dipstick.

False positive tests for ketones may be seen in the presence of:

Levodopa
Paraldehyde in the presence of ethanol
Phenformin

Bilirubin. False positives may be seen in the presence of:

Porphobilinigen
Skatole
Indole
Large quantities of bilirubin
p-aminosalicylic acid
Antipyrene
Apronalide
Bromsulfophthalein
Chlorpromazine
Phenazopyridine
Phenothiazines
Sulfadiazine
Sulfamethoxazole
Sulfanilamide
Sulfonamides

Reference: McNeely, M. D. D.: Drug Therapy, August, 1974, p. 79.

MYOGLOBINURIA, HEMOGLOBINURIA, OR PORPHYRIA?

The passage of large quantities of pigment in the urine often produces diagnostic confusion. Many substances may color the urine, but few mimic the appearance of hemoglobin. Hemoglobinuria must be distinguished from myoglobin or porphyrin compounds. Both myoglobin and hemoglobin will give positive results on the commonly employed dipstick (Labstix) for heme. The following table should provide a guide in the initial differential diagnosis of the three major causes of pigmenturia.

Physical and Biochemical Features of the Pigmenturias

PHYSICAL EXAMINATION	MYOGLOBINURIA	HEMOGLOBINURIA	PORPHYRIA
Muscles			
Weakness	+	−	±
Pain	±	−	±
Edema	+	−	−
Neuropathy (peripheral and autonomic)	−	−	+
CNS dysfunction	−	−	±
Skin lesion	−	−	±
Abdominal pain	Rare	−	+
LABORATORY TESTS			
Urine			
Color	Brown	Red-brown	Burgundy
Benzidine	+	+	−
Hematest-orthotoluidine	+	+	−
80% $(NH_4)_2SO_4$ PPT	−	+	?
80% $(NH_4)_2SO_4$ SUPER	+	−	?
Porphobilinogen	−	−	+
Spectrophotometry (α band)	582 (oxymyo)	577 (oxyhemo)	594 to 624*
Taurine	Increased	Normal	?
Immunodiffusion	Specific	Specific	−
Serum			
Appearance	Clear	Pink	Clear
Haptoglobin	Normal	Low	Normal
Creatine phosphokinases	Marked increase	Normal	Normal
Carnitine	Increased	Normal	Normal
Immunodiffusion	Specific	Specific	−
Triglycerides	↑In specific defects	−	−

*Varies with type.

The clinical circumstances may provide the most help in defining the cause of pigment in the urine. The following conditions are associated with myoglobinuria.

Causes of Myoglobinemia and Myoglobinuria

Trauma and ischemic disease
  "Crush" syndrome
  Arterial ischemia of extremities, myocardial infarction
  Pressure necrosis (comatose states)
  Surgical procedures (orthopedic, vascular, cardiac)

Exertional states
  Exertion in otherwise normal individuals (military recruits)
  Convulsive disorders

Metabolic disorders
  Alcoholic myopathy
  Anesthetic associated syndromes (malignant hyperthermia)
  Defects in carbohydrate metabolism (McArdle's disease, phosphofructokinase
    deficiency, syndrome of abnormal glycolysis)
  Defect in lipid metabolism deficiency of carnitine, palmityl transferase)
  Hypokalemia
  Toxins (heroin user's rhabdomyolysis, quail eater's disease, Haff disease,
    snake and hornet venoms)

Hereditary myopathies of unknown cause

Myositis syndromes
  Dermatomyositis, polymyositis, systemic lupus erythematosus

Other factors
  Infections?

Idiopathic rhabdomyolysis

Most hospital laboratories will make a definitive differentiation between myoglobin and hemoglobin by performing a cellulose acetate electrophoresis. Unfortunately, if it is not between 8:00 A.M. and 5:00 P.M., you may be out of luck getting the laboratory to perform this test. An alternative test, which is presumptive of the presence of myoglobin, is based on differential solubility in ammonium sulfate. This is based on the principle that myoglobin is soluble in 80 per cent saturated ammonium sulfate solution, whereas hemoglobin is not.

The test is performed as follows:

1. Clear the urine specimen by centrifugation or filtration.
2. Add 2.8 gm of $(NH_4)_2SO_4$ to 5 ml of urine, making an 80 per cent saturated solution of $(NH_4)_2SO_4$. Allow the solution to stand for 5 minutes, then filter.
3. If myoglobin is in the urine, it will remain in solution. If hemoglobin is in the urine, it will precipitate and will be detected on the filter paper.

A presumptive positive test should be followed by an electrophoresis when available. Whatever test is used, the urine must be absolutely fresh.

References: Robotham, J.L., and Haddow, J.D.: Pediatr. Clin. North Am., *23*: 279, 1976. Cifuentes, E., Norman, M.E., Schwartz, M.W., et al.: Clin. Pediatr., *15*: 63, 1976. Rosse, W.F.: *In* Williams, W.J., Beutler, E., Erslev, A.J., and Rundles, R.W. (Eds.): Hematology, 2nd ed. New York, McGraw-Hill Book Company, 1978, p. 613.

THE FE$_{Na}$ TEST: USE IN THE DIFFERENTIAL DIAGNOSIS OF ACUTE RENAL FAILURE

The physician is frequently faced with the problem of distinguishing prerenal azotemia from acute tubular necrosis in patients with acute renal failure.

In the oliguric phase of these two conditions, the renal tubule handles sodium in distinctly different fashions. In prerenal azotemia, the renal tubule avidly reabsorbs the filtered sodium; in acute tubular necrosis, the reabsorption of sodium is restricted.

These observations provide the basis for a simple test for differentiating these two conditions — the "FE$_{Na}$ test" (FE$_{Na}$ is the excreted fraction of the filtered sodium).

The test is performed by measuring both sodium and creatinine in simultaneously collected samples of plasma and urine.

The FE$_{Na}$ is calculated as follows:

$$\frac{\dfrac{[\text{Sodium}]_U}{[\text{Sodium}]_P}}{\dfrac{[\text{Creatinine}]_U}{[\text{Creatinine}]_P}} \times 100$$

U and P represent concentrations in urine and plasma, respectively.

In general, an FE$_{Na}$ of less than 1 indicates prerenal azotemia, and an FE$_{Na}$ of more than 3 indicates acute tubular necrosis.

Reference: Espinel, C.H.: J.A.M.A., *236:*579, 1976.

12

ACUTE OR CHRONIC RENAL FAILURE

When one is confronted with a patient with azotemia, it is necessary to determine quickly if the process is acute or chronic and its etiology. The following two tables should help you in this diagnostic process.

Comparison of Factors and Magnitude of Their Effect on the Concentration of Blood Urea Nitrogen and Serum Creatinine in Children

CLINICAL SETTING	BLOOD UREA NITROGEN CONCENTRATION		SERUM CREATININE CONCENTRATION	
	Magnitude of Effect	*Direction of Effect*	*Magnitude of Effect*	*Direction of Effect*
Dehydration	Marked	↑	Slight	↑
Acute renal failure	Marked	↑(rapidly)	Marked	↑ (slowly)
Chronic renal failure	Marked	↑	Marked	↑
Excessive protein intake in relation to renal function or in newborn	Marked	↑	Slight	↑
Gastrointestinal hemorrhage	Marked	↑	→	→
Catabolism	Marked	↑	Significant	↑
Starvation— relative protein deficiency	Marked	↓	Marked if muscle wasting	↓
Hepatic failure without renal impairment	Marked	↓	—	—
↓Muscle mass	—	—	Marked	↓
Muscle disease	—	—	Marked	↓(creatine ↑)

Reference: Lieberman, E. (ed.): *In* Clinical Pediatric Nephrology. Philadelphia, J.B. Lippincott, 1976, p. 50.

Major Clinical Findings and Categories of Acute and Chronic Renal Failure

	HISTORY	PHYSICAL FINDINGS	MAJOR LABORATORY ABNORMALITIES	DIAGNOSES
Acute Renal Failure (ARF)	1. Acute onset of disease 2. Known previous good health 3. ↓ urine output 4. Swelling, shortness of breath 5. Headaches 6. Nausea, vomiting, diarrhea 7. Changes in central nervous system function 8. Pallor	1. *Hydration—volume overload:* edema of eyelids, lungs, peripheral edema, ascites, congestive heart failure 2. *Central nervous system abnormalities:* generalized, not focal signs: seizures, lethargy → coma 3. *Hypertension:* hemorrhages, exudates in eyegrounds; cardiomegaly 4. *Bleeding diathesis:* petechiae, ecchymoses	1. *Chemical:* ↑BUN, ↑Cr ↑K, ↓CO_2, ↓Ca, ↑PO_4 ↑Uric acid, ↓ or Normal Na 2. *Urinary findings:* ↓S.G., protein ± Casts, ± WBC, ± RBC ± Bacteriuria 3. *Hematologic:* Normal or ↓Hgb/Hct	I. Acute circulatory insufficiency: severe dehydration; septic shock; postsurgical II. Nephrotoxic renal injury; myoglobinuria; hemoglobinuria; pharmacologic agents; poisons; hyperuricemia III. Vascular injury: renal vein or artery thrombosis IV. Glomerulopathies: acute nephritis, rapidly progressive nephritis V. Acute obstruction: calculi, tumor, blood clots
Chronic Renal Failure (CRF)	1. Insidious onset of disease 2. No clear-cut recognition of good health 3. Urine output ↓ or normal 4. Anorexia, vomiting, diarrhea 5. Fatigue, pallor, lethargy 6. Poor growth 7. Disturbances of sexual maturation 8. Bone pain, pruritis 9. Polyuria, polydipsia (in few disorders)	1. *Evidence of prolonged uremia:* pericarditis, peripheral neuropathy, osteodystrophy, malnutrition, ecchymoses and bleeding gums 2. *Skin:* pale, sallow 3. *Growth retardation:* Delayed sexual maturation 4. *Hypertension:* findings similar to those of ARF 5. *Central nervous system abnormalities:* findings similar to those of ARF	1. *Chemical:* ↑BUN, ↑Cr ↓Ca, ↑PO_4 ↑Alkaline phosphatase ↑Uric acid, ↓CO_2 2. *Urinary findings:* ↓S.G., ± RBC, + protein ± Sugar, + casts ± WBC, ± bacteriuria 3. *Hematologic:* ↓Hgb/Hct	I. Congenital malformations: cystic disorders, hypoplasia, dysplasia, ± urinary tract obstruction, ± chronic renal infection II. Glomerular diseases: chronic glomerulonephritis of known and unknown cause III. Tubulopathies, glomerular insufficiency, Fanconi's syndrome, oculocerebrorenal syndrome, distal renal tubular acidosis

12

Reference: Lieberman, E.: *In Clinical Pediatric Nephrology.* Philadelphia, J.B. Lippincott, 1976, p. 84.

PROXIMAL OR DISTAL RENAL TUBULAR ACIDOSIS

Renal tubular acidosis is a syndrome consisting of metabolic acidosis that is out of proportion to the impairment of glomerular filtration and is associated with a paradoxically alkaline urine.

Patients with this disturbance can be separated into a proximal and a distal form, either of which may be primary or secondary.

The course, complications, and treatment of the two forms of the disorder are very different. It is important to distinguish between them. The table below provides some help.

Renal Tubular Acidosis

	PROXIMAL	DISTAL
Primary	Idiopathic	Idiopathic
Usual age at diagnosis	0 to 2 years	>2 years
Sex	Male predominance	Female predominance (?)
Presenting complaint	Growth failure	Growth failure, polydipsia, polyuria, vomiting, dehydration
Secondary to	Fanconi syndrome Cystinosis Lowe's syndrome Hereditary fructose intolerance Various states of renal insufficiency	Primary hyperparathyroidism Vitamin D intoxication Amphotericin B Hyperglobulinemia Medullary sponge kidney Renal tubular necrosis
Urine pH	4.5 to 7.8, depending on plasma bicarbonate level	Always above 6.0
Bicarbonate threshold	Decreased	Normal
Hydrogen excretion	Normal, below bicarbonate threshold	Impaired, below bicarbonate threshold
Therapy	Resistant to alkali therapy; diuretics effective	Sensitive to alkali therapy; no effect of diuretics
Spontaneous remission in primary form	Yes	No
Complications	Growth failure acidemia	Nephrocalcinosis Hypokalemia Bone lesions Ricketts

Reference: Nash, M.A., Torrodo, A.D., Greifer, I., et al.: J. Pediatr., *80*:738, 1972.

THE NEPHROTIC SYNDROME IN YOUNG INFANTS

Approximately 5.5 per cent of children with nephrotic syndrome are below 6 months of age at the time of diagnosis. The following chart lists characteristics of the nephrotic syndrome in young infants and the condition that may cause the nephrotic syndrome.

PRIMARY	CHARACTERISTICS
Congenital	Family history positive
	Usually begins at less than 3 months of age
	Large placenta
	Reduced complement, elevated IgM
	Fatal illness
	Histologic findings: from minimal change to chronic glomerulonephritis; tubular changes prominent
Idiopathic infantile	Family history negative
	Later onset
	Normal placenta
	Normal complement and IgM
	Histologic findings: variable — prognosis depends on severity of glomerular lesions

SECONDARY TO:

Congenital syphilis

Nephrotoxin, e.g., mercury

Cytomegalic inclusion body disease

Renal vein thrombosis

Nephroblastoma

Reference: McDonald, R., Wiggelinkhuizen, F.C.P., and Kaschula, R.O.C.: Am. J. Dis. Child., *122*:507, 1971.

THE NEPHROTIC SYNDROME—PROGNOSIS

What is the expected course for a child with nephrosis? The following data can provide you with some reasonable expectations.

Adjusted Survival Rates

TIME FROM DIAGNOSIS	SURVIVAL RATE
1 year	94%
2 years	90%
5 years	85%
10 years	79%
15 years	77%

The nephrotic syndrome represents a diverse clinical spectrum. The clinical course can be characterized in the following manner.

20%	45%	10%	15%	10%
↓	↓	↓	↓	↓
One episode with no further activity after first year	Relapsing disease with ultimate cure	Relapsing disease with continued activity for 10 years or more	Relapsing disease with death	Death within 2 years of onset

Unfavorable prognostic factors at time of diagnosis include:

1. Azotemia (BUN >25 mg/100 ml)
2. Hematuria (>10 RBCs/HPF)
3. Hypertension (diastolic pressure >90 mm Hg)

Reference: Schwartz, M.W., Schwartz, G.J., and Cornfeld, D.: Pediatrics, *54*:547, 1974.

13
NEUROLOGY

NEUROLOGIC SIGNS OF INFANCY

The appearance and disappearance of certain neurologic signs of infancy have been well delineated. Neurologic abnormality should be suspected when these responses are not present at the appropriate time. Equal significance may be attached to the failure of certain responses to disappear. The chart below gives the age of expected appearance and disappearance of some of the more important neurologic signs in infancy.

RESPONSE	AGE AT TIME OF APPEARANCE	AGE AT TIME OF DISAPPEARANCE
Reflexes of position and movement		
Moro reflex	Birth	1–3 months
Tonic neck reflex (unsustained)	Birth	5–6 months (partial up to 2–4 years)
Neck righting reflex	4–6 months	1–2 years
Landau response	3 months	1–2 years
Palmar grasp reflex	Birth	4 months
Adductor spread of knee jerk	Birth	7 months
Plantar grasp reflex	Birth	8–15 months
Babinski response	Birth	Variable
Parachute reaction	8–9 months	Variable
Reflexes to sound		
Blinking response	Birth	
Turning response	Birth	
Reflexes of vision		
Blinking to threat	6–7 months	
Horizontal following	4–6 weeks	
Vertical following	2–3 months	
Optokinetic nystagmus	Birth	
Postrotational nystagmus	Birth	
Lid closure to light	Birth	
Macular light reflex	4–8 months	
Food reflexes		
Rooting response — awake	Birth	3–4 months
Rooting response — asleep	Birth	7–8 months
Sucking response	Birth	12 months
Handedness	2-3 years	

13

Continued

375

RESPONSE	AGE AT TIME OF APPEARANCE	AGE AT TIME OF DISAPPEARANCE
Spontaneous stepping	Birth	
Straight line walking	5–6 years	

Reference: Children Are Different. Columbus, Ohio, Ross Laboratories, 1967, p. 67.

A RATIONAL DIAGNOSTIC EVALUATION OF THE CHILD WITH MENTAL DEFICIENCY

There are hundreds of recognized disorders accompanied by mental deficiency. Given a patient with mental deficiency, what is a rational diagnostic evaluation? All too frequently, inappropriate procedures are ordered in a seemingly random fashion. One suggested approach to the problem is as follows.

A. *Appropriate History*

1. *Family history*

    About 50 per cent of patients with mental deficiency will have a genetically determined disorder. Similarly affected individuals may be present in 9 to 10 per cent of families.

    a. Pedigree: Search for a similar problem in both first and second degree relatives.

    b. Parental ages at birth of patient: Older maternal age is a factor in trisomy syndromes, while paternal age is a factor in certain fresh mutant gene disorders.

    c. Parental levels of intelligence and head circumference: Both mild mental deficiency and microcephaly may be familial.

2. *Cultural-Social History*

    Unfortunately, certain diseases occur more frequently among the poor. These include prematurity, prenatal cytomegalovirus infections, maternal alcoholism, and emotional deprivation.

3. *Prenatal History*

    Fetal activity in utero, complications of pregnancy, maternal weight gain, duration of pregnancy, and drug ingestion should all be noted.

4. *Perinatal History*

    a. Birth presentation — problems of morphogenesis and neurologic function are more common among infants who fail to assume the vertex position.

    b. Amount and character of amniotic fluid. Polyhydramnios may suggest difficulty in swallowing. Meconium staining suggests perinatal distress.

    c. Head circumference and body weight and length at birth. Small size often associated with problems of morphogenesis and brain development.

    d. Apgar score at 5 minutes.

    e. Problems such as placenta previa, traumatic delivery, prolonged hypoxia, apneic episodes, seizures, hyperbilirubinemia, hypoglycemia, and sepsis should be recorded.

   5. *Postnatal Events*
      a. Developmental progress
      b. Growth rate
      c. Postnatal events — central nervous system infections, head
         trauma.

B.   Physical Examination

   1. *Indirect assessment of brain and brain function*
         Head circumference, transillumination, scalp hair pattern (aberrant
      scalp hair pattern may be used as a clue to early fetal problems in brain
      morphogenesis), examination of ocular fundus, developmental status,
      neurologic status.
   2. *Complete non-CNS examination for major and minor anomalies*

*The combined finding of such a history and physical examination will either pro-
vide a specific diagnosis or allow one to assign the patient into one of four clinical
groupings, each of which requires a different diagnostic evaluation.*

The accompanying flow sheet illustrates this procedure.

13

After Appropriate History and Physical Examination

PRENATAL ONSET OF PROBLEM IN MORPHOGENESIS *includes*	PERINATAL ONSET OF INSULT TO BRAIN *includes*	POSTNATAL ONSET *includes*	UNDECIDED AGE AT ONSET *includes*
1. Single defect of brain development primary microcephaly hydrocephaly hydranencephaly defect of neural tube cerebral dysgenesis	hypoxic injury kernicterus hypoglycemia neonatal meningitis	trauma meningitis encephalitis hypernatremia water intoxication lead poisoning degenerative disorders metabolic errors	most patients in whom no diagnosis is made
2. Major and minor malformations in other than CNS as well as chromosomal defects syndromes of nonchromosomal cause unknown patterns of malformation			

Consider Following Diagnostic Procedures

Pneumoencephalogram or CAT scan	As indicated from history	Appropriate metabolic studies as provided from clues in history and physical examination Phenylketonuria Mucopolysaccharide disorders Galactosemia Lesch-Nyhan Homocystinuria	If male, get a buccal smear
Karyotype			
Viral titers			

Relative Frequency

This category makes up 40 to 45% of patients; it is the largest category

Accounts for 15 to 20% of all patients

About 5% of patients fall into this category; normal early development and obstetric history should make you suspect these disorders

Second largest category

13

Other laboratory studies are rarely indicated. Skull films should be obtained in patients with craniostenosis, cutaneous signs of tuberous sclerosis, or Sturge-Weber syndrome. Long bone films are justified in patients with skeletal abnormalities, and bone age studies are warranted in patients with abnormal growth. EEGs should be reserved for patients with seizures. Other blood chemistries and viral titers are justified only by pertinent findings in the history and physical examination.

Reference: Smith, D.W., and Simons, E.R.: Am. J. Dis. Child., *129*:1285, 1975.

EYE SIGNS IN THE COMATOSE PATIENT

Examination of the eyes provides valuable diagnostic information in the patient in coma. Both pupillary signs and eye movements should be noted before examining the ocular fundi.

PUPILLARY SIGNS IN COMA

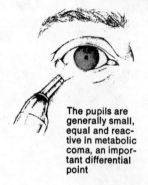

The pupils are generally small, equal and reactive in metabolic coma, an important differential point

Equal, fixed, dilated pupils result from substances like atropine; they also occur in severe anoxia or ischemia and in the terminal state

Pinpoint pupils result from opiates and also occur in patients with pontine lesions (usually hemorrhage or infarct)

FIG. 13–1A

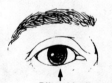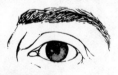

Dilated ipsilateral pupil due to:
Compression by herniated uncus
Traction of oculomotor nerve against posterior cerebral artery

A unilaterally widely dilated and fixed pupil results from pressure on the third nerve, often a sign of uncal herniation from a rapidly expanding unilateral lesion, as a rule on the side of the dilated pupil

FIG. 13–1B

EYE MOVEMENTS IN COMA

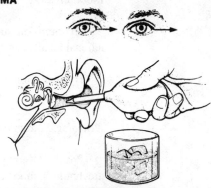

The doll's head maneu-
ver: The head is turned
rapidly from side to side
and conjugate deviation
occurs in the direction
opposite the head move-
ment as long as the
brain stem centers for
eye movement are still
intact. Loss of these
centers results in ab-
sence of doll's head
movement. These move-
ments are generally also
absent when the patient
is not comatose

The oculovestibular response: Irrigation of the
external auditory canal with ice water results in
conjugate motion of the eyes toward the side of
stimulation. This response is lost when the
pontine centers are compromised

FIG. 13-1C

Reference: Haerer, A.F.: Hosp. Med., *12*:68, 1976.

THE DIFFERENTIAL DIAGNOSIS OF COMA IN THE INFANT AND CHILD

The diagnosis of the patient in coma requires a prompt and disciplined approach. Much can be learned from the history and careful attention to the vital signs, neurologic examination, and a few carefully selected laboratory tests.

Respiration as a clue to the cause of coma

Cheyne-Stokes respiration indicates bilateral cortical lesions.

Hyperventilation may be a result of:
  Central neurogenic origin
    Seen in patients with hyperammonemia
  Metabolic acidosis
    Diabetes
    Uremia
    Fluid and electrolyte imbalance
    Lactic acidosis
    Poisoning with acidic substances (acetylsalicylic acid, acetazolamide, methyl alcohol to formic acid, ethylene glycol to oxalic acid, paraldehyde to acetic acid)
  Metabolic errors of metabolism
    isovaleric acidemia, methylmalonic aciduria, hyperglycinemia, maple syrup urine disease

Periodic breathing, ataxic breathing, and apneusis all suggest brain stem lesions.

13

Blood Pressure

Hypotension suggests that patient is in shock from septicemia, hypovolemia, adrenal insufficiency, or severe hypoxemia.

Hypertension indicates the presence of increased intracranial pressure, severe renal disease, or poisoning with sympathomimetic agents.

Neurologic Examination

Positive Kernig and Brudzinski signs suggest central nervous infection, subarachnoid hemorrhage, or posterior fossa tumor.

Eye signs (pupils should be equal and reactive to light).
  Unilateral fixed and dilated pupil suggests tentorial herniation or focal lesion in the area of third nerve nucleus.
  Bilateral dilated pupils, fixed to light, suggest irreversible brain damage or poisoning with atropine-like agents, barbiturates, or glutethimide. May also be observed with hypothermia or peripheral nerve lesions.
  Irregular pupils, unreactive to light, suggest midbrain damage.
  Pinpoint pupils indicate metabolic coma, drug intoxication (opiates, barbiturates), or pontine lesions.

Eye Movements
  VI nerve palsy — suspect increased intracranial pressure, meningeal inflammatory process, neoplastic invasion of nerve, or pontine lesion.
  III nerve palsy (eyes point down and out) suggests a tentorial herniation.

Lumbar puncture should be performed in all instances where central nervous system disease exists as a diagnostic possibility. Always measure opening pressure.

Based on the physical findings and lumbar puncture examination, the following diagnostic categories can be established.

Differential Diagnosis of Coma

No Focal Signs Normal Spinal Fluid	No Focal Signs Abnormal Spinal Fluid (cells, pressure, or protein)	Focal Signs Normal Spinal Fluid	Focal Signs Abnormal Spinal Fluid
Poisoning	Infection	Arterial occlusion	Trauma

Metabolic disorders	Lead poisoning	Demyelinating disease	Infection
			  brain abscess
			  subdural empyema
			  encephalitis

Concussion	Water intoxication	Postictal paralysis	
Postictal state	Trauma		Neoplasm
Septicemia	Subarachnoid hemorrhage		Vascular malformation
	Cerebral vein thrombosis		
	Midline tumors		
	Hydrocephalus		

Reference: Modified from a lecture by Peter Huttenlocher, M.D., May 1976.

BREATH-HOLDING SPELL OR IDIOPATHIC EPILEPSY?

About 5 per cent of infants and children will experience at least one breath-holding spell and may lose consciousness. Some features that may be used to distinguish these episodes from idiopathic epilepsy appear in the table below.

	GRAND MAL (IDIOPATHIC EPILEPSY)	ANOXIC CONVULSION (BREATH-HOLDING SPELL)
Age of onset	Rarely in infancy	Often begins in infancy
Family history	None or positive for epilepsy	Often positive for breath-holding spell or fainting
Precipitating factors	Usually absent (or specific sensory stimuli or nonspecific stresses)	Usually present (specific emotional or nociceptive stimuli)
Occurrence during sleep	Common	Never
Posture	Variable	Usually erect
Sequence and patterns	Single cry (may be absent) with loss of consciousness→tonic→clonic phases, cyanosis may occur later in attack; flushed at first, pale after attack	Long crying or single gasp, cyanosis or pallor→loss of consciousness→limpness→clonic jerks→opisthotonos→clonic jerks
Perspiration	Warm sweat	Cold sweat
Heart rate	Markedly increased	Decreased, asystole, or slightly increased
Duration	Usually >1 minute	Usually 1 minute or less
Incontinence and tongue biting	Common	Uncommon (but may occur)
Postictal state	Confusion and sleep common	No confusion. Fatigue common
Interictal EEG	Usually bilateral discharges	Usually normal
Oculocardiac activation	No response or bradycardia; 7% may have asystole of less than 4 seconds; asymptomatic	About 50% have asystole >2 seconds, usually >4 seconds; attack may be precipitated
Ictal EEG	Generalized, high-voltage polyspike discharges, gradually subsiding into slow waves and depression for several minutes	Isoelectric pattern preceded and followed by diffuse high-voltage delta waves, promptly reverting to normal pattern upon recovery of consciousness

13

Reference: Lombroso, C.T., and Lerman, P.: Pediatrics, *39*:563, 1967.

THE BULGING FONTANEL

A bulging fontanel in an infant is generally regarded as a sign of serious CNS disease, such as:

Meningitis	Subdural hematoma
Encephalitis	Lead poisoning
Hydrocephalus	Sinus thrombosis
Cerebral hemorrhage	Tumor
Intracranial abscess	

The history, however, may suggest a benign cause. A congenital subgaleal cyst over the anterior fontanel may simulate a bulging fontanel. *Benign intracranial hypertension*, a syndrome of increased intracranial pressure, normal ventricular system and CSF composition, and absence of focal neurologic signs can also produce a bulging fontanel.

The causes of benign intracranial hypertension in infancy:

Impaired CSF absorption

Obstructed inferior vena cava secondary to intrathoracic mass or obstructive lung disease

Obstruction of sagittal sinus secondary to skull fracture or other cause

Endocrine/Metabolic

Galactosemia
Addison's disease
Hypophosphatasia
Hypoparathyroidism
Hypothyroidism

Drugs

Hypervitaminosis A
Tetracyclines
Nalidixic acid

Infections

Roseola infantum
Guillain-Barré syndrome

Nutritional

Hypovitaminosis A
Rapid brain growth following starvation

Miscellaneous

Polycythemia vera
Heart disease
Allergic diseases
Anemia (severe)
Wiskott-Aldrich syndrome

References: Hagberg, B., and Silinpää, M.: Acta Paediatr. Scand., *59*:328–339, 1970. Barnett, H.L.: Pediatrics. New York, Appleton-Century-Crofts, 1972.

SKULL FILM? SKULL FRACTURE?

It is an unusual day for a pediatrician when he or she is not asked to evaluate an infant or child following head trauma. The knee-jerk response in these situations, all too frequently, is to request x-ray films of the skull. Stop and think, "Does the presence of a skull fracture in a child with a head injury indicate an increased likelihood of an intracranial complication?"

There is an abundance of facts available to answer this question. In a study involving 4465 consecutive head injuries at the Hospital for Sick Children in Toronto, the following was found:

1. 26.6 per cent of the children had skull fractures.
2. The incidence of fracture with head trauma did not vary significantly with age, but 75 per cent of all patients seen were over 2 years of age.
3. A linear fracture occurred in 73 per cent of patients with fracture; a depressed skull fracture occurred in 27 per cent.
4. The parietal bone was involved in 50 per cent of all fractures.
5. In 70 per cent of all patients with a fracture, there was external evidence of trauma. The fracture was present on the same side as the external trauma in 84 per cent of instances, and on the contralateral side in 16 per cent.
6. Cerebrospinal fluid otorrhea was observed in only 22 of 4465 children. In only one patient could a fracture of the petrous bone be demonstrated by routine films.
7. Profuse bleeding from the middle ear was observed in 241 of these 4465 patients, but in only 20 patients could a petrous fracture be demonstrated with conventional skull films.
8. Subdural hematomas occurred in 5 per cent of all children with head trauma. Only 15 per cent of these patients with subdurals had a skull fracture. The overall incidence of subdurals in children without skull fractures was 6 per cent; the incidence in children with skull fractures was 3 per cent.
9. Subdural hematomas were most common in infants 0 to 6 months of age. In this group, 28 per cent of the head injuries had associated subdural hematomas; only 7 per cent of *this group* with subdurals had skull fractures.
10. Bilateral subdural hematomas were observed in 143 children, but only 6 of these patients had bilateral fractures.
11. Extradural hematomas occurred in 1 per cent of the group. They were just as frequent in the nonfracture group as in the fracture group. Extradural hematomas occurred more frequently in children over 5 years of age.

12. Severe brain damage was observed in 3 per cent of the entire group of patients with head trauma. In this group, 65 per cent had a fracture. Of those with a fracture, approximately 80 per cent were depressed fractures.

13. In children with the most severe brain injuries and serious intracranial sequelae, fractures were frequently noted only at operation or at autopsy because clinical condition did not permit time for radiographic studies.

Conclusions

Presence of skull fracture alone is of little prognostic significance. Presence of skull fracture does not alter management except in patients with a depressed skull fracture. Virtually all depressed skull fractures are associated with a history of injury produced by local trauma by an object and can be anticipated by the findings on physical examination.

Skull films are not an emergency procedure when skull fracture is considered as a diagnostic possibility, in fact, they are rarely necessary at all. The management of an infant or child with a head injury depends on a careful assessment of the patient's neurologic status and requires periodic reevaluation.

The skull roentgenogram is a crutch that does not help you to walk.

Reference. Harwood-Nash, D.C., Hendrick, E.B., and Hudson, A.R.: Radiology, *101*:151, 1971.

THE BASAL SKULL FRACTURE

These fractures may be hard to diagnose by x-ray examination. When should you suspect them clinically? The clues include:

1. Bleeding from nose, eyes, or ears or discoloration in the mastoid area ("Battle's sign").
2. Blood behind the eardrum.
3. Cerebrospinal rhinorrhea (see below).
4. Cranial nerve palsies. These involve cranial nerves I, III, and VIII.
5. Appearance of "sinusitis."
6. Presence of pneumocephaly.

CEREBROSPINAL FLUID RHINORRHEA AND GLUCOSE TESTING

It is commonly taught that testing a nasal discharge for the presence of glucose can help to detect the presence of cerebrospinal fluid leak in the patient with head trauma. Unfortunately, this just is not true. Employing a glucose oxidase test strip, approximately 75 to 90 per cent of normal children will give a positive test in their nasal secretions.

Reference: Hull, H.F., and Morrow, G., III: J.A.M.A., *234*:1052, 1975.

BRAIN TUMORS IN CHILDREN

We frequently forget that malignancies within the central nervous system are second only to leukemia as a cause of death from cancer among children. About 31 per cent of all malignancies in children under 15 years of age are due to leukemia, while 18 per cent are central nervous system tumors.

Approximately two-thirds of the intracranial tumors of childhood are beneath the tentorium, in contrast to an incidence of only 10 per cent among adults.

The distribution of intracranial tumors in children is as follows:

INFRATENTORIAL	PER CENT OF ALL TUMORS
Cerebellar astrocytoma	20
Medulloblastoma	18
Brain stem glioma	10
Ependymoma	8
Other	10
SUPRATENTORIAL	
Astrocytoma	8
Ependymoma	6
Malignant glioma	6
Craniopharyngioma	5
Other	9

Major Symptoms

Headache. Insidious onset, intermittent, most pronounced upon arising.

Vomiting. Often occurs after head has been in dependent position, i.e., after sleeping. Not usually associated with nausea.

Easy Fatigability. Require long naps. Decrease in normal activity.

Personality Change. Irritability. Decline in intellectual function.

Seizures. Rare in infratentorial tumors. Occur in about one-third of patients with supratentorial tumors.

Characteristics of Individual Tumors

INFRATENTORIAL

Cerebellar astrocytoma	Longer duration of symptoms. Ipsilateral inco-ordination, ataxia with tendency to drift to the side of the lesion, nystagmus with slow component on ipsilateral gaze, and hyporeflexia on side of lesion.

Medulloblastoma	More common in infants. Gait disturbances and truncal ataxia. Signs of increased intracranial pressure frequent.
Brain stem glioma	Insidious onset of cranial nerve dysfunction, long tract involvement, ataxia, gait disturbance. (Seventh nerve, sixth, ninth, tenth, and facial branch of fifth.)
Ependymoma	Signs of increased intracranial pressure.
SUPRATENTORIAL	
Astrocytoma	Signs of increased intracranial pressure, focal seizures, and focal neurologic findings dependent on location.
Ependymoma	Same as astrocytoma.
Craniopharyngioma	Increased intracranial pressure and visual disturbances most common finding. Diabetes insipidus is rare.

Reference: Walker, M.D.: Pediatr. Clin. North Am., *23*: 131, 1976.

THE FLOPPY INFANT

An infant is considered "floppy" when there is decreased muscular tone. The muscular tone of infants may be assessed in the following manner:

1. Note the head and leg position in prone horizontal suspension.

2. When the infant is lying supine, pull him by the hands to a sitting position, noting resistance of arms, grasping with fingers, and the relationship of the head to the trunk.

3. With the infant supine, pick up each extremity individually, feel the resistance, and note how it falls to the mattress when released.

4. Note resistance to movement of individual joints, paying attention to resistance to rapid abduction of the flexed thighs, a common site for the first evidence of developing spasticity.

Hypotonia in the newborn commonly results from diffuse cerebral dysfunction. Asphyxia, craniocerebral hemorrhage, and congenital abnormalities of the brain are often the cause. Infants destined to develop spastic or athetoid cerebral palsy are often hypotonic during the first six months of life. The generalized conditions listed below may also make themselves manifest by hypotonia.

Chromosomal disorders, especially trisomy 21

Hypothyroidism

Inborn errors of metabolism

Generalized mental retardation syndromes, e.g., Prader-Willi syndrome and Laurence-Moon-Biedl syndrome

Ehlers-Danlos syndrome

The hypotonic infant who has cerebral abnormality or dysfunction typically demonstrates other abnormalities on physical examination, such as microcephaly, macrocephaly, or abnormal level of consciousness. There will often be a history of seizures.

It is important to remember that hypotonia in the newborn may be the result of excess depressant medication given to the mother.

In addition to the cerebral lesions mentioned above, hypotonia may result from lesions at any level in the neuromuscular system:

Cerebellum and brain stem

Spinal cord — transecting lesions

Spinal cord — diffuse lesions

Peripheral nerves

Motor end-plate region

Muscle

The table beginning on page 391 lists neuromuscular abnormalities that are characterized by hypotonia according to the site of the basic pathologic change.

Laboratory studies that will aid in making the diagnosis are listed below along with the results to be expected, depending upon the site of the lesion.

Useful Laboratory Studies in Infantile Hypotonia

	BRAIN	SPINAL CORD DIFFUSE (ANTERIOR HORN CELL)	PERIPHERAL NERVE	MUSCLE
EEG	Abnormal	Normal	Normal	Normal
CSF protein	May be increased	Usually normal	Usually increased	Normal
EMG	Normal	Abnormal	Abnormal	Usually Normal
Nerve conduction velocity	Normal	Normal or slow	Slow	Normal
Muscle biopsy	Normal	Abnormal	Abnormal	Abnormal, frequently diagnostic

References: Rabe, E.F.: J. Pediatr., *64*:422, 1964. Peterson, H. de C.: Pediatr. Ann., May 1976, p. 300.

CLINICAL SYNDROME	SITE OF PATHOLOGIC CHANGE	ASSOCIATED MENTAL RETARDATION	HEREDITARY OR FAMILIAL	DIAGNOSTIC AIDS	THERAPY AFFECTING MUSCLE FUNCTION
Congenital atonic diplegia	Brain	Yes	No	Estimation of developmental level motor and mental, repeatedly	None
Congenital cerebellar ataxia	Cerebellum: and occasionally medulla, pons, and cerebrum	Often normal	No	Estimation of developmental level motor and mental, repeatedly	None
Congenital chorea	Brain	Yes	No	Estimation of developmental level motor and mental, repeatedly	None
Kernicterus	Multiple areas of basal ganglia, pons, medulla, hippocampus	Yes	No	Estimation of developmental level motor and mental, repeatedly	None
Tay-Sachs disease	Central nervous system	Yes	Yes	Funduscopic examination	None
Infantile spinal muscular atrophy (Werdnig-Hoffmann disease)	Anterior gray horns of spinal cord	No	No	Muscle biopsy	None
Myelopathic arthrogryposis multiplex congenita	Anterior gray horns of spinal cord	No	No	Muscle biopsy	Physiotherapy
Poliomyelitis	Anterior gray horns of spinal cord	No	No	CSF examination Isolation of agent from stool	Physiotherapy
Acute infective polyneuritis (Guillain-Barré disease)	Spinal roots and peripheral nerves	No	No	Nerve conduction time CSF examination	Steroids (?) Physiotherapy

Continued

Chronic idiopathic polyneuropathy	Peripheral nerve	No	No	Nerve conduction time EMG Muscle biopsy	Steroids (?) Physiotherapy
Myasthenia gravis — neonatal, transient	Myoneural junction	No	No	Response to neostigmine or edrophonium chloride	Neostigmine
Myasthenia gravis — congenital	Myoneural junction	No	No	Response to neostigmine or edrophonium chloride	Pyridostigmine bromide
Benign congenital hypotonia	Muscle (?)	No	No	Muscle biopsy EMG	None
Universal hypoplasia of muscle	Muscle (?)	No	Yes	Muscle biopsy	None
Infantile congenital myopathy (muscular dystrophy of infancy)	Muscle	No	Yes	Muscle biopsy Serum enzyme concentrations Creatine and creatinine coefficients EMG	Not proved
Central core disease	Muscle	No	Yes	Muscle biopsy	None
Rod body myopathy	Muscle	No	?	Muscle biopsy	None
Dystrophia myotonica	Muscle, gonads	Yes	Yes	Muscle biopsy EMG	None
Polymyositis	Muscle	No	No	Muscle biopsy	Steroids (?)
Glycogen storage disease	Muscle and central nervous system	?	Probably	Muscle biopsy	None

ATAXIA, MUSCLE WEAKNESS, EXTRAPYRAMIDAL DISORDERS

The child who presents with ataxia or muscle weakness or extrapyramidal manifestations of disease may pose a difficult diagnostic problem for the pediatrician. The following tables should guide you in the right direction.

Differential Diagnosis of Chronic Progressive Ataxia

CLINICAL DISORDER	PRECEDING HISTORY	USUAL YEAR OF ONSET IN CHILDREN	EXAMINATION	USUAL LABORATORY EXAMINATION	USUAL PROGNOSIS
Arnold-Chiari malformation	Headache, dysphagia		Palatal and tongue weakness, pyramidal signs, ataxia	May have hydrocephalus, spina bifida	Slowly progressive; stationary after surgery
Hereditary spinocerebellar ataxia	Stumbling, dizziness, familial incidence	7-10	Ataxia, loss of position sense, extensor plantar responses, kyphoscoliosis, pes cavus	Frequent associated ECG changes	Progressive, with death usually by 30 years of age
Abetalipo-proteinemia	Fatty diarrhea at 6 weeks to 2 years of age	2-17	Cerebellar ataxia, posterior column signs, retinitis pigmentosa, scoliosis, pes cavus	Acanthocytosis, lack of β-lipoprotein in serum	Slowly progressive
Dentate cerebellar ataxia	Myoclonus, convulsions	7-17	Ataxia with severe intention tremor		Slowly progressive
Hereditary cerebellar ataxia	Familial incidence	3-17	Ataxia, optic atrophy, occasionally associated posterior column and pyramidal tract signs	Pneumoencephalogram: small cerebellar folia	Slowly progressive

Continued

13

CLINICAL DISORDER	PRECEDING HISTORY	USUAL YEAR OF ONSET IN CHILDREN	EXAMINATION	USUAL LABORATORY EXAMINATION	USUAL PROGNOSIS
Ataxia telangiectasia	Recurrent sinopulmonary infections in two-thirds of cases; familial incidence	1–3	Oculocutaneous telangiectasia at 4 to 6 years; ataxia, choreoathetosis, dysarthria	Chest roentgenogram: bronchiectasis; absence of IgA in serum	Death before 25 years of age
Cerebellar tumors	Headache, vomiting		Papilledema, ataxia, nystagmus	Skull roentgenogram: separation of sutures	Progressive until operated
Heredopathia atactica polyneuriti-formis	Anorexia, failing vision, unsteady, familial incidence	4–7	Retinitis pigmentosa, ataxia, deafness, polyneuropathy, ichthyosis	Elevated phytanic acid in blood, increased spinal fluid protein	Slowly progressive with death
Multiple sclerosis	Preceding neurologic symptoms	14–17	Optic neuritis; brain stem, cerebellar, pyramidal, or sensory signs	Spinal fluid may reveal increased cells, protein, or γ-globin	Exacerbations and remissions
Spinal cord tumor	May have numbness or bladder disorder		Ataxia with weakness or sensory loss	Defect on myelography	Progressive until operated

Differential Diagnosis of Acute Ataxia

DISORDER	PRECEDING HISTORY	EXAMINATION	LABORATORY EXAMINATION	USUAL PROGNOSIS
Acute cerebellar ataxia	Half have had a prodromal systemic illness, occasionally exanthems	Cerebellar ataxia	Spinal fluid usually normal	Recovery
Dilantin intoxication	Convulsions treated with phenytoin	Cerebellar ataxia, nystagmus	High serum phenytoin level	Recovery
Cerebellar tumor or abscess	Headache, vomiting	Papilledema, ataxia, nystagmus	Separation of cranial sutures	Progressive until operated
Hartnup syndrome	Skin eruptions on exposure to sun; familial incidence	Skin lesions, ataxia, nystagmus, mental disturbances	Aminoaciduria, increased indole in urine	Recurrent ataxia
Multiple sclerosis	Preceding neurologic symptoms	Optic neuritis; brain stem, cerebellar, pyramidal or sensory signs	Spinal fluid may reveal increased cells, protein, or γ-globulin	Exacerbations and remissions
Encephalitides	Headache, stiff neck, fever	Cerebral and brain stem signs; also may have ataxia	Spinal fluid: lymphocytosis; possible virus isolation or rise in antibody titer	May be fatal, or slow recovery with or without residual
Spinal cord tumor	May have numbness or bladder disorder	Ataxia with weakness or sensory loss	Defect on myelography	Progressive until operated
Infectious polyneuropathy	Half have a prodromal systemic illness	Ataxia with motor and sensory loss	Spinal fluid: normal cells, increased protein	May be fatal, but recovery usually complete

13

Differential Diagnosis of Disorders of Muscle, Anterior Horn Cell, and Peripheral Nerves

CLINICAL AND LABORATORY FEATURES	MUSCLE	ANTERIOR HORN CELL	PERIPHERAL NERVES
Site of predisposition	Usually proximal and axial musculature	Proximal and/or distal extremity musculature	Usually distal extremity musculature
Deep tendon reflexes	Preserved until late in course	Reduced to absent early in course	Reduced to absent early in course
Sensation deficit	Rarely observed	Not observed	Usually present
Fasciculations	Usually absent	Frequently present	Occasionally present
CSF protein	Normal	Normal or elevated	Elevated or normal
Electromyography Interference pattern	Normal until late in disease	Reduced	Reduced
Fibrillation potentials	Not usually present	Usually present	Present
Action potentials	Short duration	Prolonged with occasional giant potentials	Prolonged with normal or polyphasic potentials
Evoked sensory and mixed nerve potentials	Normal	Normal	Absent, diminished amplitude, or prolonged conduction time

Differential Diagnosis of Extrapyramidal Disorders

DISORDER	FAMILIAL	SIGNS	ASSOCIATED FINDINGS
Hepatolenticular degeneration	Autosomal recessive	Rigidity, tremor, dystonia, dementia, corneal ring, jaundice	Increased urinary and hepatic copper, low serum ceruloplasmin
Juvenile parkinsonism	Rarely	Resting tremor, rigidity, bradykinesia	Decreased dopamine level in substantia nigra
Kernicterus	No	Athetosis, deafness, occasional intellectual impairment	Neonatal hyperbilirubinemia
Huntington's disease	Autosomal dominant	Rigidity, chorea, convulsions, dementia	
Torsion dystonia	Autosomal dominant or recessive	Dystonia, involuntary movements, normal intellect	
Chorea minor (Sydenham's)	No	Involuntary choreic movements, possibly carditis	Group A streptococcal infections
Absence of hypoxanthine-guanine phosphoribosyl transferase (Lesch-Nyhan syndrome)	X-linked recessive	Choreoathetosis, mental retardation, self-mutilation	Increased urinary and blood uric acid

Reference: Farmer, T.W. (Ed.): Pediatric Neurology. New York, Harper & Row, 1975, pp. 400, 403, 411, and 466.

MUSCULAR DYSTROPHIES AND MYOTONIAS

It is very hard to remember all the characteristics of the various muscular dystrophies and myotonias. The accompanying table should provide you with most of the essential facts.

DISEASE	GENETIC PATTERN	AGE AT ONSET	EARLY MANIFESTATIONS	INVOLVED MUSCLES
Muscular dystrophies Duchenne's muscular dystrophy (pseudohypertrophic, infantile)	X-linked recessive; autosomal recessive unusual. Thirty to 50% have no family history	2–6 years; rarer in infancy or at birth.	Clumsiness and easy fatigability on walking, especially on running and climbing stairs. (Climbing upon legs when rising from supine position—Gowers' maneuver). Waddling gait. Lordosis.	Axial and proximal before distal. Pelvic girdle; pseudohypertrophy of gastrocnemius (90%), triceps brachii, and vastus lateralis. Shoulder girdle usually later. Sometimes mild articulation difficulties. Eventually, cardiac muscle (50%).
Becker's muscular dystrophy (late onset)	X-linked recessive.	Childhood (usually later than in Duchenne's).	Similar to Duchenne's.	Similar to Duchenne's.
Limb-girdle muscular dystrophy A. Pelvifemoral (Leyden-Möbius) B. Scapulohumeral (Erb's juvenile)	Autosomal recessive in 60%; high sporadic incidence. A. Relatively common. B. Rare.	Variable: early childhood to adulthood.	Weakness, with distribution according to type. Waddling gait, difficulty climbing stairs. Lordosis.	A. Pelvic girdle usually involved first and to greater extent. B. Shoulder girdle often asymmetric. Quadriceps and hamstrings may be weakest. Pseudohypertrophy of calves uncommon.
Facioscapulohumeral muscular dystrophy (Landouzy-Déjèrine). Scapuloperoneal variant	Autosomal dominant; sporadic cases not uncommon.	Usually late childhood and adolescence; rare in infancy; not uncommon in twenties.	Diminished facial movements with inability to close eyes, smile, or whistle. Face may be flat, unlined. Difficulty in raising arms over head. Lordosis. Tripping in scapuloperoneal type.	Facial muscles followed by shoulder girdle with occasional spread to hips or distal legs (scapuloperoneal variant).
Distal myopathies A. Gowers' type B. Welander's	Autosomal dominant.	A. Gowers': Some early; usually adult. B. Welander's: usually adult; occasionally adolescence.	Gowers': Wasting of cranial musculature. Welander's: weakness of hands and feet; rarely, muscles of face and tongue.	Distal muscle weakness, especially small muscles of hands and feet.

Continued

13

DISEASE	GENETIC PATTERN	AGE AT ONSET	EARLY MANIFESTATIONS	INVOLVED MUSCLES
"Oculocraniosomatic syndrome" (ophthalmoplegia and "ragged reds"; progressive external ophthalmoplegia)	(?) Acquired; 80% female; other hereditary neurologic disorders may be found in patient or family.	Variable: from infancy to adult life; most at about 10 years of age.	Ptosis and limitation of eye movements; hearing and visual loss (retinitis pigmentosa); intellectual loss; cerebellar disturbances (ataxia).	Extraocular muscles, often asymmetric. Variable involvement of axial muscles; cardiac muscles with conduction defect.
Congenital myopathies: Central core	Generally, autosomal dominance with variable penetrance.	Onset generally prenatal.	Infantile hypotonia, delay in attaining motor milestones. Mild weakness.	Often diffuse and variable, mainly proximal, legs more than arms.
Nemaline (rodbody) Myotubular (centronuclear) Congenital fiber type disproportion	Autosomal recessive also reported. Genetics unclear.	Onset usually in infancy, occasionally later childhood.	Nemaline: associated dysmorphism (face, spine, feet, pigeon chest). Myotubular: may show ptosis, facial weakness.	Nemaline: some diffuse muscle wasting. May include extraocular muscles.
Myotonias Myotonia congenita (Thomsen)	Autosomal dominant (autosomal recessive cases reported).	Early infancy to late childhood.	Difficulty in relaxing muscles after contracting them, especially after sleep; aggravated by cold, excitement.	Hands especially; muscles may be diffusely enlarged, giving patient Herculean appearance.
Myotonic dystrophy (Steinert)	Autosomal dominant.	Late childhood to adolescence; neonatal and infantile forms increasingly recognized.	Myotonia of grasp, tongue; worsened by cold, emotions. "Hatchet-face." In infancy, floppiness with facial diplegia; arthrogryposis multiplex. Thin ribs on chest x-ray. Myotonic phenomena: "bunching up" of muscles of tongue, thenar eminence, finger extensors after tapping with percussion hammer. Mild to moderate MR in about 80% may precede muscular symptoms.	Wasting of facial muscles, including muscles of mastication; sternocleidomastoids, hands.

REFLEXES	MUSCLE BIOPSY FINDINGS	OTHER DIAGNOSTIC STUDIES	TREATMENT	PROGNOSIS
Knee jerks ± to 0; ankle jerks ++ to +; occasionally, extensor plantar response (Babinski sign)	Degeneration and variation in fiber size; proliferation of connective tissue. Basophilia, phagocytosis. Poor differentiation of fiber types on ATPase reaction; deficiency of type 2B fibers.	EMG myopathic. CPK (4000–5000 IU), aldolase, SGOT very high with decrease toward normal over the years. ECG. Chest x-ray.	Physical therapy, braces, wheelchair eventually, weight control.	Ten percent show nonprogressive mental retardation. Death from pneumonia 10–15 years after diagnosis with 75% of patients dead by age 20.
Similar to Duchenne's	Similar to above, except type 2B fibers present.	Similar to above, although muscle enzymes may not be as elevated.	As above. Wheelchair in late childhood or early adult life.	Slower progression than Duchenne's, with death usually in adulthood.
Usually present	Variation in muscle fiber size with many very large fibers. Fiber splitting and internal nuclei common. Many "moth-eaten" whorled fibers.	EMG myopathic. CPK, other enzymes variable: often normal but may be elevated. ECG.	Physical therapy, weight control.	Mildly progressive: spread from lower to upper limbs may take 15–20 years. Life expectancy mid to late adulthood.
Present	Predominantly large fibers with scattered tiny atrophic fibers, "moth-eaten" and whorled fibers. Inflammatory response. Little or no fiber-splitting, fibrosis, or type 1 fiber predominance.	EMG myopathic. Muscle enzymes usually normal.	Physical therapy where indicated. Wheelchair in old age.	Very slowly progressive, often with plateaus, except in infantile form where there may be difficulties in walking by adolescence. Usually normal lifespan.
Present	Nonspecifically myopathic.	EMG myopathic. Muscle enzymes may be mildly elevated.	None.	Normal life expectancy.
Depressed to ± or 0	Mitochondrial abnormalities. "Ragged red" fibers. Changes in fiber size, usually due to type 2 fiber atrophy.	Muscle enzymes usually normal. ECG with conduction block. Rule out myasthenia gravis, Refsum's disease. CSF protein elevated. Nerve conduction studies.	Plastic retraction of eyelids. Support of cardiac defect. Where there is evidence of denervation, corticosteroids may be helpful.	Dysphagia may develop (50%) as well as generalized muscle weakness. Prognosis fair if disease is confined to ocular muscles.

Continued

13

REFLEXES	MUSCLE BIOPSY FINDINGS	OTHER DIAGNOSTIC STUDIES	TREATMENT	PROGNOSIS
Normal to ± or 0	Specific histochemical findings determine diagnosis. Central core: amorphous areas in fiber devoid of oxidative enzymes.	Muscle enzymes usually normal.	Physical therapy to prevent contractures and strengthen existing muscles. Correction of dislocated hips or other deformities.	Usually very slowly progressive or nonprogressive, with plateaus and improvements possible, depending on type. Weakness occasionally increases in adolescence.
	Nemaline: red rods with trichrome stain. Myotubular: central nuclei in areas devoid of myofibrils; type 2B fibers hypertrophy.	CPK may be slightly elevated.		
Normal	Nonspecific and minor changes; type 2B fibers may be absent.	EMG "myotonic."	Usually none. Phenytoin, especially in cold weather, may improve muscle functioning.	Normal life expectancy, with only mild disability.
In infantile form, marked hyporeflexia	Type 1 fiber atrophy, type 2 hypertrophy, sarcoplasmic masses, internal nuclei, phagocytosis, fibrosis, and cellular reaction.	EMG markedly "myotonic." Hormonal studies, especially testosterone, glucose tolerance test, thyroid tests. ECG. Chest x-ray and pulmonary function tests. Immunoglobulins.	Procainamide, 250 mg 3 times daily orally, increased to tolerance; phenytoin, 5–7 mg/kg/day orally.	Frontal baldness, cataracts (85%), gonadal atrophy (85% of males), thyroid dysfunction, diabetes mellitus (20%). Cardiac conduction defects; impaired pulmonary function. Low IgG. Life expectancy normal to slightly decreased, though severely handicapped in late adult life.

Reference: Nellhaus, G.: *In* Kempe, C.H., Silver, H.K., and O'Brien, D. (Eds.): Current Pediatric Diagnosis and Management. Los Altos, California, Lange Medical Publications, 1978, pp. 608–609.

Chorea—Greek for dance, the term may appear incongruous with the grotesque twitching and movements that characterize this disease of the central nervous system.

DISORDERS OF MOVEMENT

The patient is observed to be making unusual involuntary movements. Is it a tic, a tremor, chorea, athetosis, or some other involuntary movement? The recognition and classification of the movement disorder is essential for the establishment of a correct diagnosis.

Athetosis refers to a writhing, irregular movement associated with increased tone in the distal extremities. These movements are primarily around the long axis of the limb. Hyperextension of the digits is common. The movements are often continuous, with the amplitude increased by volition or excitement. It is usually the result of birth injury or kernicterus.

Ballismus refers to rapid movements occurring usually at the shoulder, but they may also be observed at the hip. They are irregular and consist of violent hurling, flinging, and throwing in the upper extremity and kicking or circumduction in the lower extremity. It is usually unilateral (hemiballismus). In the adult the lesion in the contralateral subthalamic nucleus is of vascular origin, while in children it represents a severe form of chorea.

Chorea consists of rapid, involuntary, nonrhythmic jerks of various parts of the body. They involve both proximal and distal portions of the limbs but may involve the face and trunk as well.

Dystonia refers to a movement disorder characterized by simultaneous contraction of agonist and antagonist muscles. The muscular contraction occurs prior to the onset of movement, leading to a tightening and stiffening of the affected parts of the anatomy. The end position, following a movement, is maintained for a prolonged period.

Myoclonus is an involuntary, repetitive, instantaneous, irregular contraction of a group of muscles, or more rarely, a single muscle.

Tremor is a rhythmic, oscillatory movement of a body part. It may be distinguished from myoclonus and tics by the regularity and the equal force and speed of the movement in both directions.

Tic, the most common movement disorder, consists of rapid stereotyped movements in areas about the face, neck, and shoulder that are usually directed away from the midline. They occur irregularly and last less than a second or may occur repetitively over several minutes. They are most obvious during excitement or emotional stress.

The table below summarizes the characteristic features of these movement disorders:

Reference: Lockman, L. A.: *In* Swaiman, K. F., and Wright, F. S. (Eds.): The Practice of Pediatric Neurology. St. Louis, C. V. Mosby, 1975.

Characteristics of Abnormal Movements

MOVEMENT	SPEED	LOCATION	DIRECTION	STEREOTYPE	RHYTHMICITY	INTERVAL
Athetosis	Slow	Most prominent in distal limbs	Axial rotations (writhing) and hyperextension	Common; continuous movement in extremity	Not rhythmic	Continuous, amplitude increased by excitement
Ballismus	Rapid	Proximal, especially at shoulder; also at hip; sometimes trunk, face, and muscles of respiration	Hurling, flinging, throwing, kicking, circumducting	Constant location; movements vary	Not rhythmic	0.5 to 120 seconds
Chorea	Rapid	Generalized; may be unilateral	Primarily at right angles to axis; also facial grimacing; flexion and extension	None; movements generally dance from joint to joint; when proximal and severe may appear semipurposeful	Not rhythmic	0.5 to 5 seconds
Dystonia	Rapid, slow; very slow relaxation	Trunk, head, extremities	Any, often twisting	Common; because of location of movements, relative strength of contracting muscles	Irregular	Irregular
Myoclonus	Very rapid	Localized or generalized	Any	Stereotyped	Irregular	0.5 to 5 seconds
Tic	Rapid	Usually in area supplied by motor cranial nerve (face, shoulder, neck)	Rotational; away	Stereotyped	Irregular	1 second to minutes
Tremor	Variable	Usually localized, often in hand	Complex or simple	Extreme stereotype	Very rhythmic; may be irregular	0.1 to 1 second

DIZZINESS AND VERTIGO IN CHILDREN

Every now and then we see children with dizziness and vertigo without obvious cause. Most but not all causes are due to ear problems. The most common causes of vertigo include:

1. Ear disorders with ear symptoms
   Acute otitis media
   Chronic suppurative otitis media
   Labyrinthitis
   Endolymphatic hydrops
   Otic capsule fracture
   Perilymphatic fistula
   Ototoxicity (e.g., gentamicin)
   Postmeningitis labyrinthitis
   Acoustic neuroma (intracanalicular)
2. Ear disorders without ear symptoms
   Benign postural vertigo
   Vestibular neuronitis
   Ototoxicity (streptomycin)
3. Associated with systemic disorders
   Intoxication (drugs, alcohol, etc.)
   Hypoglycemia
   Hyperventilation
   Psychogenic
4. Associated with CNS disorders
   Seizures
   Posttraumatic
   Neoplasm
   Demyelinating disease
   Vestibulogenic migraine

Reference: Chasin, W. D.: Hosp. Pract., *12:*103, 1977.

Vertigo is the sudden sensation of spinning of the individual or the surroundings. The cause may be the central nervous system (central vertigo) or the vestibular system (peripheral vertigo).

Evaluation of the child who complains of vertigo includes:

1. A detailed family and personal history with particular attention to a history of seizures, loss of consciousness, or migraine headaches.
2. Ear, nose, and throat examination with a hearing test.
3. Complete neurologic examination with particular emphasis on balance testing.
4. Electroencephalogram.
5. Electronystagmographic recording to determine whether one labyrinth responds to hot and cold water stimulation with a greater intensity of nystagmus than the other (labyrinthine preponderance).

The diagnoses made in 50 children complaining of vertigo, along with the characteristics of each diagnosis, are listed below.

	DIAGNOSIS	NUMBER	CHARACTERISTICS
Central Vertigo	Vertiginous seizures (idiopathic)	25	The clinical history included attacks of vertigo sometimes accompanied by headaches, nausea, vomiting, loss of postural control, loss of consciousness, sometimes ending in a generalized seizure. Hearing is normal.
			The EEG may or may not be normal. There may be positional nystagmus and/or labyrinthine preponderance.
			Response to anticonvulsants is good.
	Postmeningitic vertigo	3	There is a history of meningitis or meningoencephalitis. Vertigo may be accompanied by sensorineural hearing loss, tinnitus, seizures.
			There may be seizure activity evident on EEG, and there may be labyrinthine preponderance with thermal stimulation.

	DIAGNOSIS	NUMBER	CHARACTERISTICS
	Posttraumatic	4	These children have a history of brain concussion or contusion. The EEG may be abnormal. Anticonvulsants may be required.
	Migraine	5	The vertigo occurs as an aura to migraine attacks. There is usually a strong family history of migraines, the EEG is normal, but response to bithermal caloric stimulation may be abnormal.
	Psychosomatic	5	These are tense, nervous individuals who are usually adolescents. They complain of headaches and vertigo without nausea, vomiting, or loss of consciousness. All physical and laboratory tests are normal.
Peripheral Vertigo	Vestibular vertigo	5	The history includes an upper respiratory infection and earache a few days prior to the acute onset of attacks, a loss of postural control and nausea without impairment of hearing or central nervous system disturbance. Vestibular examination may be abnormal temporarily. If the condition does not resolve spontaneously within 2 weeks, patients may be treated with dimenhydrinate.
	Paroxysmal benign vertigo	2	This condition is characterized by attacks of unsteadiness during which patients appear pale and frightened. Ataxia and dysmetria are often present during the attack. Nystagmus may be observed. The EEG is normal, and vestibular testing may be normal as well. The attacks may subside spontaneously or they may be treated with dimenhydrinate.
	Congenital deafness	1	Vertigo may accompany sensorineural hearing loss. Attacks of vertigo may precede upper respiratory infections.

Reference: Eviatar, L., and Eviatar, A.: Pediatrics, *59*:833, 1977.

EVALUATIONS OF CEREBROSPINAL FLUID SHUNTS

The figure below is a diagram outlining the approach to cerebrospinal fluid (CSF) shunts which do not appear to be working properly. The first step, after a history and physical examination have been obtained, is to decide if "overt shunt dysfunction" is occurring. Obvious signs of this include fluid collections around the shunt, palpable disconnections of shunt components, flushing device permanently depressed or incompressible, erosion of the shunt through the skin, or x-ray evidence of malposition or disconnection. If any of these signs are present, the shunt must be revised. If no overt shunt infection is present, ascertain by the history (vomiting, lethargy, etc.) or physical examination (increased head circumference, prominent scalp veins, papilledema, etc.) whether the patient has a significantly high intracranial pressure. Symptomatic increased pressure mandates shunt revision.

Revising a shunt in the presence of CSF infection may result in continued and often more severe infection. When infection and shunt dysfunction occur together, it is often best to treat with antibiotics for several days prior to replacing the shunt apparatus. Intraventricular antibiotics may be necessary in addition to intravenous antibiotics, depending on the organism. Temporary CSF drainage with a ventriculostomy is used to control intracranial pressure. After 3 to 7 days of antibiotic administration and external drainage, the new shunt is inserted and the course of antibiotics is finished over the next 2 to 5 weeks. If the shunt is functional and only infection is present, a course of antibiotic therapy is carried out. If, following this course, the CSF remains clear of infection, the shunt may be left in. If the infection persists or quickly returns, the shunt apparatus should be replaced even though it is operative. Some feel (Fig. 13–2) that if a gram-negative infection is present, the shunt must be replaced early in the initial treatment with antibiotics.

Some patients will not demonstrate evidence of infection or of overt shunt dysfunction. In these patients, an expectant approach is best.

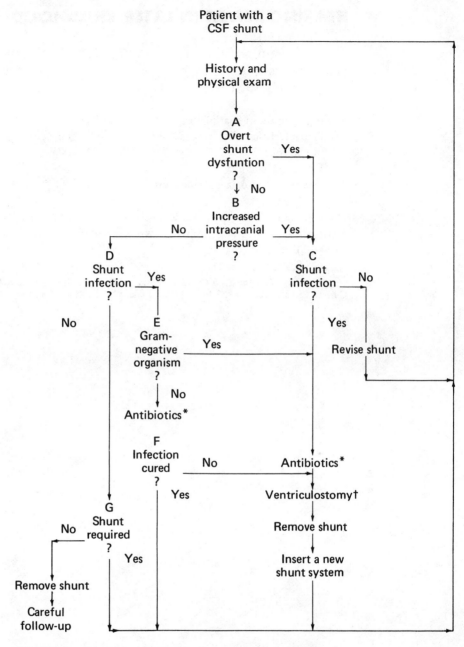

*Choice of antibiotic(s) and route of administration depend upon organism, focus of infection, and type of shunt.

†Proximal portion of shunt can serve as ventriculostomy if obstruction is distal.

FIG. 13-2

Flow diagram illustrating steps in the evaluation of a patient with a cerebrospinal fluid shunt.

Reference: Loeser, J.D., Sells, C.J., and Shurtleff, D.B.: J. Family Practice, 6:285, 1978.

HEARING DEFICIT IN LATER CHILDHOOD

The severity of the handicap associated with hearing deficit during childhood is a function of several factors in addition to the child's hearing levels, such as:

Age at onset of hearing loss
Characteristics of hearing loss (especially abilities in speech discrimination)
Intelligence
Emotional stability
Presence of associated handicaps

The accompanying table outlines the degree of handicap usually associated with given hearing losses, as well as some potentially useful remedial procedures.

Reference: Goodman, A.C., and Chasin, W.D.: *In* Gellis, S.S., and Kagan, B.M. (Eds.): Current Pediatric Therapy. 7th Ed. Philadelphia, W.B. Saunders Company, 1976, p. 518.

HEARING LEVEL IN DECIBELS (DB)	PROBABLE HANDICAP	HAS DIFFICULTY HEARING:	SUSTAINED ATTENTION	SPEECH/ LANGUAGE	MAY BENEFIT FROM
-10 to 26 db normal limits	None for most children; may have some if at upper limits	In classroom for some	May be difficult if at upper limits	Normal	Sitting near front of class or hearing aid, if at upper limits
27–40 db mild loss	Slight for some but significant for many	Faint or distant speech	May be difficult		All above plus instruction in speech reading
41–55 db moderate loss	Significant for most	Conversation beyond 3 to 5 feet, classroom or group discussion	Very difficult	May be defective	All above plus auditory training speech conversation; speech and language therapy
56–70 db moderately severe loss	Marked	Classroom and group discussion	Very difficult	Defective	All above plus special teaching in language skills and perhaps tutoring in academic subjects
71–90 db severe loss	Severe	Anything but shouted or amplified speech; consonants	Very difficult	Severely defective	All above plus school for or classes for deaf children
>90 db profound loss	Extreme	All but some loud sounds		Severely defective	All above

13

DERMATOMES IN DIAGNOSIS

Knowledge of the cutaneous distribution of the dermatomes plays an important role in determining the level of the lesion in patients with neurologic disorders.

The man in Figure 13-3 with his unusual wrinkles should help you in interpreting your neurologic findings.

Dermatome Areas   Dermatome Areas

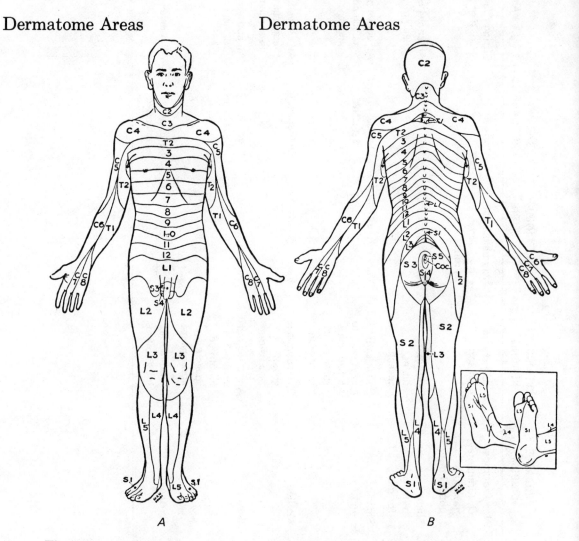

A   *B*

The dermatomes from the anterior view.   The dermatomes from the posterior view.

FIG. 13-3

14
ENDOCRINOLOGY

DIAGNOSIS OF THYROID DISORDERS WITH TRH

With the recent release of synthetic thyrotropin releasing hormone (TRH) by the FDA, a new avenue in the diagnosis of thyroid disorders has developed. The interpretation of thyroid stimulating hormone (TSH) response to TRH stimulation can determine the etiology of four types of thyroid disease: primary, secondary, and tertiary ("hypothalamic") hypothyroidism as well as hyperthyroidism.

TRH is a tripeptide hormone produced by the hypothalamus which stimulates the pituitary to release TSH as well as prolactin. TSH, of course, stimulates the thyroid to make T_3 and T_4.

Figures 14-1 and 14-2 demonstrate how TRH administration may aid in the diagnosis of thyroid disorders.

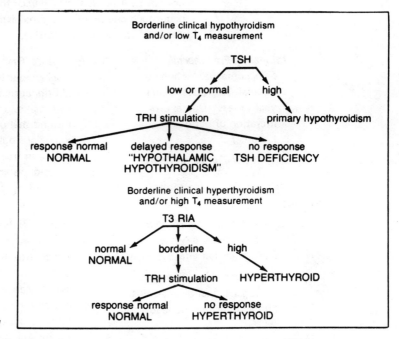

FIG. 14-1

14

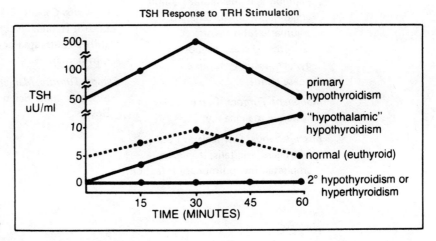

FIG. 14-2

Reference: Wilson, K.: Laboratory Management, 16:38, 1978.

CAUSES OF BREAST ENLARGEMENT

The causes of breast enlargement range from innocent and benign to serious and occasionally fatal. The enlargement seen in newborns isn't worrisome since 60 per cent of all neonates have some degree of enlargement. The evaluation of the older child requires some skill, as the following list indicates.

PREPUBERTAL CHILDREN

Boys

Idiopathic Prepubertal Gynecomastia: Isolated or familial. Regresses in one year or less. (Ductal proliferation or periductal fibrosis.)

Interstitial Tumor of Testis

Adrenal Tumor (secreting estrogen).

Congenital Adrenal Hyperplasia with 11-β-Hydroxylase Deficiency (adrenal estrogen).

Exogenous Causes: Estrogens, androgens, anabolic steroids, human chorionic gonadotropin (HCG).

Benign Tumors: Lipoma, keratoma, papilloma, hemangioma, lymphangioma, neurofibroma, posttraumatic fat necrosis, cellulitis, abscess, pseudogynecomastia (= fat in an obese child).

Malignant Tumors: Carcinoma, systemic malignancy.

Miscellaneous. Cirrhosis of liver (estrogen), digitalis, isoniazid, amphetamine, pulmonary infection.

Girls

Neonatal Breast Hypertrophy: With or without galactorrhea. Occurs in 60% of normal newborns. A residual may persist for months or through childhood (maternal estrogens and possibly endogenous prolactin).

Premature Thelarche: Asynchronous or synchronous breast development without additional signs of sexual maturation. May regress or remain stationary until normal puberty. May herald precocious puberty (transient elevations in free or total serum estradiol observed, transient activation of hypothalamic-pituitary-ovarian axis postulated).

Precocious Puberty: Idiopathic (80%); CNS disorders (5–10%)—brain tumor, encephalitis, hydrocephalus, McCune-Albright syndrome, tuberous sclerosis, neurofibromatosis; hypothyroidism; ovarian tumors (5%)—granulosa cell tumor, theca cell tumor, teratoma, choriocarcinoma; adrenal tumor (secreting estrogen).

Exogenous Causes: Estrogen or stilbestrol (tablets, meat from stilbestrol-treated poultry or cattle, ointments).

Benign Tumors, Malignant Tumors, Miscellaneous: See under Prepubertal Boys.

ADOLESCENTS

Boys

Adolescent Gynecomastia. 70% of prepubertal boys have 1- to 2-cm breast nodules. A more extensive breast enlargement is common. At times, familial male limited autosomal dominant inheritance.

Testicular Tumor: Interstitial cell, choriocarcinoma.

Adrenal Tumor.

3-β-Hydroxysteroid Dehydrogenase Defect.

Primary Testicular Failure, Related Syndromes, Hypergonadotropic States. Klinefelter's syndrome, XX males, syndromes of incomplete male pseudohermaphroditism with defects in testosterone metabolism or action, familial true hermaphroditism (failure to inhibit the female breast anlage due to fetal and androgen deficiency?).

Chromophobe Adenoma of pituitary, hyperprolactinemia, galactorrhea.

Tuberous Sclerosis with hyperprolactinemia.

Liver Cancer (HCG production, conversion of androgens to estrogen).

Benign Tumors, Malignant Tumors, Miscellaneous: See under Prepubertal Boys.

Conditions Associated with Adult Gynecomastia: Recovery from malnutrition with or without systemic disease; drug exposure (estrogen, testosterone, HCG, phenothiazines, meprobamate, hydroxyzine, reserpine, marihuana, spironolactone); trophoblastic tumors; bronchogenic carcinoma; pituitary and CNS tumors and metastases.

Girls

Benign Tumors: Fibroadenoma, cystosarcoma phylloides, lipoma, keratoma, papilloma, granular cell myoblastoma.

Mastopathies: Fibrosis, cystic ductal hyperplasia, lobular hyperplasia, cysts, fibrocystic disease.

Inflammatory Causes: From infection, fat necrosis, and trauma.

Malignant Tumors: Carcinoma, sarcoma, systemic malignancies.

Juvenile Breast Hypertrophy.

14

Reference: Hochman, H.I.: *In* Reece, R.M. (ed.): Manual of Emergency Pediatrics. Philadelphia, W.B. Saunders Company, 1978, p. 565.

SEXUAL MATURITY RATING AND THE SERUM ALKALINE PHOSPHATASE

Tanner has suggested a rating system using sequential acquisition of secondary sexual characteristics, which provides a logic for the highly variable rates (and ages) at which adolescents mature during puberty. This system is outlined below.

Boys

STAGE	PUBIC HAIR	PENIS	TESTES
1	None	Preadolescent	
2	Scanty, long, slightly pigmented	Slight enlargement	Enlarged scrotum, pink, texture altered
3	Darker, starts to curl, small amount	Penis longer	Larger
4	Resembles adult type, but less in quantity; coarse, curly	Larger. Glans penis increased in size	Larger, scrotum dark
5	Adult distribution, spread to medial surface of thighs	Adult	Adult

Girls

STAGE	PUBIC HAIR	BREASTS
1	Preadolescent	Preadolescent
2	Sparse, lightly pigmented, straight, medial border of labia	Breast and papilla elevated as small mound; areolar diameter increased
3	Darker, beginning to curl, increased amount	Breast and areola enlarged, no contour separation
4	Coarse, curly, abundant but amount less than in adult	Areola and papilla form secondary mound
5	Adult feminine triangle, spread to medial surface of thighs	Mature; nipple projects, areola part of general breast contour

Among the physiologic measurements shown to correlate with this rating system is the serum alkaline phosphatase (SAP) level. Elevation of SAP may be a perplexing problem in children in this age group. This elevation has been shown to be a normal phenomenon, related to the child's sexual maturity rating. As illustrated in Figure 14–3, SAP values tend to peak at stages 1 and 3, fall during stage 4, and approach adult norms during stage 5.

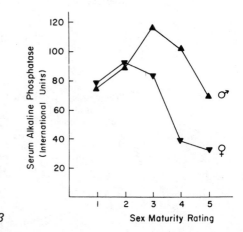

FIG. 14–3

Elevations in SAP seen during normal puberty are due primarily to increases in the bone isoenzyme of alkaline phosphatase. Other causes of elevated SAP, both during puberty and at other times, can be grouped under these broad headings:

Obstructive jaundice
Hepatocellular liver disease
Abnormal bone (calcium/phosphorus) metabolism
Metastatic malignancy in the liver

Reference: Bennett, D.L., Ward, M.S., and Daniel, W.A.: J. Pediatr., *88*:633, 1976.

14

PRECOCIOUS SEXUAL DEVELOPMENT (ISOSEXUAL)

Adolescent sexual development may begin in normal children as early as 8 to 10 years of age in girls and 10 to 11 years in boys. Precocious onset of this process may result from the early secretion of gonadotropic hormone (complete sexual precocity) or from secretion of sex hormones by the gonads or adrenals. The following chart lists the types and etiology of sexual precocity in males and females.

ETIOLOGY	LESION IN MALES	LESION IN FEMALES	CHARACTERISTICS
Gonadotropin Secretion			
Neurogenic	Brain tumor Encephalitis Obscure disorder — hypothalamus	Brain tumor Encephalitis Obscure disorder — hypothalamus Albright's syndrome — (bone dysplasia and pigmentation)	Gonads mature normally Spermatogenesis or ovulation may occur
"Idiopathic" activation of pituitary	None found	None found	Sex hormones excreted in normal adolescent or adult amounts
Gonadotropin-secreting tumor	Hepatoma Teratoma (?) Other (?)	Hepatoma (?) Teratoma (?) Chorioepithelioma (?)	Leydig cell hyperplasia of testes without spermatogenesis
Sex Hormone Secretion			
Gonadal	Interstitial cell tumor of testis	Granulosa cell tumor or (?) cyst Luteoma or thecoma	Tumor usually in one gonad, other gonad may be immature or atrophic Sex hormones *sometimes* excreted in excess amounts
Adrenal	Virilizing adrenal hyperplasia Virilizing tumor	Feminizing adrenal tumor (rare)	Gonads usually immature (some exceptions) 17–KS increased

The cause of sexual precocity must be determined by careful history, physical examination, and laboratory studies. The approach will differ depending upon whether the patient is male or female.

Females

Precocious sexual development occurs twice as frequently in females as in males. Approximately 80 to 90 per cent of females with sexual precocity have the idiopathic (constitutional, cryptogenic) form, and the diagnosis must be one of exclusion. Others will have small undiagnosable hamartomas or other small and benign hypothalamic lesions. Exclusion of other causes is essential, however, and the following list includes the conditions to be considered along with the clinical associations of those conditions.

CONDITION	CLINICAL ASSOCIATIONS
Neonatal estrinization	Breast development and vaginal secretion may occur during the newborn period. They are probably due to maternal and placental hormone stimulation during the prenatal period, and vaginal bleeding may result from estrogen withdrawal following birth.

CONDITION	CLINICAL ASSOCIATIONS
Bleeding due to foreign bodies or lesions in the vagina	Vaginal bleeding without breast development may be due to the presence of a foreign body or a rectovaginal fistula. Vaginal inspection under anesthesia may be necessary.
Estrogen ingestion	Breast development and vaginal changes may be a result of accidental ingestion of estrogen or stilbestrol. Cosmetic creams may be an unsuspected source of estrogens. Ingestion of stilbestrol is often accompanied by blackish pigmentation of the areolae.
Premature thelarche	Early breast development may occur without accompanying development of the labia minora or changes in the vaginal smear. It may be due to oversensitivity of the breast tissue to low levels of circulating estrogen. This condition is entirely benign.
Premature pubarche	Increased sensitivity of sexual hair follicles or early elaboration of adrenal androgens may cause the growth of coarse sexual hair without other sexual changes. These patients eventually mature normally. This condition may suggest the adreno-genital syndrome, but with the latter syndrome there would be rapid progression of sexual maturation and greatly elevated 17-ketosteroids.
True sexual precocity due to intracranial lesions	Urinary gonadotropins are not always elevated. Skull roentgen-ogram and careful neurologic evaluation will usually rule out cerebral tumors in girls, because neurologic symptoms are almost always present prior to signs of sexual development. A history of encephalitic disease points to a cerebral origin of precocity. Cerebral lesions causing early puberty may also occur in tuberous sclerosis and neurofibromatosis.
Gonadotropin-secreting tumor	Chorioepithelioma, teratoma, or hepatoma may cause precocious puberty. The finding of greatly elevated gonadotropins should suggest this diagnosis.
Ovarian neoplasms	Abdominal and rectal examination will usually reveal the presence of a granulosa cell tumor. Urinary estrogens may be elevated in the presence of a granulosa cell tumor. Elevated urinary pregnanediol may accompany a luteoma. In the absence of palpable tumor or elevated hormones, there is little likelihood of feminizing neoplasm.
Adrenal tumor	This diagnosis should be suggested by the presence of elevated urinary 17-ketosteroids.
Fibrous dysplasia (Albright's syndrome)	History may reveal skeletal fractures, and physical examination may reveal pigmented skin lesion. The entire skeleton and skull should be included in an x-ray search for bone lesions.
Hypothyroidism	Sexual precocity has been found along with hypothyroidism in a few cases. The sella turcica may be enlarged. Symptoms and signs abate with treatment of the hypothyroidism.

14

Males

Idiopathic sexual precocity is more unusual in boys than in girls. If the male patient has a family history positive for the condition, he is more likely to have the idiopathic form. Sexual precocity in boys is more likely to be of cerebral origin. Other forms are listed below along with their clinical associations.

CONDITION	CLINICAL ASSOCIATION
Premature pubarche	This is much less frequent in boys than in girls. It includes growth of the penis and testes without accompanying pubic hair. There may be slight elevation of 17-ketosteroids, and epiphyseal development and growth may be slightly accelerated.
Iatrogenic virilization	Anabolic steroids and androgens given to promote growth may be virilizing. Careful history should be taken to ascertain accessibility of androgens to a sexually precocious male child.
True sexual precocity due to intracranial lesion	Gonadotropins are not always elevated with this condition, and 17-ketosteroids are normal or only slightly elevated. Careful neurologic evaluation should be undertaken, and in the absence of another explanation for precocious sexual development, diagnostic radiologic studies should be carried out.
Interstitial cell tumor of the testis	Very high or moderately elevated levels of 17-ketosteroids are present, and they do not decrease with dexamethasone suppression. One testis may be larger than the other.
Virilizing adrenal hyperplasia	Elevated 17-ketosteroids suppress with dexamethasone. There is enlargement of the penis without concomitant testicular enlargement. Testicular biopsy shows no spermatogenesis.
Virilizing adrenal tumor	Elevated 17-ketosteroids do not suppress with dexamethasone. High levels of dehydroepiandrosterone are almost pathognomonic of adrenal tumor.
Teratoma-secreting androgen	Increased levels of chorionic gonadotropin.
Hepatoma	There may be elevated 17-ketosteroids that do not suppress with dexamethasone. Levels of chorionic gonadotropin are exceedingly high. Testicular biopsy shows tremendous Leydig cell hyperplasia with underdeveloped or degenerated seminiferous tubules.
Chorioepithelioma	Increased chorionic gonadotropin.

Reference: Wilkins, L.: *In* The Diagnosis and Treatment of Endocrine Disorders in Childhood and Adolescence. Springfield, Illinois, Charles C Thomas, 1965.

> *Hymen*—The vaginal membrane may owe its name to Hymen, the god of marriages. On the other hand, it may simply derive from *hymen*, Greek for membrane.

THE GIRL WITH DELAYED MENARCHE

The girl who is 14 years old and has not experienced menarche must be further evaluated, even if there is a family history of late onset of menses. Evaluation may be conducted by the pediatrician initially. The largest number of patients will be found to have physiologic delay, anatomic abnormalities, or primary ovarian failure.

The steps to be followed in the initial evaluation are as follows:

1. Physical examination.
   a. Thelarche — The development of the breast bud is the first indication of puberty in the female. If breast buds are present they indicate release of endogenous estrogen by the ovary and indirectly point to the presence of pituitary gonadotropins.

   b. Adrenarche — Pubic hair usually appears shortly after thelarche. Its presence indicates that the ACTH-adrenal androgen axis is functional. Axillary hair does not appear until pubic hair growth in complete. In some females axillary hair never develops.

   c. Growth spurt — A growth velocity chart should be used to determine the patient's growth rate. The peak growth rate for girls during puberty is about 9 cm per year. Menarche occurs after the growth rate has decelerated. The increment in linear growth at menarche is about 5 cm per year, and slower growth rates occur thereafter. The girl who is experiencing the adolescent growth spurt has a good prognosis for the onset of physiologic menarche.

   d. Palpation of the cervix — Palpation of the cervix on rectal or vaginal examination ensures the presence of the uterus. At the same time the examiner can be sure that the hymen is perforate. Other than imperforate hymen and transverse vaginal septum, the most common cause of anatomical delay of menarche is total vaginal agenesis (as is seen in the Rekitansky syndrome in which there are also bilateral, rudimentary, nonfunctional intra-abdominal uteri). Delay of menses because of genital tract obstruction is almost always accompanied by cyclic or constant pelvic pain with bladder irritation.

2. Vaginal smear for hormonal cytology. The smear should be taken from the upper lateral vaginal wall. It should be stained promptly with pinacyanole or

14

Sedi-stain. In girls who are close to menarche, it should show an increase in superficial cells and the presence of Döderlein's bacilli, which indicate that the pH of the vagina has dropped into the adult range. If the patient has no breast development, the vaginal smear is not necessary, since it is extremely unlikely that it will show any estrogen effect. If, on the other hand, the patient has evidence of developing breasts and the vaginal smear shows no estrogen effect, the physician must explain why the ovaries stopped producing hormones. A pituitary tumor may interfere with the release of ovarian steroids after the initiation of breast development.

3. Lateral skull x-ray. Since a pituitary tumor (usually a craniopharyngioma or chromophobe adenoma) may be the cause of delayed onset of menses, the sella turcica should be examined in all girls with menarchal delay. Failure to make this diagnosis early is life-threatening to the patient.

4. Follow-up every 6 months for a year. On return visits repeat height determination and vaginal smear should be performed. Normal phenotype, slight increase in secondary sex characteristics, and a normal cervix and vagina indicate physiologic menstrual delay.

Further Evaluation

5. Buccal smear for chromatin mass. Buccal smear should be obtained on any patient who presents with delayed menarche, short stature, and sexual infantilism.

6. X-rays for bone age. The finding of delayed bone age verifies the diagnosis of physiologic delay of puberty. In addition to the usual anterior-posterior views of the hand, an anterior-posterior view of the pelvis will help predict the onset of the first menstrual period. (*Pelvic x-rays should be performed only after you are certain that the patient is not pregnant.*) The ossification center above the iliac crest is visible radiologically 6 months before to 6 months after the menarche. Pelvic x-rays also aid in detecting tumor calcification that may be present in the patient with gonadal dysgenesis.

7. Gonadotropins, T_4. If the vaginal smear shows no estrogen effect, follicle stimulating hormone (FSH) and luteinizing hormone (LH) should be determined. Serum gonadotropins should be high in primary ovarian failure (FSH over 75 to 80 mI.U./ml of serum). The diagnosis of primary ovarian failure should only be made after elevation of gonadotropins has been determined on two or three consecutive serum samples.

Remember that hyperthyroidism may be a cause of amenorrhea.

8. Cytogenetic studies. Patients with growth retardation and sexual infantilism should have chromosomal determination made because of the risk of primary ovarian failure secondary to gonadal dysgenesis. These patients may have a few menstrual periods followed by secondary amenorrhea, since the streak gonads may occasionally secrete estrogen.

Patients with chronic systemic disease may experience delayed menarche. Although in many cases it is due to primary ovarian failure, careful and complete evaluation should be carried out in any case. If ovarian failure is found, development of secondary sex characteristics may be brought about by cyclic estrogen and progesterone. Patients who receive estrogen substitution therapy for a prolonged period of time should have endometrial biopsies done periodically when they reach adulthood.

Reference: McDonough, P.G.: Adolescent Gynecology, *In* Ross Round Table on Critical Approaches to Common Pediatric Problems, 1977, p. 16.

DIABETES INSIPIDUS — DIAGNOSIS AND TREATMENT

Normally, antidiuretic hormone (ADH) is released from the posterior pituitary at a rate that maintains plasma osmolality between 281.7 and 287.3 mOsm/liter. A defect in this precise regulation may result from any of the following:

> Lack of synthesis of ADH
> A blunted response to osmotic stimuli
> Renal tubular insensitivity to ADH (nephrogenic diabetes insipidus)

Diabetes insipidus of pituitary origin may have the following etiologies:

> Congenital (autosomal dominant)
> Trauma to the posterior pituitary or hypothalamus
> Neoplasm (including craniopharyngioma, glioma, histiocytosis)
> Sarcoidosis
> Surgery

Nephrogenic diabetes insipidus is inherited as an X-linked trait and presents shortly after birth with vomiting, anorexia, constipation, failure to thrive, and retarded psychomotor development.

Diagnosis

Step 1: Initiate fluid deprivation for a 6- to 8-hour period.

Step 2: Obtain urine and plasma at the conclusion of this period for determination of osmolality. In normal individuals the urine osmolality should plateau between 500 and 1400 mOsm/liter, and the plasma osmolality should remain between 288 and 291. The patient with diabetes insipidus will be able to concentrate the urine only to 100 to 200 mOsm/l, while the plasma osmolality may rise to 320 to 330 mOsm/l.

Step 3: Administer 5 units aqueous vasopressin subcutaneously. The normal patient will respond with no increase in urine osmolality. The patient with nephrogenic diabetes insipidus will also have no response to vasopressin because of renal tubular insensitivity. In the patient with diabetes insipidus on a pituitary basis, urine osmolality will approximately double after administration of vasopressin.

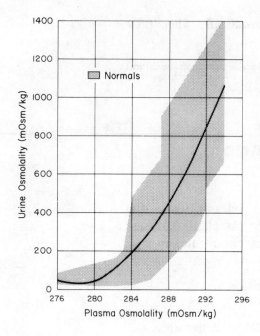

FIG. 14-4

In the normal person the plasma osmolality increases as urine osmolality increases, but plasma osmolality remains within a small range because of normally active ADH.

Caution

1. In patients suspected of having a severe form of diabetes insipidus, the water deprivation test should not be done overnight because of the risk of hypovolemic shock. In these patients, initiate water deprivation in the morning. Collect hourly urines until the osmolality of three urines shows a plateau. At that point collect a blood sample for plasma osmolality. Give aqueous vasopressin, and measure the osmolality of the next two urine samples at half-hour intervals. An increase in urine osmolality of 9 per cent or more following vasopressin administration indicates that the patient has diabetes insipidus.

2. Some patients with diabetes insipidus may be able to prevent a diuresis only at the expense of increased plamsa osmolality. These patients have an intact thirst mechanism and prevent large increases in plasma osmolality by drinking large amounts of fluid. In these patients a plasma osmolality should be determined during water deprivation at a time when the urine osmolality has reached a plateau and before the administration of aqueous vasopressin.

3. In patients who are overhydrated, 12 to 18 hours may be required for urine osmolality to reach a plateau.

Treatment

Treatment of diabetes insipidus depends upon the degree of ADH dysfunction observed.

A. Patients who are essentially devoid of ADH will exhibit no antidiuresis even though plasma osmolality may reach 330 mOsm/l. These patients must be treated with synthetic vasopressin.

B. Patients who do not respond with antidiuresis when plasma osmolality rises to 297 to 300 mOsm/l, but who produce hypertonic urine when stressed to the point of dehydration, show some residual ability to release ADH. These patients may not need hormonal treatment and may respond to chlorpropamide or clofibrate, alone or in combination. These drugs promote ADH release from the neurohypophysis.

C. Patients with diabetes insipidus of renal origin do not respond to hormonal drugs or to clofibrate or chlorpropamide. Thiazide diuretics have been found to produce antidiuresis in these patients by causing sodium depletion and enhanced reabsorption of fluid in the proximal tubule on that basis. Because of this mechanism of action, patients with nephrogenic diabetes insipidus who are being treated with thiazide diuretics should be sodium restricted.

Remember: Some patients may have polyuria and polydipsia on a psychogenic basis. These patients have low serum sodium, low plasma and urine osmolalities, and a normal response to the water deprivation test.

Reference: Moses, A.M.: Hospital Practice, July, 1977, p. 37.

THE PROBLEM OF AMBIGUOUS EXTERNAL GENITALIA

The finding of ambiguous external genitalia in the newborn is a diagnostic challenge to the physician and a great source of anxiety for parents. The more expeditious the approach to a diagnosis, the better. Figure 14–5 illustrates one such approach.

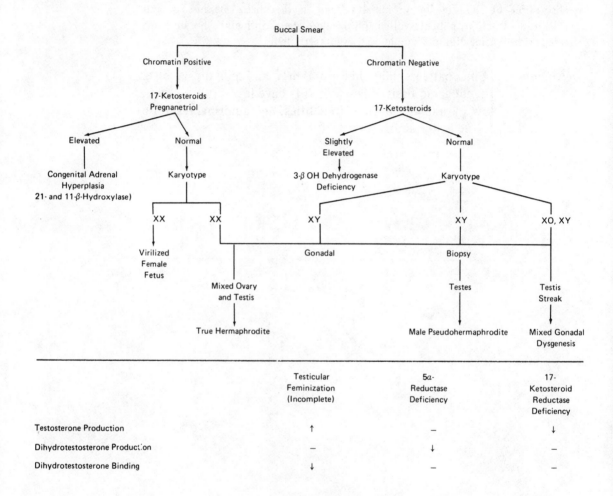

	Testicular Feminization (Incomplete)	5a-Reductase Deficiency	17-Ketosteroid Reductase Deficiency
Testosterone Production	↑	–	↓
Dihydrotestosterone Production	–	↓	–
Dihydrotestosterone Binding	↓	–	–

FIG. 14–5

Reference: Yannone, M.E.: Continuing Education, Oct., 1980, p. 89.

15
SURGERY/ ORTHOPEDICS

LOEB'S LAWS OF MEDICINE

A. If what you're doing is working, keep doing it.
B. If what you're doing is not working, stop doing it.
C. If you don't know what to do, don't do anything.
D. Above all, never let a surgeon get your patient.

Reference: Gottlieb, A.J., Zamkoff, K.W., Jastremski, M.S., Scalzo, A., and Imboden, K.J.: The Whole Internist Catalog. Philadelphia, W.B. Saunders Company, 1980, p. 25.

INTUSSUSCEPTION

The pediatrician is usually the first physician to see a child with an intussusception. Prompt recognition of this acute disorder will reduce morbidity and mortality. Remembering the following facts will facilitate early diagnosis and improve management.

Age of Patients	% Presenting at Given Age
Under 12 months	52%
1 – 2 years	24%
2 – 3 years	10%
3 – 7 years	11%
Over 7 years	3%

Signs and Symptoms	% Presenting with Given Sign or Symptom
Pain	94%
Vomiting (at least once)	91%
Gross blood with stool	66%
Abdominal mass	59%

Patients typically are healthy infants and children with no previous history of gastrointestinal disease. Nearly all infants present with recent onset of abdominal pain and at least one episode of vomiting. The pain is characterized by the child's crying and drawing his legs into his abdomen. Males are affected about twice as often as females. The mass is usually sausage-shaped and is palpable along the course of the colon. On occasion one may elicit Dance's sign — an emptiness in the right lower quadrant that reflects the fact that the intussuscepting bowel has moved out of this portion of the abdomen.

Etiology of Intussusception

In less than 10 per cent of patients will an etiologic factor be determined. Specific causes include Meckel's diverticulum (most common), ileal polyp, ileal granuloma, inspissated meconium in patients with cystic fibrosis, Henoch-Schönlein purpura, and lymphosarcoma.

Although the barium reduction will successfully reduce approximately 75 per cent of all intussusception, *it is advisable for all patients over 6 years of age to have elective exploratory laparotomy because of the high probability that intussusception at this age has a specific cause; it is frequently produced by an intestinal lymphosarcoma.*

Reference: Wayne, E.R., Campbell, J.B., Burrington, J.D., and Davis, W.S.: Radiology, *107*:597, 1973.

APPENDICITIS IN INFANCY

Less than 2 per cent of children treated for appendicitis are under 2 years of age. It is in the infant, however, that the diagnosis may be the most difficult to make. Common symptoms and signs of infantile appendicitis are listed below in decreasing order of frequency.

Symptoms

Vomiting
Pain
Lethargy
Nausea
Feeding problems
Diarrhea

Signs

Tenderness
Fever
Spasm
Guarding
Positive rectal findings
Absent bowel sounds
Mass
Urinary retention

The clinical findings may often be verified by radiographic abnormalities. Approximately 80 per cent of infants in whom the diagnosis of appendicitis is made at surgery will have one or more of the following x-ray findings if both upright and supine films of the abdomen are obtained preoperatively:

Abnormal gas pattern (paucity of gas in RLQ, diffuse
    small bowel dilatation, gas-fluid levels)
Free peritoneal fluid or air
Scoliosis
Obscuration of psoas margin by excessive bowel gas
Thickened abdominal wall
Fecalith
Abscess

Reference: Wilkinson, R.H., Bartlett, R.H., and Eraklis, A.J.: Am. J. Dis. Child., *118*:687, 1969.

"Children are like grown people; the experience of others is never of any use to them."

Daudet

MANAGEMENT OF RESPIRATORY FOREIGN BODIES

Foreign bodies of the ear or respiratory tract are therapeutic as well as diagnostic problems. These guidelines for removal of foreign bodies of various types may help you and your patient.

SITE	FOREIGN BODY DESCRIPTION	SUGGESTION FOR REMOVAL
Ear	Smaller than external canal	Hartman or alligator forceps
	Larger than external canal	Insert loop behind object, then withdraw
	Nonvegetable object	Stream of water
	Vegetable object	Do *not* irrigate (may cause object to swell)
	Attached to drum or associated with perforation	ENT consultation; do not irrigate
	Insect	Irrigate with alcohol before removal
	Metallic object	Use magnet

SITE	SUGGESTIONS FOR REMOVAL
Nose	1. Explain situation to parents; sedate child p.r.n. 2. Spray nasoconstrictor into nostril. 3. Examine local area after cleaning with gentle suction. 4. Remove soft object with forceps; pass loop behind larger or harder objects. 5. If above unsuccessful, try blowing into child's mouth while compressing uninvolved nostril.
Pharynx	Foreign body (e.g., fish bone) imbedded in soft palate or tonsil may be removed with tonsil hemostat. Other foreign body in other pharyngeal sites requires ENT consultation.
Trachea or bronchial tree	Foreign body here requires ENT and/or surgical consultation.
Esophagus	Foreign body at cardioesophageal junction may be observed for 24 to 48 hours. ENT consultation is indicated if no passage by that time. Foreign body at other esophageal sites requires immediate ENT consultation.

Reference: Stool, S.E., and McConnel, C.S., Jr.: Clin. Pediatr., *12*:113, 1973.

TORTICOLLIS

Torticollis, or wryneck, is a sign of a disorder in and around the cervical spine. Pediatricians, all too often, are aware of congenital muscular torticollis but are unfamiliar with a variety of other disorders that may also produce wryneck. The table below describes the types of torticollis and their features.

Types of Torticollis

BASIC PATHOLOGIC PROCESS	UNDERLYING ABNORMALITY	SPECIAL FEATURES
Osseous	Congenital defect of the odontoid process. Hypoplastic odontoid process may result in posterior dislocation of anterior ring of axis	
	Failure of odontoid process to fuse with body of axis	Seen in a variety of forms of dwarfism and in mucopolysaccharidosis.
	Rotary subluxations	May follow "horseplay," upper respiratory infections, sleeping in a draft, a blow to the mandible, and infections in the pharynx.
	Congenital anomalies of the cervical vertebrae, e.g., hemivertebrae	Look for in patients with Klippel-Feil syndrome or Sprengel's deformity.
Ligamentous	Seen rarely in patients with congenital absence of transverse ligament. Results in subluxations or dislocations	Ligamentous laxity observed in patients on high-dosage, long-term steroids.
Muscular	Congenital form appears within 10 days of birth. Fibrous mass present at base of sternocleido-mastoid muscle	Head tilts toward affected muscle-face, rotated to the opposite side. Uncorrected may produce under-development of face on involved side.
	Traumatic injury to muscle	
Neurologic	Posterior fossa tumor	
	Phenothiazine intoxication	May be accompanied by trismus and opisthotonos.
	Syringomyelia	
	Myasthenia gravis	
Ocular	Vertical strabismus as a result of fourth nerve palsy	Patching eye corrects torticollis.
	Congenital nystagmus	
Functional	Rare in children	Disappears with sleep.

Reference: Clark, R.N.: Pediatr. Ann., 5:231, 1976.

15

WHERE IS THE COIN — IN THE ESOPHAGUS OR TRACHEA?

Unfortunately, young children frequently swallow or aspirate foreign bodies. Some of the favorite objects placed in the mouth and subsequently swallowed are coins. Opaque foreign bodies, such as coins, are accurately localized with radiography.

Foreign bodies lie in the plane of least resistance. If a coin enters the esophagus it will lie in a frontal plane and thus appear head-on in the anterior-posterior film of the chest. In contrast, a coin in the trachea will come to rest in the sagittal plane and will appear end-on in the anterior-posterior view of the chest.

Get the x-ray, so you will be prepared to respond when you are asked, "Have you noticed any change in your patient?"

Reference: Holinger, P. H., and Johnson, K. C.: Pediatr. Clin. N. Am., *1:*827, 1954.

INCARCERATED INGUINAL HERNIA IN CHILDREN

Acute incarceration of an inguinal hernia is one of the commonest reasons for emergency surgical admission of young children. Figure 15-1 illustrates the age incidence of both reducible and incarcerated hernias in early childhood. Of hernias appearing in the first 6 months of life, most are incarcerated except in the immediate newborn period. Incarcerated hernias appear to be rare after the age of 3. Young girls are as likely as young boys to have incarcerated hernias. Overall, a predominance of right-sided hernias exists, with 72 per cent of all hernias appearing on the right side alone, while only 19 per cent are on the left side alone. Infarction and necrosis of bowel is actually very uncommon, even with nonreducible hernias. In fact, infarcted testes are more common than infarcted bowel with incarcerated hernias in boys.

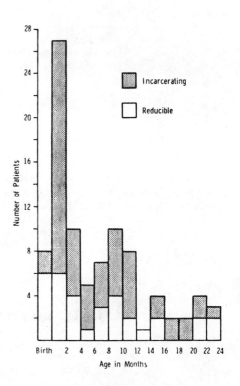

FIG. 15-1

Reference: Palmer, B.V.: Ann. Roy. Coll. Surg., 60:121, 1978.

THE HYDROCELE

A hydrocele is a fluid collection at the bottom of a hernial sac. A hydrocele may represent a physiologic event if the processus vaginalis closed before birth, trapping peritoneal fluid in the scrotal portion of the patent processus vaginalis. This trapped fluid is absorbed, and such a hydrocele will slowly disappear during the first 3 months of life. If an infant over 4 months of age has a hydrocele, it is no longer a physiologic phenomenon but represents an inguinal hernia of the indirect type. The presence of a hydrocele in an infant of 4 months is an indication for an inguinal herniorraphy.

In general, at 35 to 36 weeks gestation the left processus vaginalis is normally closed; about 7 to 10 days later the right processus vaginalis closes. Therefore, it is logical to expect that if a young infant has a visible or palpable hernia on the left side, he probably has a similar lesion on the right side, even if it is not seen or palpated — yet the contrary is not true.

Reference: Koop, C.E.: *In* Visible and Palpable Lesions in Children. New York, Grune & Stratton, 1976, pp. 70-71.

I would like to see the day when somebody would be appointed surgeon somewhere who had no hands, for the operative part is the least part of the work.
Harvey Cushing *(1869–1939)*
Letter to Dr. Henry Christian,
November 20, 1911

LOCAL ANESTHETICS

The choice of a local anesthetic should depend on how rapidly you want it to work and for how long. The onset and duration of selected local anesthetics are as follows:

DRUG	ONSET (MIN)	DURATION (MIN)
Procaine	3	19
Lidocaine	5	40
Mepivacaine	4	99
Tetracaine	7	135
Bupivacaine	8	415

Reference: Mofenson, H.C., and Greensher, J.: N.Y.State J. Med., *80:*57, 1980.

THE THREE MODES OF ONSET
OF JUVENILE RHEUMATOID ARTHRITIS

The onset of juvenile rheumatoid arthritis (JRA) takes three general forms: the acute febrile onset, the monoarticular onset, and poly-articular onset. All three forms may be confused with other diseases, and the diagnosis is often difficult. Awareness of the clinical character-istics of the three presentations of this disease may help avoid the devastating effects of misdiagnosis.

15

	ACUTE FEBRILE ONSET	MONOARTICULAR ONSET	POLYARTICULAR ONSET
Per cent	20	30	50
Joint manifestations	One-half have no joint swelling at onset. The other one-half have only arthralgia. Pain may be inferred from the flexed-knee position in which these children tend to lie.	The knee is most common site of onset. Other sites are ankle, elbow, wrist and finger joints. Swelling, stiffness, and pain are usually minimal. Painful tendinitis or bursitis, especially of the heel, may be the presenting symptom. In early stages, the arthritis may be asymmetrical and migrating.	Four or more joints are involved. May have abrupt onset with painful swelling of knees, ankles, feet, and hands. May have insidious onset with no complaint of pain. Joint involvement must be inferred from guarding movements and knee-flexed position. Arthritis may be migratory at first. Cervical spine may be involved. Subcutaneous nodules are not present.
Fever	Daily spikes to 105° F or higher with temperature falling sometimes to subnormal levels. Fever may precede arthritis by weeks, months, or years.	There may be low-grade daily fever spikes.	Low-grade fever with daily spikes.
Rash	90% have macular or slightly maculopapular rash usually on the trunk and extremities, occasionally on the neck and face. Rash is rarely pruritic, is usually fleeting with macules appearing for a few hours during the day or week, usually in conjunction with fever. Rash is more florid when the skin is rubbed or scratched (Köbner phenomenon).	Rash is sometimes present, but is rarely of diagnostic help.	Maculopapular rash is sometimes present.

	ACUTE FEBRILE ONSET	MONOARTICULAR ONSET	POLYARTICULAR ONSET
Iridocyclitis	Rarely occurs in patients presenting in this way.	This group is most susceptible to ocular disease. It is often asymptomatic and may smolder for weeks or months. It may be the first manifestation of the disease. If undetected and untreated, it may lead to blindness from band keratopathy and cataracts. Diagnosis may be made only by slit lamp examination.	Rarely occurs in patients presenting in this way.
Lymphadenopathy	May be generalized. Splenomegaly may be present. Enlarged mesenteric nodes may lead to abdominal pain and vomiting. Lymphadenopathy may suggest lymphoma or leukemia.	Infrequent.	Infrequent.
Cardiac manifestations	10% have pericarditis clinically. Pericarditis may last 2 to 12 weeks and may recur years later. Myocarditis and resulting heart failure may occur.	—	Infrequent.
General appearance	Patient is usually irritable, listless, anorectic, and suffers from weight loss.	May have generalized symptoms.	Patient is usually listless, anorectic, and underweight.
Laboratory	Neutrophilic leukocytosis with WBC of 15,000 to 50,000/mm^3. There may be a moderate normocytic, normochromic anemia.	CBC and ESR may be normal. X-ray examination may reveal accelerated maturation or early closure of epiphyses, periosteal proliferation, metaphyseal	WBC may be elevated, but is rarely higher than 20,000. ESR is elevated, usually corresponding roughly to the intensity of the arthritis.

Continued

15

overgrowth of long bones, especially about the knee.

The ESR is usually elevated.

Synovial fluid aspiration reveals clear to opalescent fluid with good to poor mucin clot, 15,000 to 25,000 WBC/mm^3 with 50 to 90% neutrophils. Glucose of synovial fluid is about 25 mg/100 ml less than the serum glucose.

Differential diagnosis

Must be differentiated from other connective tissue diseases by absence of antinuclear antibody, difference in the nature of the rash, and age of onset (peak onset of JRA is 1 to 3 years of age, while SLE is rare in children under 5 years of age).

Must be differentiated from traumatic injury and from infectious arthritis by synovial fluid analysis. (Onset of symptoms commonly follows trauma.)

Must be differentiated from rheumatic fever by difference in fever pattern (fever of rheumatic fever is remittent or sustained), by x-ray findings, and by arthritis persisting longer than a few weeks.

Differentiation from the arthritis sometimes accompanying rubella is made by detection of an increase in the HI antibody to rubella in acute and convalescent sera. The synovial fluid of rubella arthritis has a predominance of mononuclear cells.

Reference: Calabro, J.J.: Hospital Practice, February 1974, p. 61.

BONE TUMORS IN CHILDREN AND ADOLESCENTS—THE DIFFERENTIAL DIAGNOSIS

Malignant tumors of bone are rare in the experience of most pediatricians and thus one frequently forgets their diagnostic features. Unwarranted pessimism accompanies their diagnosis. Recent advances in treatment have dramatically improved the prognosis in some of these tumors. Early and precise diagnosis is now more critical than ever for appropriate treatment. The accompanying table describes the salient features of the more common malignant tumors encountered in children and adolescents.

EWING'S SARCOMA	OSTEOGENIC SARCOMA	METASTATIC NEUROBLASTOMA	NON-HODGKIN'S LYMPHOMA	EMBRYONAL RHABDOMYOSARCOMA
Most common in second decade — occurs below age 10	Most common of the bone tumors. Peak incidence in early teens	Usually in children under age 5	No age predilection	Systemic symptoms are rare
Rare in blacks		Long bones symmetrically involved	Long bones most common site	Soft tissue swelling usually initial complaint
Pain most common presenting symptom	Pain most common presenting complaint. Often follows trivial trauma	Lytic lesions can be extensive without soft tissue masses	Diffuse metaphyseal lesions	Lesions of trunk or extremely frequently involve bone as a result of invasion
Flat bones common site (ribs, scapula, pelvis)	Occurs most commonly in long bones (distal femur, proximal tibia, proximal humerus)	Bone marrow often displays tumor cells	Lymphadenopathy and splenomegaly often present	
Femur most common site		Presence of primary tumor. Paraspinal or suprarenal mass most common		Lesions in head and neck usually primary, not metastatic
Diaphyseal lesions in long bones	X-ray films show both lytic and sclerotic changes	Urine positive for VMA and/or catecholamines	Diffuse bone marrow involvement may be seen	
Diffuse osteolytic lesion	Involves metaphysis of bone			
Large soft tissue mass often present — originating in bone	Tissues mass late sign			

15

Reference: Rosen, G.: Pediatr. Clin. North Am., 23:183, 1976.

GROWING PAINS

"Growing pains" are a frequent complaint in children, and knowledge of their usual characteristics may help in differentiating these pains from those associated with other illnesses. Notable features of growing pains are as follows:

Frequency – intermittent.

Intensity – generally mild; however, a few children complain of severe pain that provokes crying.

Location – muscular, *not articular*. The legs are more frequently affected.

Onset – usually in late afternoon or evening. Not provoked by walking. The gait is always normal.

Other findings – pain is occasionally accompanied by restlessness, but never by tenderness, erythema, or local swelling.

Outcome – pain is usually gone by the following morning. It is not associated with organic disease.

Growing pains occur in approximately 15 per cent of children. They are more frequent in girls (18 per cent of girls; 13 per cent of boys). There is a decreasing incidence in boys after age 13, but they may persist in both boys and girls until young adulthood.

Children who have growing pains are more likely to complain of periodic headache and/or abdominal pain as well.

There is no relationship between the rate of growth and the occurrence of growing pains.

Reference: Oster, J., and Nielsen, A.: Acta Paediatr. Scand., *61*:329, 1972.

CONGENITAL DISLOCATION OF THE HIP

"Do you feel that click?" The student who is learning to examine an infant's hips is often not sure of the significance of that question. The more experienced examiner, as well, may feel a click without being sure exactly what it means or what should be done about it.

Some statistics

1. Congenital dislocation of the hip occurs in 1.5 per 1000 live births.
2. The right hip alone is dislocated in 20 percent of cases.
3. Both hips are affected in 25 per cent of cases.
4. Sixty-five per cent of affected infants are females.
5. Fifteen per cent of affected infants are born breech.
6. Frank dislocation is present in 1 of every 35 female infants who are born breech.
7. Younger siblings of an affected child are affected 2.2 per cent of the time.

Definitions

1. Subluxable — the femoral head lies within the acetabulum but can be partially displaced by the examiner.
2. Dislocatable — the femoral head lies within the acetabulum but can be completely dislocated by the examiner.
3. Dislocated — the femoral head lies completely outside the femoral head.

Diagnosis

Newborn. Most congenital hip dislocations occur at or near the time of birth. There is no soft tissue contracture. The proximal femur is normal except for an occasional mild increase in anteversion. The skin creases are most often symmetrical. Roentgenographic changes are subtle in the newborn because no soft tissue contractures or bony abnormalities have developed. The x-ray examination serves only to ensure that there are no other congenital abnormalities of the hips and proximal femurs.

Since the diagnosis rests on the clinical examination and since early treatment is the only insurance against residual morbidity, every newborn should be carefully examined.

It is extremely important that the infant be lying quietly during the examination to avoid muscular tightness.

The Ortaloni maneuver (Fig. 15–2) tests whether the hip is dislocated. The hand of the examiner opposite the hip to be examined is placed with the palm across the infant's back and the thumb gently resting on the anterior pelvis. The examining hand flexes the knee and hip of the side to be examined. The thumb is placed at the mid-thigh (not in the femoral angle), and the long finger lies just over the greater trochanter. If the hip is dislocated, the examiner can feel a slight displacement on gentle abduction of the hip as the femoral head is lifted from the lateral dislocation position to the reduced position.

15

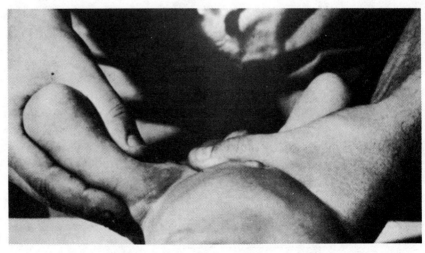

FIG. 15–2

The Barlow maneuver (Fig. 15–3) is used to detect a subluxable or dislocatable hip. The hands are placed in the same position as in the Ortaloni maneuver. The thigh is moved into the abducted position slightly past the midline, and gentle outward force is exerted on it. In a dislocatable hip the femoral head can be felt to displace completely from the acetabulum.

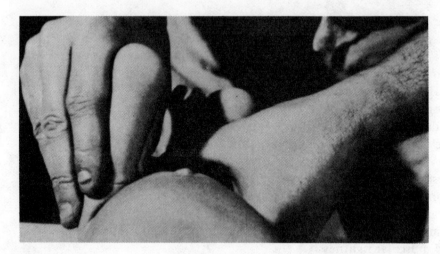

FIG. 15–3

Older infants. Soft tissue contractures and bony abnormalities are present after the infant is 2 to 3 months of age. Femoral shortening may cause asymmetrical flexion creases on the legs.

The walking child. Femoral shortening and limited abduction are present. The leg is held in external rotation. If there is bilateral dislocation, the awkward gait may appear to be simply the waddling of a toddler.

Treatment

Dislocation or dislocatable hips in the infant under 6 months of age may be treated with a harness that maintains the hip in a stable flexed position yet prevents avascular necrosis of the femoral head. Hips that sublux with pressure by the examiner may be treated with triple diapering.

The older child and some young infants in whom soft tissue contractures have developed must be treated with traction followed by reduction under anesthesia.

The child with dislocated or dislocatable hips should be treated only by an orthopedist or a physician who has experience in this area.

Reference: Ramsey, P.L.: Postgrad. Med. *60*:115, 1976.

16
DERMATOLOGY

SKIN LESIONS

You may have had an easier time with the Latin, French, German, or Spanish you learned in high school and college than you have with the language of dermatology. Description of skin lesions, however, is impossible without some knowledge of the dermatologist's vocabulary. The following list defines some of the more commonly useful terms for describing skin lesions. Memorize them, and then see if you can make a sentence using each one.

Types of Lesions

Macule — A circumscribed area of change in normal skin color without elevation or depression of the surface in relation to the surrounding skin.

Telangiectases — Permanent dilatations of blood capillaries that may or may not disappear with the pressure of a glass slide.

Papule — A solid elevated lesion generally understood to be less than 1 cm in diameter.

Plaque — Elevation above the skin surface that occupies a relatively large surface area in comparison with its height above the skin.

Lichenification — A proliferation of keratinocytes and stratum corneum forming a plaque-like structure. The skin appears thickened, and the skin markings appear accentuated. The process results from repeated rubbing.

Nodule — A palpable, solid, round or ellipsoid lesion; it can be located in the epidermis or extend into the dermis or subcutaneous tissue.

Wheal — A rounded or flat-topped elevation in the skin that is characteristically evanescent, disappearing within hours. Lesions are the result of edema in the upper layers of the dermis.

Bulla — A relatively large vesicle (diameter 0.5 cm).

Pustule — A circumscribed elevation of skin that contains a purulent exudate. (Follicular pustules are conical and usually contain a hair in the center.)

Furuncle — A deep necrotizing form of folliculitis with pus accumulation.

Carbuncle — Coalescence of several furuncles.

Abscess — A localized accumulation of purulent material so deep in the dermis or subcutaneous tissue that pus is usually not visible on the surface of the skin.

Cyst — A sac that contains liquid or semisolid material.

Atrophy — Thin, almost transparent epidermis which may or may not retain normal skin lines.

Sclerosis — Circumscribed or diffuse hardening or induration in the skin.

16

ATOPIC DERMATITIS

The diagnosis and treatment of atopic dermatitis requires careful evaluation on the part of the physician and cooperation and understanding between physician and parent (as well as the patient in the years past infancy).

The *infantile stage* rarely begins before 2 to 3 months of age and presists for 2 years. The typical areas of involvement at this stage are the extensor surfaces of the arms and legs and the scalp and face. Vesiculation, erythema, and crusting are usually present.

The *childhood stage* occurs after a remission until 2 to 4 years of age. This stage is characterized by less redness with increased dryness and lichenification. The trunk and flexural areas of the extremities are typically involved. The hands or feet or both may exhibit localized involvement. (Though the involvement of the feet may look like athlete's foot, this is unusual in a preadolescent. Contact dermatitis or atopic dermatitis is the more likely diagnosis for a rash in this area.)

In the *adolescent and adult stage* dermatitis is found on the face, neck, and in the flexural areas of the extremities. Lichenification is common. Dermatitis may resolve in this age group, to be replaced by other forms of atopy such as hay fever or asthma.

The diagnosis may be simplified by the following criteria:

Must have each of the following:

1. Pruritus
2. Typical morphology and distribution:
    a. Flexural lichenification in adults
    b. Facial and extensor involvement in infancy
3. Tendency toward chronic or chronically relapsing dermatitis

plus

Two or more of the following:

1. Personal or family history of atopic disease (asthma, allergic rhinitis, atopic dermatitis)
2. Immediate skin test reactivity
3. White dermographism and/or delayed blanch to cholinergic agents
4. Anterior subcapsular cataracts

or

Four or more of the following features:

1. Xerosis/ichthyosis/hyperlinear palms
2. Pityriasis alba
3. Keratosis pilaris

4. Facial pallor/infraorbital darkening
5. Dennie-Morgan infraorbital fold
6. Elevated serum IgE
7. Keratoconus
8. Tendency toward nonspecific hand dermatitis
9. Tendency toward repeated cutaneous infections

These criteria may be of little value in infancy. At that age the differentiation must be made between seborrheic dermatitis and atopic dermatitis. Seborrhea tends to appear earlier in life, characteristically involves the scalp and postauricular and intertriginous areas, and is not pruritic.

Treatment

Acute phase

1. Burow's solution (one Domeboro packet per pint or per quart in infancy) applied with a soft dish towel one layer thick for 5 to 10 minutes 4 to 6 times a day. The towel should be kept moist during the entire time it is applied.

2. If there is any sign of secondary infection, systemic antibiotics should be used.

3. A potent steroid should be applied thinly following the treatment with Burow's compress. Fluorinated steroids should never be used on the face because of the side effect of permanent, unsightly atrophy, permanent striae, thinning of the skin, and telangiectasia. The following chart lists local steroids in order of potency. Initial treatment should be with the creams or lotions in group IV except on the face. The preparations in groups V and VI should be used on the face. The use of fluorinated steroids in the intertriginous areas should be discontinued as soon as possible. Avoid the use of ointments during the acute, weeping stage because of their occlusive effects.

LOCAL STEROIDS IN ORDER OF POTENCY

Group I	Halog Cream 0.1 per cent
	Lidex Cream 0.05 per cent
	Lidex Ointment 0.05 per cent
	Topsyn Gel 0.05 per cent
Group II	Diprosone Cream 0.05 per cent
	Valisone Ointment 0.1 per cent
	Flurobate Gel (Benisone gel) 0.025 per cent
	Aristocort Cream 0.5 per cent
	Valisone Lotion 0.1 per cent
Group III	Synalar Ointment 0.025 per cent
	Cordran Ointment 0.05 per cent
	Kenalog Ointment 0.1 per cent
	Aristocort Ointment 0.1 per cent
	Synalar Cream (HP) 0.2 per cent

Group IV	Kenalog Cream 0.1 per cent
	Synalar cream 0.025 per cent
	Cordran Cream 0.05 per cent
	Kenalog Lotion 0.025 per cent
	Valisone Cream 0.1 per cent
Group V	Locorten Cream 0.03 per cent
	Tridesilon Cream 0.05 per cent
Group VI	Topical steroids with hydrocortisone, dexamethasone, flumethasone, prednisolone, and methylprednisolone

From Stoughton, R.B.: Bulletin of the Dermatology Foundation, Sept., 1975. There is significant difference of potency of agents within any given group.

4. Aveeno baths may help reduce pruritus. Add ½ cup of this processed oatmeal to ½ tub of tepid water. Hot baths and soap are contraindicated.

5. Sedation may be achieved with Benadryl, 5 to 25 mg, or Atarax, 5 to 25 mg at night.

6. Systemic steroids are seldom necessary. If they are to be used, Prednisone in a single morning dose for 7 to 10 days is the drug of choice.

Chronic phase (two regimens are presented here)

1. Bathing with soap and water is stopped entirely except for the use of a moist wash cloth to cleanse the anus, groin, and axillae.

2. Cetaphil Lotion or Rainbath Dry Skin Bath Gel (Neutrogena) mixed 1:9 with water is used to cleanse the entire skin surface twice a day. The lotion is applied liberally and then removed gently, leaving a thin film on the skin.

3. No oily or greasy lubricants are used.

4. Pruritic areas are treated with a topical steroid as described above.

or

1. Oilated Aveeno bath (½ to 1 cup per tub of tepid water) may be used. If the patient wishes to use bath oil, it should be added near the end of the bath. If it is added initially, it prevents rather than enhances hydration.

2. The patient is dried immediately, and a lubricating lotion is applied to the skin to produce water trapping (Lubriderm Lotion, Nivea Lotion, or Nutraderm Lotion may be used).

3. Appropriate steroid creams are applied to pruritic areas as described above.

Special Notes

1. The patient and the parents must be dealt with gently and carefully. They should be reminded that they are dealing with a condition which cannot be cured but may be controlled with attention to daily detail. They should be reassured that the condition is not contagious, that it does not leave scars, and that hyperpigmentation or hypopigmentation is temporary. They should also be informed that the disease may remit, but that it may be replaced by hay fever or asthma.

2. Because of the complications of eczema herpeticum and vaccinatum, all patients with atopic dermatitis should be isolated from patients with herpes simplex

or patients who have been recently vaccinated. A patient with atopic dermatitis should never receive a smallpox vaccination. Patients with atopic dermatitis are also subject to infection with *Staphylococcus aureus.*

3. Because of the danger of atopic cataracts, it is imperative that an ophthalmologic consultation be obtained if systemic steroids are to be used over an extended period of time.

4. The amount of fluorinated steroid used in the treatment of atopic dermatitis should be kept to a minimum because of possible systemic absorption. Potent topical steroids used with occlusion may also lead to significant systemic absorption.

Reference: Moss, E.M.: Pediatr. Clin. N. Amer., *25*:225, 1978.

ATOPIC DERMATITIS OR SEBORRHEIC DERMATITIS

Do you have trouble distinguishing these two common entities? The following facts may help you in remembering the differences.

	SEBORRHEIC DERMATITIS	ATOPIC DERMATITIS
Family history of allergy	15–25%	40–60%
Character of individual lesions	Dry, scaly, "potato chip" lesion which may or may not appear greasy	Erythema, papules, vesicles, weeping, scales, lichenification, or a combination. May have super-imposed pyoderma
Color of lesion	Only slightly erythematous, but more often of a salmon, yellow, or brown color	In acute phase, always red and often of an intense redness
Feature of lesion	More intense color at periphery — clearing at center. Appears sharply demarcated	More red at center. Gradually tapers out at periphery, fading into normal skin
Vesicles	Never present	Present in acute phase
Weeping and edema	Absent	Always present at some time in evolution of disease
Lichenification	Absent	Characteristic of late stage
Pruritus	Mild or moderate	Paroxysmal and severe

16

Reference: Perlman, H.H.: Ann. Allergy, *23*:583, 1965.

ERYTHEMA NODOSUM

Erythema nodosum is an inflammatory cutaneous manifestation of certain systemic or local inflammatory diseases. These painful lesions are most commonly found on the legs between the knees and the ankles. They also may be found over the elbows, forearms, wrists, or anterior thighs. Although in the past tuberculosis and streptococcal infections were their most frequent cause, other diseases now are also recognized to be associated with these lesions. Remembering them may provide an early clue to diagnosis.

Infection
  Bacterial
    Streptococcus
    Neisseria gonorrhoeae
    Neisseria meningitidis
    Streptococcus pneumoniae
    Yersinia
  Mycobacterial
    Tuberculosis
    Leprosy
  Fungal
    Coccidioidomycosis
    Histoplasmosis
    Blastomycosis
    Monilia
  Other Infectious Agents
    Psittacosis
    Lymphogranuloma venereum
    Influenza

Systemic
  Ulcerative colitis and regional ileitis
  Sarcoidosis
  Systemic lupus erythematosus
  Glomerulonephritis

Drugs
  Iodides
  Bromides
  Sulfa drugs, including acetazolamide and tolbutamide
  Birth control pills

Miscellaneous
  Behçet's syndrome
  Secondary to positive skin test
  Pancreatitis

References: Blomgren, S.E.: N.Y. State J. Med., *72*:230, 1974. Beachler, K.J.: Brooke Army Medical Center Progress Notes, *18*:13, 1974.

IS IT REALLY KAWASAKI'S DISEASE?

Motorcycle jokes aside, Kawasaki's disease (mucocutaneous lymph node syndrome) has become as much an American disease as McDonald's hamburgers have become a fast-food item in Japan. Every house officer seems to make this diagnosis five times more frequently than that of scarlet fever and other more common red rashes. Is it really Kawasaki's disease? Figure 16-1 shows us what to expect if and when we are to make this diagnosis, and the table below helps us to distinguish this disorder from its imitators.

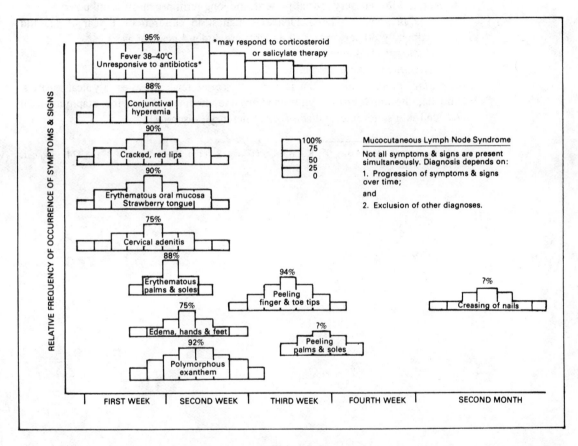

FIG. 16-1

Familiarity with its features will help you to make the diagnosis.

Major Manifestations

Fever in excess of 38.5° C for five days
Redness and induration of palms and soles
Desquamation of skin over fingers during convalescence
Polymorphous exanthem over trunk; no vesicles
Conjunctivitis
Redness and fissuring of the lips
Strawberry tongue
Diffuse redness of oropharynx
Acute, nonpurulent swelling of cervical lymph nodes

Other features of the disease may include tachycardia, gallop rhythm, distant heart sounds, heart murmurs, EKG changes, diarrhea, proteinuria, pyuria, leukocytosis, mild anemia, elevated platelet count, increased erythrocyte sedimentation rate, and increasing level of IgE during period of illness.

Less frequent manifestations include arthralgia, arthritis, aseptic meningitis, and mild jaundice.

Mortality is approximately 1 to 2 per cent. Deaths are due primarily to coronary artery thrombosis and resultant myocardial infarction, and occur late in the course of the disease. Coronary angiography during the illness may reveal abnormalities in as many as 60 per cent of patients. These include aneurysms, dilatation, stenosis, tortuosity, and irregularity of arterial vessel walls. These appear to regress with recovery, but at present, the long-term prognosis is unknown.

Age Incidence: The incidence is highest in children of 1 year of age and approximately 80 per cent of all patients are under 4 years of age.

Etiology: Unknown.

Treatment: None that is effective.

May mimic some of the features of scarlet fever, measles, atypical measles, rubella, Stevens-Johnson syndrome, juvenile rheumatoid arthritis, staphylococcal scalded-skin syndrome, and acrodynia (mercury poisoning).

References: Kawasaki, T., Kosaki, F., Okawa, S., et al.: Pediatrics, *54*:271, 1974. Lancet, *1*:675, 1976.

CLINICAL FEATURES OF MUCOCUTANEOUS LYMPH NODE SYNDROME (MCLS) AND OTHER MUCOCUTANEOUS SYNDROMES

	MCLS	Infantile Polyarteritis Nodosa	Erythema Multiforme Minor	Erythema Multiforme Exudativum	Streptococcal Scarlet Fever	Staphylococcal Scarlet Fever	Toxic Shock Syndrome	Leptospirosis	Tick Typhus	Reiter's Syndrome
Age, yr	Usually <5	Usually <1	All ages	Usually 3-30	Usually 2-8	Usually 2-8	Usually adolescent	Usually >2	Usually >5	Usually >10
Fever	Prolonged	Prolonged	Prolonged	Prolonged	Variable	Variable	Usually <10 days	Variable	Usually 5-10 days	Prolonged
Eyes	Hyperemia of the ocular conjunctivae	Hyperemia of the ocular conjunctivae	Hyperemia of the ocular conjunctivae; palpebral edema	Catarrhal conjunctivitis; chemosis; iritis; uveitis; panophthalmitis	No change	Hyperemia of the ocular conjunctivae	Hyperemia of the ocular conjunctivae	Hyperemia of the ocular conjunctivae; uveitis	Hyperemia of the ocular conjunctivae; palpebral edema	Hyperemia of the ocular conjunctivae; keratitis; iritis; uveitis
Lips	Red, dry, fissured	Red	Erosions; ulcerations	Erosions; crusted, fissured, bleeding	No change	No change	Red	No change	No change	No change
Oral cavity	Diffuse erythema; "strawberry tongue"	Diffuse erythema	Erosions, aphthous-like ulcerations	Erythema; bullae, ulcers, pseudomembrane formation	Pharyngitis; palatal petechiae; "strawberry tongue"	Pharyngitis	Erythema; pharyngitis	Pharyngitis	Erythema	No change
Peripheral extremities	Erythema of palms and soles; indurative edema; periungual desquamation	Erythema of palms and soles; swelling of hands and feet; dry gangrene (rare)	No change	No change	Periungual membranous desquamation	No change	Swelling of the hands and feet; dry gangrene	Gangrene of the hands and feet (rare)	Swelling of the hands and feet	No change
Exanthem	Erythematous, polymorphous	Erythematous, polymorphous	Erythematous, polymorphous; iris lesions	Erythematous, polymorphous; iris lesions, vesicles, bullae, crusts	Finely papular erythroderma; Pastia's lines, circumoral pallor	Finely papular erythroderma; Pastia's lines	Erythroderma	Erythematous, maculopapular, petechial, or purpuric	Maculopapular, petechial; centrifugal	Erythematous, evanescent

Continued

16

CLINICAL FEATURES OF MUCOCUTANEOUS LYMPH NODE SYNDROME (MCLS) AND OTHER MUCOCUTANEOUS SYNDROMES (Continued)

	MCLS	Infantile Polyarteritis Nodosa	Erythema Multiforme Minor	Erythema Multiforme Exudativum	Streptococcal Scarlet Fever	Staphylococcal Scarlet Fever	Toxic Shock Syndrome	Leptospirosis	Tick Typhus	Reiter's Syndrome
Cervical lymph nodes	Nonpurulent swelling; unilateral (frequent)	Nonpurulent swelling (frequent)	No change	Nonpurulent swelling (occasional)	Nonpurulent or purulent swelling (frequent)	Nonpurulent or purulent swelling (occasional)	No change	Nonpurulent swelling (infrequent)	No change	No change
Other	Meatitis; diarrhea; arthralgia and arthritis; meningitis; rhinorrhea (uncommon); ECG changes	Rhinorrhea and cough (common); diarrhea; ECG changes	Malaise; rhinorrhea; arthralgia; recurrent episodes	Malaise; cough, rhinorrhea, pneumonitis; vomiting; arthralgia; recurrent episodes	Malaise; vomiting		Headache; confusion; hypotension; icteric hepatitis; diarrhea; coagulopathy; renal injury	Headache; myalgia; abdominal pain; icteric hepatitis; meningitis	Headache; myalgia; photophobia; arthralgia; splenomegaly; stupor	Dysuria and urethritis; arthralgia and arthritis

Reference: Yanagihara, R., and Todd, J.K.: Acute febrile mucocutaneous lymph node syndrome. Am. J. Dis. Child., *134:*603, 1980. Copyright 1980, American Medical Association.

SIGNS OF NEUROFIBROMATOSIS

Neurofibromatosis may present in unusual ways. The clues are often missed on repetitive routine examinations. Apparently isolated findings such as scoliosis occurring at an unusual age or the early onset of breast development may, in fact, be indicative of neurofibromatosis. A careful dermatologic examination will detect the vast majority of children within the first year of life. The most common findings in neurofibromatosis include:

1.	Café au lait spots and cutaneous fibromas	72%
2.	Positive family history	46%
3.	CNS lesions	26%
4.	Retarded development	24%
5.	Skull or facial deformities	22%
6.	Scoliosis	20%
7.	Breast enlargement	13%
8.	Seizures	13%
9.	Hemihypertrophy	13%
10.	Isolated benign tumors	11%
11.	Extracranial malignancy	11%
12.	Vascular disease	9%

Reference: Fienman, N. L., and Yakovac, W. C.: J. Pediatr., *76:*339, 1970.

WHITE SPOTS IN TUBEROUS SCLEROSIS

Adenoma sebaceum is present in 80 to 90 per cent of patients with tuberous sclerosis, but only 13 per cent of children manifest this finding in the first year of life when seizures may have already developed. Shagreen patches are noted in 20 to 50 per cent of patients but usually appear between the second and fifth birthday. Café au lait spots are fairly common (26 per cent), but their significance is unknown since it is rare to see more than one or two in tuberous sclerosis. Periungual and gingival fibromas do not appear until puberty and thus are of little value in the early diagnosis of this disorder.

White spots (leukoderma), rare in normal children, are seen in 78 per cent of cases with tuberous sclerosis. These may be small (white freckles measuring 2 to 3 mm) or large (7 to 8 cm), but only 18 per cent of white spots are the typical ash leaf shape. Parents of children with tuberous sclerosis uniformly comment that these white spots were present at birth. They neither increase in size or number as the child becomes older nor do they disappear. Their detection is facilitated by the use of a Wood's lamp. The white spots of tuberous sclerosis must be differentiated from vitiligo. This may be accomplished by following the criteria in the table below.

Reference: Hurwitz, S., and Braverman, I. M.: J. Pediatr., *77:*587, 1970.

Differential Criteria Between White Spots and Vitiligo

CRITERIA	LEUKODERMA IN TUBEROUS SCLEROSIS	VITILIGO
Age of onset	Birth or neonatal period	Any age; rare in infants
Location	Trunk, arms, and legs	Face, neck, hands, feet, body folds, and around the body orifices
Depigmentation	Partial	Usually complete
Color	Dull white	Ivory white
Course	Does not change with age	Frequently spreads; sometimes repigments spontaneously
Melanocytes	Normal in number with reduction in size of melanosomes and melanin granules within them	Absent or decreased in number

RELIEVING THE STING OR THE ITCH

Although a number of drugs and lotions are available for the treatment of bites and rashes, home remedies are often as good or even better in producing relief. Here are some tried and true home remedies:

FOR	TRY
Bee stings, wasp stings, and jellyfish bites	Adolph's meat tenderizer. Add a little water to the powder and rub into the bite. Expect relief in minutes.
Poison ivy	Ban roll-on deodorant. Just rub on the rash and rub away the itch.
Chickenpox	Spray starch. Just spray the lesions with this laundry starch.
Chigger bites	Clear nail polish. Paint each bite with nail polish. The chigger suffocates and the itch disappears.

All these remedies, which have a long history of success in the South, were suggested by Barbara Davis, Dr. P. Charlton Davis, Ann Derrick, and Dr. Warren Derrick. If they don't work you can write to them in Columbia, South Carolina.

Pruritus—This often seems to be misspelled with *-itis* at the end. The word is Latin and comes from the verb to *itch, prurire,* as does the word *prurient,* with the sense of itching for or yearning for something sexual. Interestingly, other Latin words ending *-itus,* such as *detritus, decubitus,* and of course *cubitus,* are almost never misspelled.

16

CUTANEOUS REACTIONS TO DRUGS

The Boston Collaborative Surveillance Program estimated the rates of allergic skin reactions to commonly employed drugs in 22,227 patients admitted consecutively to participating hospitals. Reactions to penicillin or blood products affected 38 per cent of the patients and accounted for 70 per cent of the skin reactions observed.

Once these patients were subtracted from the data base, the detection of individual drugs that produced skin reactions was based on two criteria: the frequency of reactions in the patients receiving the drug in question had to be at least twice as high as the frequency of reactions in the remaining patients at large, and a characteristic cluster of rashes had to appear in the days after the first exposure to the drug.

Clearly the data are firmer for the drugs received by at least 1000 patients. The list is also a good indication of drug utilization in a hospitalized population.

DRUG	NO. OF REACTIONS	NO. OF RECIPIENTS	REACTION RATE PER 1000 PATIENTS
Trimethoprim-sulfamethoxazole	10	169	59
Ampicillin	156	2988	52
Semisynthetic penicillin	27	760	36
Whole blood	32	908	35
Corticotropin	3	106	28
Platelets	4	145	28
Erythromycin	11	481	23
Sulfisoxazole	8	462	17
Penicillin G	51	3286	16
Practolol	2	128	16
Gentamicin sulfate	10	607	16
Cephalosporins	17	1308	13
Plasma protein fraction	3	245	12
Quinidine	8	652	12
Dipyrone	10	876	11
Mercurial diuretics	6	630	9.5
Nitrofurantoin	2	219	9.1
Packed red blood cells	11	1366	8.1
Chloramphenicol	2	292	6.8
Trimethobenzamide hydrochloride	5	752	6.6
Phenazopyridine hydrochloride	1	153	6.5
Methenamine	1	157	6.4
Nitrazepam	7	1118	6.3
Cyanocobalamin	3	486	6.2

DRUG	NO. OF REACTIONS	NO. OF RECIPIENTS	REACTION RATE PER 1000 PATIENTS
Barbiturates	22	4658	4.7
Glutethimide	1	221	4.5
Indomethacin	1	229	4.4
Chlordiazepoxide	9	2161	4.2
Metoclopramide hydrochloride	1	247	4.0
Diazepam	18	4692	3.8
Propoxyphene	10	2976	3.4
Isoniazid	2	675	3.0
Guaifenesin and aminophylline	7	2440	2.9
Nystatin	1	342	2.9
Chlorothiazide	2	707	2.8
Furosemide	9	3497	2.6
Isophane insulin	1	777	1.3
Phenytoin	1	905	1.1
Phytonadione	1	1111	0.9
Flurazepam hydrochloride	1	1862	0.2
Chloral hydrate	1	4809	0.2

Reference: Arndt, K.A., and Jick, H.: J.A.M.A., *235:*918, 1976.

16

17
GENETICS

THE RISK OF PRODUCING A CHILD WITH CYSTIC FIBROSIS

At the present time there is no convenient, reliable method for detecting either the heterozygote for cystic fibrosis or the homozygote in utero.

Genetic counseling, at present, is limited to providing risk calculations. The table below should assist you in such counseling. It is based on the assumption that the prevalence of cystic fibrosis is 1 in 1600 in the Caucasian population, and its mode of inheritance is autosomal recessive with complete penetrance. The risk in blacks and Orientals is very much lower.

ONE PARENT	THE OTHER PARENT	RISK OF CYSTIC FIBROSIS IN EACH PREGNANCY
No CF history	No CF history	1 in 1600
No CF history	With first cousin with CF	1 in 320
No CF history	With aunt or uncle with CF	1 in 240
No CF history	With sib with CF	1 in 120
No CF history	With CF child by previous marriage	1 in 80
No CF history	With parent having CF	1 in 80
No CF history	Has CF	1 in 40
With sib with CF	With sib having CF	1 in 9
With CF child	With CF child	1 in 4

Reference: Bowman, B.A., and Mangos, J.A.: N. Engl. J. Med., *294*:937, 1976.

"Man, discontented with the present, imagines for the past a perfection that never existed. He praises the dead out of contempt for the living, and beats the children with the bones of their ancestors."

Comte de Volney, Constantin
François de Chasseboeuf

17

THE FETAL ALCOHOL SYNDROME

It is now quite clear that infants born to mothers with severe chronic alcoholism display a recognizable pattern of malformations as well as abnormalities of growth and development. It is important to be aware of these abnormalities. When they are present, a careful and nonthreatening discussion should be held with the parents in an attempt to determine if alcohol abuse might be responsible for the patient's problems.

The more common abnormalities include the following.

ABNORMALITY	PER CENT OF PATIENTS
Growth and Performance	
Prenatal growth disturbance	97
Postnatal growth deficiency	97
Microcephaly	93
Developmental delay or mental deficiency	89
Fine-motor dysfunction	80
Craniofacial	
Short palpebral fissures	92
Midfacial hypoplasia	65
Epicanthic folds	49
Limb	
Abnormal palmar creases	49
Minor joint anomalies	41
Other	
Cardiac defects	49
Minor anomalies of external genitalia	32
Hemangiomas	29
Minor ear anomalies	22

Other defects that may be present include microphthalmos, intraocular defects, strabismus, ptosis of eyelids, cleft palate, pectus excavatum, diaphragmatic anomalies, hypoplastic nails, pigmented nevi, and hirsutism.

These abnormalities can be recognized at birth. Be suspicious of the fetal alcohol syndrome in infants who are born small for gestational age or who fail to thrive. Two examples of patients with characteristic facies are shown in Figure 17-1.

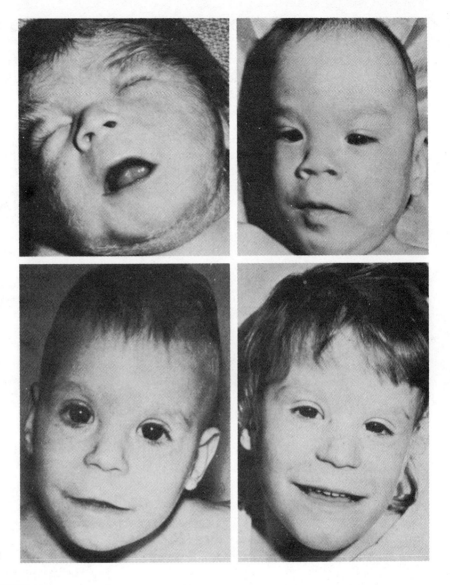

FIG. 17-1

Reference: Hanson, J.W., Jones, K.L., and Smith, D.W.: J.A.M.A., *235*:1458, 1976.

17

THE HAND AS AN AID TO DIAGNOSIS

Although the art of palmistry may be dead, there is still much to learn from the examination of the hand. A careful look at the hands may provide a clue to a long list of syndromes or disease states. The hand should be examined in a systematic fashion. These steps include:

1. Inspection of the dorsum of the hand, paying particular attention to the texture of the skin and hair.
2. Flex the hand to determine the length of the metacarpals. Normally, a line drawn across the tips of the metacarpals of the little and ring fingers will be distal to the tip of the metacarpal of the long finger. If this is not the case the patient may have brachymetacarpalia.
3. Examine finger shape.
4. Examine the finger joints and test their range of motion.
5. Examine the nails.
6. Examine the palm, note the size of the thenar and hypothenar eminences. Ask the patient to squeeze your fingers to determine muscle strength.
7. Determine the length and width of the fingers.
8. Examine the palmar creases.
9. Check the wrist for range of motion.
10. Palpate the radial pulse.

The lists that follow are provided to help you interpret the significance of your findings.

Abnormalities Associated with Clinodactyly of the Little Finger

Absent pectoral muscle
Acral-renal syndrome
Ankyloglossum superins syndrome
Bird-headed dwarf (Seckel's)
Bloom's syndrome
Brachydactyly (type A^3)
Cornelia de Lange syndrome
Familial brachydactyly
Fanconi's syndrome
Focal dermal hypoplasia
Holt-Oram syndrome
Kirner's deformity
Larsen's syndrome
Laurence-Moon-Biedl syndrome
Meckel's syndrome

Myositis ossificans progressiva
Oculodentodigital syndrome
Oral-facial-digital syndrome
Osteoonychodysplasia
Otopalatodigital syndrome
Popliteal pterygium syndrome
Prades-Willi syndrome
SC syndrome
Silver's syndrome
Smith-Lemli-Opitz syndrome
Symphalangism
Thrombocytopenia-absent radius (TAR)
Treacher-Collins syndrome
Turner's syndrome
Zellweger's syndrome

CHROMOSOMAL DISORDERS

Extra metacentric chromosome
4p-
Trisomy 6-12
Ring 13
Mosaic trisomy 15
Partial deletion of chromosome #5

Pseudo 18
Translocation 17-18
Trisomy 21
XXXXX
XXXXY-Klinefelter

Abnormalities Associated with Clinodactyly and Short, Little Fingers

Cornelia de Lange syndrome
Embryo poisoning with Cytoxan
Gargoylism
Nail patella syndrome
Oral-facial-digital syndrome

Papillon-Léage-Psaume syndrome
Proximal symphalangism
Russel dwarf
Silver's syndrome
Turner's syndrome

CHROMOSOMAL DISORDERS

Partial deletion of #5 chromosome

Trisomy 21 (Down's syndrome)
XXXXY

Abnormalities Associated with Syndactyly

Absent ulna
Acrocephalosyndactylism
Aglossia-adactylia
Alopecia congenita
Apert's syndrome
Aplasia cutis congenita
Bloom's syndrome
Brachydactyly
Cleft hand
Cleft lip
Cleft palate
Congenital heart disease
Corradi's disease
Crouzon's disease
Cryptophthalmia
Deficiency of long bones
Ectodermal dysplasia (hypohydrotic)
Focal dermal hypoplasia
Glossopalatine ankylosis
Goltz syndrome
Hallermann-Streiff syndrome
Hemihypertrophy
Hereditary abnormalities
Hypertelorism
Incontinentia pigmenti
Klippel-Trenauney syndrome
Lateral facial cleft
Laurence-Moon-Biedl syndrome

Lip pits
Maternal radiation
Maternal riboflavin deficiency
Meckel's syndrome
Micrognathia-polydactyly-genital
  anomalies
Möbius' syndrome
Multiple congenital deformities
Neurofibromatosis
Oblique facial cleft
Oculodentodigital dysplasia
Orodigitofacial dysostosis
Osteogenesis imperfecta
Papillon-Léage-Psauma syndrome
Pectoral muscle absence
Pierre Robin syndrome
Pili annulati
Poland's syndrome
Polydactyly
Popliteal pterygium
Prader-Willi syndrome
Pseudoainhum
Silver's syndrome
Synostosis
Thalidomide poisoning
Thrombocytopenia — absent radius
Ventriculoseptal defect
Waardenburg's syndrome

CHROMOSOMAL DISORDERS

B-D translocation
Extra metacentric chromosome
  triploidy

Trisomy 18
Trisomy 21 (Down's syndrome)

17

Abnormalities Associated with Polydactyly

Absence of abductor muscles
Acral-renal syndrome
Albinism
Anophthalmia microphthalmia
Apert's syndrome
Aplasia cutis congenita
Aplasia of tibia
Biemond's syndrome
Bifid tongue
Blepharoptosis
Bloom's syndrome
C syndrome
Cebocephaly
Cheilognathoglossoschisis
Cleft hand
Cleft lip
Cleft palate
Congenital ichthyosiform erythroderma
Conradi's syndrome
Cyclops
Ectodermal hypohydrotic dysplasia

Ellis-van Creveld syndrome
Epidermolysis bullosa
Familial brachydactyly
Focal dermal hypoplasia
Goltz syndrome
Hereditary abnormalities
Hydrometrocolpos
Ichthyosis simplex
Klippel-Trenannay-Webber syndrome
Lateral facial cleft
Laurence-Moon-Biedl syndrome
Lissencephaly
Maternal radiation
Meckel's syndrome
Medial and oblique facial cleft
Milroy's disease
Orodigitofacial dysostosis
Pili annulati
Smith-Lemli-Opitz syndrome
Syndactyly
Ventriculoseptal defect

CHROMOSOMAL DISORDERS

Trisomy 15

Abnormalities Associated with a Single Palmar Crease

Acrocephalosyndactyly X
Anencephaly
BBB syndrome
C syndrome
Cleft lip/palate (4%)
Coffin-Siris syndrome
Cornelia de Lange syndrome
Epilepsy
First arch syndrome
Hirschsprung's disease
ISC syndrome
Kidney-liver-hand syndrome
Lenz's syndrome
Lissencephaly
Manic-depressive psychosis
Maple syrup urine disease

Mental retardation (10%)
Nonmongol mental defectives (13%)
Noonan's syndrome
PKU (25%), institutionalized
Pseudohypoparathyroidism
Psoriasis
Rubella syndrome
Rubinstein's syndrome
Schwartz's syndrome
Seckel's dwarf
Smith-Lemli-Opitz syndrome
Thalidomide poisoning
Thrombocytopenia, absent radius
Treacher-Collins syndrome
Zellweger syndrome

CHROMOSOMAL DISORDERS

Autosomal isochromosome	12 (C autosomy)
2 D translocation	Partial trisomy 13-15 (isochromosome)
4 short arm deletion	Trisomy 15
Long 4-5 chromosome	Trisomy 18
4-5/? 6-X-12	Trisomy 21 (Down's syndrome)
4-5/? and partial trisomy of ?	Trisomy 22
donor chromosome	XO-Turner's syndrome
4-5/13-15 reciprocal translocation	XO/XX/XXX
4-9 translocation and partial trisomy	XXXXX
5 ?/?	
6-partial deletion	

Abnormal Thumbs and Physical Diagnosis

Thumb hypoplasia (radial dysplasia)	Skeletal, renal, central nervous, cardiovascular (Oram-Holt syndrome), gastrointestinal, ear, palate, lip, face, genital, pulmonary and ophthalmologic abnormalities. Thalidomide, mandibulofacial dysostosis, trisomy 18, ankyloglossum superius syndrome, Rothmund-Thomson syndrome
Fingerlike thumb	Fanconi's syndrome, congenital heart disease, congenital anemia.
Short thumbs	Smith-Lemli-Opitz syndrome, myositis ossificans progressiva, popliteal pterygia syndrome, aglossia-adactylia syndrome
Short broad thumbs	Rubinstein-Taybi syndrome, oto-palatodigital syndrome, Larsen's syndrome, Leri's pleonosteosis
Retroflexible thumbs	Trisomy D_1, partial trisomy D_1, diastrophic dwarfism, Rothmund-Thomson syndrome
Low-set thumbs	Trisomy 22, Cornelia de Lange syndrome
High-set thumbs	Trisomy 18, partial trisomy 18 (4/18 translocation)
Bifid thumbs	Focal dermal hypoplasia syndrome, translocation 3/13, cyclopia, familial absence of middle phalanges with nail dysplasia
Flexed thumbs	Arthrogryposis, whistling-face syndrome, trigger thumb
Thumb sign	Marfan's syndrome

17

Reference: Johnson, C. F.: The Child's Hand. A Key to Diagnosis. MEDCOM, 1973.

OPHTHALMOLOGIC MANIFESTATIONS OF INHERITED DISORDERS

The examination of the eye is often a clue to the diagnosis of a wide variety of inherited disorders. Did you know that long eyelashes may be suggestive of hereditary spherocytosis? The table below outlines various parts of and disorders affecting the eye. Details of the specific anomalies may be seen in the reference.

TISSUE	INHERITED DISORDERS
Eyelids	Amyloidosis
	Cornelia de Lange syndrome
	Maple syrup urine disease
	Porphyria, hepatic
	Hereditary spherocytosis
	Urbach-Wiethe syndrome (lipid proteinosis)
	Zeroderma pigmentosa
Corneal epithelium	Familial dysautonomia (Riley-Day syndrome)
	Fabry disease
	Tyrosinemia
Corneal stroma	Cystinosis
	Hyperlipoproteinemia, type II
	Lecithin: choline acyltransferase (LCAT) deficiency
	Muscular dystrophy
	Lattice dystrophy
	Schnyder crystalline dystrophy
	Mucopolysaccharidosis (Hurler, Scheie, Hunter, Morquio, and Maroteaux-Lamy)
	I-cell disease
	Tangier disease
	Wilson's disease
Conjunctiva and Sclera	Alkaptonuria
	Ataxia-telangectasia
	Porphyria (erythropoietic)
Lens: Cataract forming	Galactosemia
	Galactokinase deficiency
	Glucose-6-phosphate-dehydrogenase deficiency (G-6-PD)
	Lowe's syndrome
	Pseudohypoparathyroidism
	Pseudo-pseudo-hypoparathyroidism
Lens dislocation	Homocystinuria
	Hyperlysinemia
	Sulfite oxidase deficiency
	Marfan's syndrome

TISSUE	INHERITED DISORDERS
Pigment Epithelium	Abetalipoproteinemia Albinism Gangliosidosis GM_1 type II GM_2 type III Mucopolysaccharidosis (Sanfilippo) Neuronal ceroid lipofuscinosis (Batten disease) Refsum's syndrome
Macula	Farber lipogranulomatosis Gangliosidosis (Tay Sachs, Sandhoff and generalized) Glycogen storage disease type I (Von Gierke) Goldberg-Cottier syndrome Lactosyl ceramidosis Metachromatic leukodystrophy Niemann-Pick disease Sea-blue histocyte syndrome Wolman disease
Retinal vessels	Diabetes mellitus Hemoglobinopathies (sickling) Hyperlipoproteinemia Types I, III, IV, V Porphyria, acute – intermittent
Optic nerve	Globoid cell leukodystrophy (Krabbe disease) Hyperphosphatasia Hypophosphatasia

Reference: Berman, E. R.: The eye and inborn errors of metabolism. The National Foundation-March of Dimes, Birth Defects: Original Article Series, *12*(3), 1976. New York, Liss Co., 1976, p. 15.

17

RECURRENCE RISKS AND SEX FOR COMMON CONGENITAL MALFORMATIONS

When a child is born with a congenital malformation, the obvious question that will be asked is whether this will occur again. The first table below lists the recurrence rates of many of the more common congenital malformations based on the presence of the same anomaly in a parent or other sibling. The risk of repetition, however, also varies with respect to the sex of the next child since each of these malformations varies in relative sex incidence (see second table).

Overall Risk for Recurrence in Future Children When Affected Person Is:

ANOMALY	SIBLING	PARENT	PARENT AND SIBLING	2 SIBLINGS
Cleft lip and palate		4%	17%	9%
Cleft lip		6%	15%	
Club foot	2%		10%	
Dislocation of hip	3–8%			
Meningomyelocele	5%			
Anencephaly	3.9%			
Pyloric stenosis	5.8%	(9.8% for future male; 1.7% for female)		

Relative Sex Incidence

ANOMALY	MALE:FEMALE
Pyloric stenosis	5:1
Club foot	2:1
Cleft lip and palate	2:1
Cleft lip	1:127
Meningomyelocele	1:1.5
Anencephaly	1:2
Dislocation of hip	1:5.5

Reference: Smith, D.: Alabama J. Med. Sci., *3:*130, 1966.

That they bred in and in, as might be shown,
Marrying their cousins—nay, their aunts, and nieces,
Which always spoils the breed, if it increases.

George Gordon, Lord Byron *(1788–1824)*
Don Juan, Canto I, Stanza 57

CHROMOSOMAL ABNORMALITIES

There are two ways in which a chromosomal abnormality may occur: (1) there may be an error in meiosis, leading to chromosomal nondysjunction and trisomy or monosomy, or (2) single chromosomes may break, resulting in translocations and depletion of chromosomal fragments. Chromosomal anomalies occur at a rate of 0.56/100 live-born infants. The table may help suggest a possible diagnosis the next time you see a child with congenital anomalies.

17

Clinical Syndromes Due to Chromosome Abnormalities

SYNDROME	INCIDENCE	TYPE OF ANOMALY	CLINICAL AND LABORATORY FEATURES
Down's (mongolism)	1.8:1000 births	47,XX,G21+ and/or translocation involving D and G chromosomes	G trisomy is the most common autosomal anomaly.
Klinefelter's	1:400 male births	47,XXY or variants XY/XXY or XX/XXY	One of the most common causes of male hypogonadism. Clinical features do not become obvious until after puberty.
XYY	0.5:100 male births	47,XYY	Phenotypically male; behavioral problems; increased height, elevated plasma testosterone levels
Triple-X	1:1000 female births	47,XXX	May show mental retardation, irregular menses, reduced fertility.
XXXY	Unknown	48,XXXY	Retardation, hypertelorism, epicanthus, strabismus, hypoplastic scrotum, small testes, radioulnar synostosis, scoliosis, and kyphosis.
Turner's (gonadal dysgenesis)	1:2500 female births, 5:100 aborted fetuses	45,X or variant XO/XX	Triad of (1) short stature, (2) multiple malformations (left-sided cardiac lesion, short or webbed neck, peripheral, lymphedema, shield chest, cubitus valgus), and (3) sexual infantilism—primary amenorrhea and sterility.
Trisomy 8	Unknown	Usually mosaic for 47,8+/46	Mild-to-moderate mental retardation; delayed, poor speech; delayed motor development; abnormal head shape and ears; strabismus; prominent everted lower lip; clinodactyly; camptodactyly; joint contractures; bone abnormalities of vertebra and patella; hydronephrosis.

SYNDROME	INCIDENCE	TYPE OF ANOMALY	CLINICAL AND LABORATORY FEATURES
Trisomy 9	Unknown	Mostly mosaic	Microcephaly; small, palpebral fissures; prominent nose; low-set ears; genital abnormalities.
Trisomy 13, D1 trisomy (Patau's)	0.2:1000 births	47,XX,D1+ 47,XY,D1+	Incomplete development of forebrain and olfactory and optic nerves; minor motor seizures; mental retardation; microcephaly; wide sagittal suture and fontanels; capillary hemangiomata of forehead; localized scalp defects; microophthalmia; cleft lip and palate; low-set, misshapen ears; abnormalities of extremities; cardiac and renal anomalies; persistence of fetal or embryonic hemoglobin. Fatal outcome within 2 years.
Trisomy 18 (Edwards')	0.3:1000 births	47,XX,E18+	Polyhydramnios; small placenta; single umbilical artery; low birth weight; mental retardation; deafness; prominent occiput; low-set malformed ears; small mouth; narrow palatal arch; characteristic position of hand (clenched, index finger overlapping third, fifth over fourth); abnormal dermatoglyphics; skeletal muscle hypoplasia, associated cardiac, gastrointestinal, and renal anomalies. Fatal outcome within 2 years. Risk of recurrence is low (2–3%)
Trisomy 22	Unknown	47,XX,22+ 47,XY,22+	Mental retardation, growth retardation, microcephaly, coloboma, finger-like thumbs, multiple other defects.
4p–	Unknown	46,XX,4p– 46,XY,4p–	Midline scalp defects, carplike mouth, beaklike nose, hypospadias, and markedly delayed ossification centers. Similar to 5p– in phenotype but no cri du chat (can be differentiated from 5p– by autoradiographic studies).

Continued

17

Clinical Syndromes Due to Chromosome Abnormalities (Continued)

SYNDROME	INCIDENCE	TYPE OF ANOMALY	CLINICAL AND LABORATORY FEATURES
5p– (cri du chat)	Unknown, usually occurs in females	46,XX,5p– or, less commonly, 46,XY, 5p–	Cry similar to meowing of cat; low birth weight; mental retardation; microcephaly; hypertelorism; epicanthus; low-set, abnormally shaped ears; micrognathia; round face; failure to thrive; short stature; large frontal sinuses; premature graying of hair; seizures. About 1 in 7 cases is the result of a translocation transmitted from a phenotypically normal parent who has a balanced translocation.
9p–	Unknown	46,XX,9p– 46,XY,9p–	Mental retardation, hypotonia, trigonocephaly, anteverted nostrils, long upper lip, congenital heart disease.
9p+	Unknown	46,XX,9p+ 46,XY,9p+ May be translocated to some other chromosome	Mental retardation, microcephaly, brachycephaly, enophthalmos, prominent nose, inverted nostrils, protuberant ears.
13q–	Unknown	46,XX,13q– 46,XY,13q–	Mental retardation, microcephaly, facial asymmetry, ptosis of eyelids, coloboma, retinoblastoma, hypospadias, congenital heart disease, imperforate anus.
18q–	Unknown	46,XX,18q– 46,XY,18q–	Low birth weight; mental retardation; seizures; dysplasia of the midface (characteristic); long, tapering fingers; abnormal dermatoglyphics. Risk of recurrence is low.
18p–	Unknown	46,XX,18p– 46,XY,18p–	Multiple malformations, but no well defined syndrome.

Reference: Bingol, N.: Genetics. *In* Wasserman, E., and Gromisch, D.S. (eds.): Survey of Clinical Pediatrics, 7th ed. New York, McGraw-Hill Book Company, 1981, pp. 89–90.

18
THERAPEUTICS/
TOXICOLOGY

THE SYMPTOMATIC TREATMENT OF FEVER

The rational treatment of fever requires an understanding of its pathophysiologic basis. This requires some knowledge of the principles of temperature regulation, heat production, and conservation, and a recognition of the fact that fever has different causes and thus different treatments.

No symptom in pediatrics is more inappropriately treated than fever. Most febrile states in children result from an abnormal elevation in the hypothalamic setpoint. This occurs when a pyrogen released at the site of illness reaches the hypothalamus and causes alterations in the chemical environment. Heat production is increased and heat loss is minimized. Much less commonly, fever is a result of excessive heat production alone or when heat production is normal but heat loss is faulty.

The table on the next page examines the pathophysiologic basis for fever and the corresponding appropriate treatment.

18

Pathophysiologic Basis for Symptomatic Treatment of Fever

DISEASE PROCESS CAUSING FEVER	PATHOPHYSIOLOGY OF FEVER	CLINICAL FINDINGS	APPROPRIATE NONSPECIFIC TREATMENT	INAPPROPRIATE NONSPECIFIC TREATMENT
Infection, malignancy, allergy, steroid fever, collagen disease	Endogenous pyrogen causes rise in hypothalamic setpoint	Patient complains of feeling cold; piloerection; cold extremities; absent or minimal sweating; body positioned to minimize surface area, shivering	Drug-induced lowering of hypothalamic setpoint (e.g., with aspirin, acetaminophen); supply sufficient clothing and covers for maximal comfort; avoid shivering	Physical removal of heat, e.g., sponging, ice blanket, ice water enemas; without change in setpoint; these measures will cause discomfort, increase metabolic rate and will only lower body temperature for brief period
CNS lesion, DDT poisoning, scorpion venom, radiation, epinephrine and norepinephrine overdose	Agent or illness acts directly on hypothalamus to raise setpoint	Same as above	Drug-induced lowering of hypothalamic setpoint theoretically indicated as above; it is not clearly established, however, as possible with presently available drugs	Same as above
Malignant hyperthermia, hyperthyroidism, hypernatremia, primary defect in energy metabolism, aspirin overdose	Heat production exceeds heat loss mechanisms	Patient complains of feeling hot; no piloerection; hot extremities; active sweating; body positioned to maximize surface area	Undress patient; physical removal of heat, e.g., ice blanket, sponging	Attempt to lower setpoint (which is already set normally) with drugs, e.g., aspirin — possible toxicity of drug without potential benefit
Overuse of sauna, exposure to industrial heat, over dressing	Environmental heat load exceeds normal heat loss mechanisms	Same as above	Eliminate heat source; undress patient; physical removal of heat is effective but is not usually necessary	Same as above
Ectodermal dysplasia, burns, phenothiazine, anticholinergic overdose, heat stroke	Defective heat loss mechanisms cannot cope with normal heat load	Patient complains of feeling hot; sweating decreased (secondary to disease process); hot extremities; body positioned to maximize surface area	Provide cool environment; undress patient; physical removal of heat may be necessary	Same as above

Reference: Stern, R.: Pediatrics, *59:*92, 1977.

THE ANTIPYRETIC EFFECTS OF ASPIRIN AND ACETAMINOPHEN

Is aspirin any better than acetaminophen (Tylenol) for reducing fever? Studies indicate that used in equivalent doses, they do the same job.

The table below gives you some indication as to how fast these agents act and how much reduction in temperature you can expect.

Fall in Temperature (C°) After Treatment

DRUG	TIME (HR)			
	½	1	1½	2
Aspirin	0.4	0.8	1.2	1.5
Acetaminophen	0.6	1.1	1.5	1.6

Maximum temperature depression occurs 2 to 3 hours after ingestion. The effect of the drug begins to disappear within 3 to 4 hours and is totally gone by 6 hours.

Reference: Hunter, J.: Arch. Dis. Child., *48*:313, 1973.

18

ASPIRIN SENSITIVITY IN CHILDREN WITH ASTHMA

Intrinsic asthma, nasal polyps, and aspirin intolerance form a constellation that has been well recognized in adults. Aspirin sensitivity has recently been detected in 14 (28 per cent) of a group of 50 children with atopic asthma. This sensitivity was manifested by a 30 per cent reduction in FEP (maximal midexpiratory flow rate) lasting four hours or more. Characteristics of the children who demonstrated aspirin sensitivity included the following:

Most were female
Most had experienced onset of asthma before the age of 2 years
They had·more frequent episodes of sinusitis than other
   children with asthma

None of these children were aware of their aspirin sensitivity, although all of them had taken aspirin in the past. This failure to detect sensitivity may be due to the delay in onset of manifestations by 30 minutes to one hour. Another reason for failure to identify aspirin as a cause for worsening symptoms may be the presence of salicylates in a wide variety of preparations that the asthmatic child may ingest. In addition to many pain relievers not identified as "aspirin," salicylates are also contained in indomethacin and tartrazine (a yellow coloring material found in soft drinks, canned vegetables, and, until recently, in Marax, a drug used frequently in the treatment of asthma).

There is little evidence for the genetic transmission of aspirin sensitivity, and the mechanism for the sensitivity is not known.

It seems reasonable to avoid aspirin administration in any child who suffers from asthma.

Reference: Rachelefsky, G.S., Coulson, A., Siegel, S.C., et al.: Pediatrics, 56:443, 1975.

A SIMPLETON'S GUIDE TO DIURETICS

AGENT	MECHANISM OF ACTION	SIDE-EFFECTS
Sulfonamide derivatives Thiazide diuretics and their congeners	Inhibit sodium reabsorption in the cortical portion of the ascending tubule and the distal convoluted tubule (site of 10% of all sodium reabsorption). Possess a flat dose-response curve beyond the upper limits of dosage.	Hypokalemia and hypochloremic alkalosis Hyperuricemia Hyperglycemia Azotemia (avoid in patients with impaired renal function) Hypercalcemia Hyponatremia (Gastrointestinal upset, weakness, dry mouth, bad taste in mouth, leukopenia, thrombocytopenia, pancreatitis, skin rash, photosensitivity.)
Loop diuretics Furosemide (Lasix) Ethacrynic acid (Edecrin)	Inhibit sodium reabsorption in the ascending limb of the loop of Henle, where almost 20% of all sodium is reabsorbed. More potent than the "thiazide" diuretics. Possess an infinite dose-response curve, therefore more dangerous. Will work in volume-depleted patient. Should be used only in refractory edema or in presence of renal failure.	Similar to side-effects listed above. Exceptions are: Do not cause hypercalcemia. Ethacrynic acid unlikely to produce photosensitivity but produces more gastrointestinal upset. May produce temporary nerve deafness when given intravenously and rapidly to azotemic patients.
Distal tubular diuretics Spironolactone (Aldactone) Triamterene (Dyrenium)	Prevent exchange of sodium for potassium in distal tubule. Only 5% of sodium reabsorption occurs here. Spironolactone is a specific inhibitor of aldosterone.	Hyperkalemia (drug contraindicated in patients with renal failure). Gastrointestinal side-effects. Spironolactone may produce gynecomastia, hirsutism, and menstrual irregularities.

18

The Diuretic of Choice in Patients without Edema

DIAGNOSIS	DIURETIC
Primary (essential) hypertension	
Normal renal function	Thiazide class
Impaired renal function	Loop class
Primary aldosteronism	Spironolactone
Hypercalcemia	Loop class
Idiopathic hypercalciuria	Thiazide class
Nephrogenic diabetes insipidus	Thiazide class

The Diuretic of Choice in Patients with Edema

DIAGNOSIS	DIURETIC
Congestive heart failure	Thiazide class (take precautions to avoid hypokalemia if patient receiving digitalis)
Nephrotic syndrome	Thiazide and spironolactone
Cirrhosis and ascites	Thiazide and spironolactone
Acute and chronic renal failure	Loop class
Chronic lymphedema	Thiazide class

STEROIDS — HOW AND WHEN TO TAPER

Patients being treated with glucocorticosteroids should be tapered from the drug to avoid exacerbation of their underlying disease and to avoid the manifestations of adrenal insufficiency. The following is a step by step protocol for tapering steroids.

Step I. Reduce the dose gradually every three to seven days until the physiologic dose (20 mg/m^2 of hydrocortisone per day) has been reached. Raise the dose again temporarily for exacerbations of the underlying disease. If the disease remains quiescent, cover the patient with increased doses in times of stress.

If steroid treatment has been brief (less than five to seven days), tapering may continue at the above rate until the drug is discontinued.

Step II. If the patient has had prolonged or high dose treatment, the physiologic dose should be continued in the form of a single oral morning dose of the short-acting hydrocortisone. After two to four weeks, a fasting, 8 A.M. cortisol level should be drawn before the morning cortisol dose. Further tapering should then begin with a reduction in dose of 2.5 mg hydrocortisone per day each week until the patient is taking half the physiologic dose. Supplementation should be provided in times of stress.

Step III. Morning cortisol levels should be obtained prior to the morning dose every four weeks. When the morning cortisol is greater than 10 μg/dl, daily hydrocortisone may be discontinued with continued glucocorticoid coverage for stress.

Step IV. The responsiveness of the adrenal gland to pituitary stimulation may be tested in the following way: (1) Obtain a baseline plasma cortisone level. (2) Administer 250 μg of ACTH intramuscularly. (3) Obtain a plasma cortisol 30 to 60 minutes later. An increment of greater than 6 and up to greater than 20 μg/dl shows a normal response.

Once the normal adrenal response to ACTH stimulation is demonstrated, the physician may assume that the pituitary-adrenal axis is no longer suppressed. Routine glucocorticoid coverage in times of stress may be discontinued; however, treatment must be reinstituted and reevaluation of the patient undertaken if manifestations of chronic or acute adrenocortical insufficiency appear.

Note: In times of minor stress (infection to be treated at home, minor surgery, or dental work) glucocorticoid coverage should consist of increasing the daily dose to five times the physiologic dose, given in two doses per day. With major stress (major trauma, surgery) the patient should receive a dose of five times the physiologic dose every six to eight hours for three to four days, followed by tapering to the physiologic dose.

When patients are taking physiologic doses of glucocorticoids at home, the parents should be instructed to contact a physician at the first sign of vomiting, so that intramuscular steroid may be administered.

18

Reference: Byyny, R. L.: N. Engl. J. Med., *295:*30, 1976.

SIDE-EFFECTS OF ANTICONVULSANTS

Awareness of potential side-effects of anticonvulsants is important for their safe long-term use. The following two tables describe specific side-effects and include comments on detection and management of the more common side-effects.

GENERIC NAME	TRADE NAME	DROWSINESS	NYSTAGMUS, DIPLOPIA, AND/OR ATAXIA	HYPERACTIVITY, BEHAVIOR CHANGE	HEPATITIS	RENAL INVOLVEMENT	RASH	BLOOD DYSCRASIA	GASTRO-INTESTINAL UPSET	LUPUS-LIKE SYNDROME	OSTEO-MALACIA	MISCELLANEOUS
Phenobarbital	Many	X	X	X			X				X	Rash uncommon
Phenytoin	Dilantin	X	X		X		X	X	X	X	X	Drowsiness uncommon; hypertrichosis and/or gingival hyperplasia
Mephenytoin	Mesantoin	X			X			X		X		
Ethosuccimide	Zarontin	X		X			X	X	X	X		
Carbamazepine	Tegretal	X	X		X	X	X	X	X	X		Neuropathy or cardiac problems may be seen
Trimethadione	Tridione	X			X	X	X	X		X		Visual problems (hemeralopia)
Primidone	Mysoline	X	X			X	X	X	X	X	X	
Mephobarbital	Mebaral	Similar to phenobarbital.										
Paramethadione	Paradione	Similar to trimethadione.										

Side Effects of Anticonvulsants

SIDE-EFFECT	COMMENT
Drowsiness	Usually dose-related; try dosage adjustment.
Nystagmus, diplopia, and/or ataxia	Frequently encountered with phenytoin; usually dose-related; often manageable by dose reduction.
Hyperactivity and/or behavioral changes	Most often encountered with phenobarbital; an idiosyncratic reaction; dosage adjustment *not* helpful.
Gingival hyperplasia	Most common with phenytoin; maximal after 9 to 12 months of therapy; can be minimized — but *not* eliminated — by fastidious oral hygiene; gingivectomy may be indicated.
Hepatic involvement	Periodic liver function studies indicated when using drug associated with hepatitis; parents should be asked to notify you of any symptoms (e.g., jaundice, malaise, fever, dark urine) possibly referable to the liver; stop drug immediately if hepatic involvement found.
Renal involvement	Periodic urinalyses and renal function studies indicated if drug associated with renal problems (e.g., trimethadione).
Skin rash	May be accompanied by lymphadenopathy, fever, and hematopoietic disorders (particularly leukopenia); anticonvulsants should be stopped immediately upon noting rash (remember to substitute another drug); if the rash is mild and disappears completely, is not associated with the above, or other systemic signs, *and* is not hemorrhagic, exfoliative or bulbous in character, a cautious trial of the same drug may be tried.
Hematologic involvement	May affect platelets, neutrophils, or red cells; periodic CBC indicated when using drug known to be associated with this problem.
Lupus-like syndrome	Usually resolves some time after drug discontinued; antinuclear antibodies may persist for months or years.
Gastrointestinal upsets	Usually dose-related; often manageable by dividing dose or giving with meals. *Rule out hepatic involvement.*
Osteomalacia	*May* be related to duration of therapy; serum calcium and phosphorus usually normal; alkaline phosphatase may be elevated.

References: Livingston, S.: *In* Gellis, S.S., and Kagan, B.M. (Eds.): Current Pediatric Therapy. 6th Ed. Philadelphia, W.B. Saunders Company, 1973. Guinane, J.E.: *In* Gellis, S.S., and Kagan, B.M. (Eds.): Current Pediatric Therapy. 7th Ed. Philadelphia, W.B. Saunders Company, 1976.

PENICILLIN ALLERGY

What should be done about the patient with a history of penicillin allergy and a problem for which penicillin or its synthetic derivatives is clearly the best therapy? How reliable is a history of penicillin allergy?

Patients with a history of penicillin allergy should be skin tested with both penicillin G and penicilloyl polylysine (PPL) before administering penicillin in situations in which doubt exists and therapy with this group of antibiotics is necessary. With this approach, many patients with a false-positive history of penicillin allergy, or patients who have lost their hypersensitivity, can be identified and treated if necessary.

Here are some statistics that may help you place the problem in perspective.

Incidence of positive skin tests	
History of penicillin allergy	19%
No history of penicillin allergy	7%
Incidence of positive skin tests as related to allergic symptoms	
Previous anaphylactic reactions	45%
Previous maculopapular eruption	7%
Reactions with penicillin challenge	
With positive history and skin test	67%
With positive history alone	6%
With negative history	2%

No test presently available can detect 100 per cent of patients at risk from penicillin therapy. When penicillin hypersensitivity is highly suspected, and the drug is necessary for treatment, skin testing should be performed. Initial testing should be done by the scratch technique; if this is negative, intradermal testing should be employed. If testing is negative, then penicillin can be administered with careful observation.

Reference: Greene, G.R.: Hospital Practice, June 1976, p. 28.

HEMATOLOGIC MANIFESTATIONS OF CHLORAMPHENICOL THERAPY

Chloramphenicol is again being used to treat infants and children as a result of the emergence of ampicillin-resistant strains of *Hemophilus influenzae*. A generation of physicians has grown up without experience with the hematologic effects of this drug.

The drug produces characteristic pharmacologic effects on hematopoiesis and may also produce "idiosyncratic reactions." The pharmacologic effects are dose-related and are more common in patients with hepatic or renal disease. These pharmacologic events are self-limited and are completely reversible when the drug is discontinued. Effects are generally gone and recovery is complete within 7 to 10 days after cessation of therapy. The hematologic manifestations include:

	TIME	FREQUENCY
Delayed iron clearance from plasma	Early	Common
Rise in serum iron	Early	Common
Reticulocytopenia	3-5 days	Common
Increase in myeloid: erythroid ratio	3-5 days	Common
Vacuolization of marrow precursors	5-7 days	Common
Mild fall in hemoglobin	7-10 days	Common
Mild fall in platelets	10-14 days	Common
Neutropenia	10-14 days	Uncommon

The drug should only be used when necessary, employed in the lowest effective dose, and should not be administered for prolonged periods of time. It should not be used in patients who have developed aplastic anemia as a result of previous exposure. Patients on therapy should have reticulocyte counts and hemoglobin determinations performed weekly, platelet counts and white cell counts at 0, 7, 10, and 14 days. The drug should be discontinued if the patient's platelet count falls below $100,00/mm^3$ or if the patient develops an absolute neutropenia (polymorphonuclear count of less than $1500/mm^3$). Reticulocytopenia is not an indication for stopping therapy.

The "idiosyncratic reactions" that result in the development of aplastic anemia are unrelated to dose or duration of therapy. Aplastic anemia appears after the medication is discontinued; in fact, weeks to months may pass. Genetic predisposition appears to play a large part in its development. It occurs with an incidence of 1 in 60,000 to 1 in 200,000 patients. This form of reaction resulting in aplastic anemia has been seen in twins, an uncle, and a niece, is more common in children, affects females more commonly than males, and may occur after the administration of a single dose of the drug. It has been reported to occur even after the use of chloramphenicol eyedrops. Aplastic anemia when it occurs is serious and frequently fatal. Because of the risk of this type of unpredictable reaction, the drug should only be used when no other satisfactory alternative antibiotic is available. Once drug therapy is initiated, it should be continued as necessary, employing the guidelines previously described.

Keep your fingers crossed each time you write an order for this antibiotic. If you try this, it makes order writing more difficult.

ANTIBIOTICS — THE DOSE AND THE KIDNEY

Most antibiotics are primarily excreted via the kidney. For this reason it is important to consider lowering the dose in patients with renal impairment. Many antibiotics, particularly the penicillins, have a very short half-life that is not appreciably modified by mild-to-moderate degrees of renal disease. The table below lists the major excretory route and the dose modification required for patients whose renal function is compromised.

ANTIBIOTIC	MAJOR EXCRETORY ROUTE	DOSAGE MODIFICATION
Little or No Change		
Cloxacillin, dicloxacillin	Kidney (Liver)	None
Chloramphenicol	Liver	
Doxycycline	Liver	
Isoniazid	Liver (Kidney)	
Erythromycin	Liver	
Oxacillin	Kidney (Liver)	
Penicillin (low dose)	Kidney	
Minor Alteration		
Ampicillin	Kidney (Liver)	In anuric patients
Carbenicillin	Kidney (Liver)	give full dose on
Cephalothin	Kidney and liver	first day followed
Lincomycin, clindamycin	Liver and kidney	by half-doses
Methicillin	Kidney (Liver)	thereafter
Penicillin G (high dose)	Kidney	
Nafcillin	Liver (Kidney)	
Major Alteration		
Amphotericin B	Liver and kidney	Serum concentrations should be
Cefazolin	Kidney	measured if these
Colistimethate	Kidney	antibiotics are to
Gentamicin	Kidney	be used in
Kanamycin	Kidney	patients with
Tobramycin	Kidney	renal impairment
Amikacin	Kidney	
Polymyxin B	Kidney	
Streptomycin	Kidney	
Vancomycin	Kidney	

Relatively Contraindicated in Renal Insufficiency

Nitrofurantoin
Nalidixic acid
Absorbable sulfonamides
Methenamine mandelate
Para-aminosalicylic acid
Tetracycline other than doxycycline

Optimal therapy with minimal toxicity may be achieved with the cephalosporins and the penicillins (except nafcillin) only with frequent measures of serum antibiotic concentrations. The following table gives a recent recommendation for the alteration of cefazolin doses in patients with varying degrees of renal impairment.

Dose Recommendations for Use of Cefazolin in Children with Renal Failure

CREATININE CLEARANCE (ml/min/1.73 m²)	DOSE OF CEFAZOLIN (mg/kg)	INTERVAL BETWEEN doses (hr)
≥50	7 (up to 500 mg/dose)	6–8
25–50	7	12
10–25	7	24–36
<10	7	48–72

A "loading" dose of aminoglycosides must be administered during the first 24 hours regardless of the degree of renal impairment. This dose should be the same as that administered to a patient with normal renal function. After the first 24 hours, serum levels are mandatory.

References: Graef, J.W., and Cone, T.E., Jr. (eds.): Manual of Pediatric Therapeutics, Boston, Little, Brown & Company, 1974. Nelson, J.D.: Pocketbook of Pediatric Antimicrobial Therapy. Waco, TX, Hill Printing and Stationery Company, 1979. Hiner, L.B., Baluarte, H.J., et al.: J. Pediatr., *96:*335, 1980.

METABOLIC EFFECTS OF CERTAIN DRUGS

1. *Drugs with a high sodium content*
   Carbenicillin (4.7 mEq/gm)
   Penicillin G (1.7 mEq/million units)
   Ampicillin (3 mEq/gm)
   Cephalothin (2.5 mEq/gm)
   Kayexalate (65 mEq/16 gm)
   Fleet's Phospho-Soda (24 mEq/5 ml)
   Antacids (variable amounts of sodium depending on the preparation)

2. *Drugs with a high potassium content*
   Penicillin G (1.7 mEq/million units)
   Salt substitutes

3. *Drugs with a high magnesium content*
   Antacids (absorbable)
   Laxatives

4. *Magnesium depletion*
   Diuretics

5. *Drugs with a high calcium content*
   Antacids (absorbable)

6. *Hypocalcemia*
   Anticonvulsants
   Heparin

7. *Acidosis*
   Methenamine mandelate
   Para-aminosalicylic acid
   Phenformin
   Isoniazid
   Ethanol
   Paraldehyde
   Nitrofurantoin
   Ammonium chloride
   Acetazolamide

8. *Alkalosis*
   Absorbed antacids
   Large doses of penicillin G and carbenicillin

9. *Elevation of the blood urea nitrogen*
   Tetracyclines
   Androgenic steroids
   Glucocorticoids
   Diuretics
   Hydroxyurea

10. *Fluid retention*
    Indomethacin
    Phenylbutazone
    Clofibrate
    Carbamazepine
    Vincristine
    Vinblastine
    Cyclophosphamide
    Chlorpropamide
    Thioridazine
    Diazoxide
    Ibuprofen

11. *Fluid depletion*
    Lithium carbonate
    Demeclocycline

Reference: Anderson, R.J., Gambertoglio, J.G., and Schrier, R.W.: Fate of drugs in renal failure. *In* Brenner, B.M., and Rector, F.C. (eds.): The Kidney. Philadelphia, W.B. Saunders Company, 1976, p. 1917.

Poisons and medicine are oftentimes the same substance given with different intents.

Peter Mere Latham *(1789–1875)*
General Remarks on the Practice
of Medicine, Ch. IV

"BLACK TONGUE FEVER"

Pepto-Bismol is used frequently in the treatment of gastroenteritis. It is well recognized that this medication may cause black stools (pseudomelena), which results from the oxidation of bismuth, possibly enhanced by fever. Patients taking Pepto-Bismol for the treatment of gastroenteritis may also develop a black discoloration of the tongue and buccal mucosa. If the cause of this finding is unrecognized, it may be quite alarming to both patient and physician.

Reference: William H. Dietz, Jr.: Personal communication, 1976.

INGESTIONS OF LOW TOXICITY

Knowledge of substances that cause little or no toxicity when ingested can be helpful both in immediately allaying parental (and your own) anxiety as well as in preventing iatrogenic problems associated with unnecessary hospitalization, induced emesis, gastric lavage, or other measures used in treatment of ingestions. The table lists those substances that are nontoxic or toxic only in large amounts.

NO TREATMENT REQUIRED	REMOVAL NECESSARY ONLY IF LARGE AMOUNTS INGESTED
Ball-point inks	After-shave lotion
Bar soap	Body conditioners
Bathtub floating toys	Colognes
Battery (dry cell)	Deodorants
Bubble bath soap	Fabric softeners
Candles	Hair dyes
Chalk	Hair sprays
Clay (modeling)	Hair tonic
Crayons with AP, CP or CS 130–46 designation	Indelible markers
Dehumidifying packets	Matches (greater than 20 wooden matches or two books of paper matches)
Detergents (anionic)	No Doz
Eye makeup	Oral contraceptives
Fish bowl additives	Perfumes
Golf balls	Suntan preparations
Hand lotion and cream	Toilet water
Ink (blue, black, red)	
Lipstick	
Newspaper	
Pencils (lead and coloring)	
Putty and Silly Putty	
Sachets	
Shampoo	
Shaving cream and shaving lotions	
Shoe polish (occasionally aniline dyes present)	
Striking surface materials of matchboxes	
Sweetening agents (saccharin, cyclamate)	
Teething rings	
Thermometers	
Toothpaste	

The minimal toxicity associated with these substances should not preclude investigation of the circumstances of the ingestion or advice regarding future preventive measures.

Reference: Mathies, A.W.: *In* Gellis, S.S. and Kagan, B.M. (Eds.): Current Pediatric Therapy. 6th Ed. Philadelphia, W.B. Saunders Company, 1973, p. 730.

THE ANATOMY OF POISONING

The ingestion of drugs or toxins by children is frequently not an "accident." The physician should always gather all the facts surrounding an ingestion because it may indicate the presence of chronic stress in a household. If efforts are not directed to correct such circumstances, a repeat ingestion can occur.

A study of 94 episodes of aspirin poisoning in children 1 to 5 years of age revealed the following three patterns of ingestion.

Transient Unusual Episode in Home

In such circumstances, the normal family routine was disrupted by a nonfamily visitor or the presence of illness in a member of the family. In this setting, the aspirin was unusually available because it had been used to treat a member of the family.

Unusual Resourcefulness by Child

In these instances, the majority of incidents were social in nature, with several children sharing the drug as "play medicine" or candy. Children often displayed unusual skill and curiosity in obtaining the medicine.

Serious Chronic Family Situations

These instances were characterized by one-parent homes, marital discord, working mothers, inadequate play space, and other signs of strife.

Try to categorize the circumstances of ingestion in your patients so that appropriate advice and guidance can be offered.

Reference: Meyer, R.J.: Am. J. Dis. Child., *102*:47, 1961.

18

THE EPIDEMIOLOGY OF DRUG POISONING

Aspirin continues to head the list of commonly ingested drug products among pediatric patients. In some centers, plants are a more common source of concern than drugs, but accidental ingestion of pharmacologic agents is still a risk for young children. Figures 18–1 and 18–2 depict the 12 most commonly reported drugs responsible for drug overdose as recorded by the Massachusetts Poison Control System. Figure 18–2 represents the incidence of symptoms that developed as a result of overdose. It is noteworthy that 25 per cent of the children under 5 years of age who accidentally ingested a toxic drug became symptomatic.

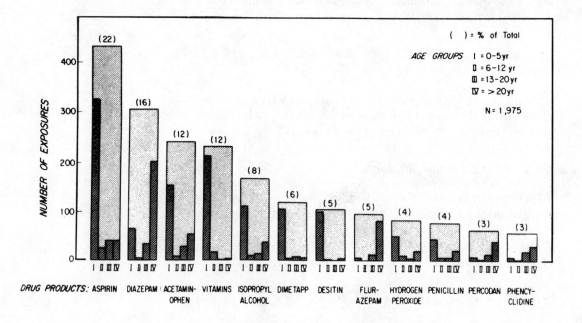

FIG. 18-1

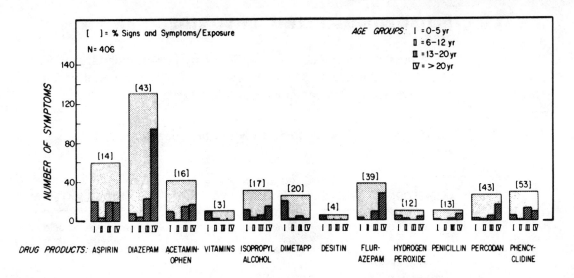

FIG. 18-2

Reference: Saracino, M., Flowers, J., and Lovejoy, F.H.: Am. J. Dis. Child., 134:763, 1980.
Copyright 1980, American Medical Association.

18

POISONING—FERRIC CHLORIDE

A possible aid to diagnosis in potentially poisoned children is 10 per cent ferric chloride solution. A few drops of this material in 5 ml of urine (or serum) may provide an additional clue to diagnosis.

Conditions and Drugs Associated with Color Reaction of Ferric Chloride

CONDITION OR DRUG	COLOR WITH FERRIC CHLORIDE	REACTING MATERIAL
Phenylketonuria	Blue-green	Phenylpyruvic acid
Oasthouse urine disease (methionine malabsorption)	Purple to red-brown	Alpha-ketobutyrate
Odor of rancid butter syndrome (tyrosinemia)	Transient blue-green	Para-hydroxyphenylpyruvate
Maple syrup urine disease	Greenish gray	Branched chain keto acids
Histidinemia	Blue-green	Imidazole pyruvic acid
Alkaptonuria	Blue or green transient	Homogentisic acid
Ketosis	Reddish brown	Acetoacetic acid
Pyruvic acid	Deep yellow	
Xanthurenic acid	Dark green	
3-Hydroxyanthranilic acid	Dark brown	
Bilirubin	Blue-green	
Melanin	Gray precipitate	
Alpha-ketobutyric acid	Purple	Faint purple
Salicylates	Purple	Purple salicylate
Para-aminosalicylic acid	Purplish brown	PAS
Isonicotinic hydrazide	Gray	INH
Phenothiazines	Purple-brown	
Lysol ingestion	Green	
Antipyrine or acetophenetidin	Cherry red	
Normal urine	Brown-white precipitate	Phosphates, other anions

Reference: Snyderman, S.: Pediatr. Clin. North Am., *18*:199, 1971.

POISONING—UNKNOWN POISON

Situations sometimes arise where a possible poisoning has occurred but the amount and nature of the ingested substance are unknown. Features that should suggest poisoning in an ill child include:

1. Abrupt onset of illness
2. Child's age 1 to 4 years
3. History of previous ingestion
4. Multiple organ system involvement that does not fit single disease

Sometimes a combination of symptoms will suggest the drug or poison involved:

SYMPTOMS AND SIGNS	POSSIBLE POISON
Agitation, hallucinations, dilated pupils, bright red color to the skin, dry skin, and fever	Atropine-like agents LSD
Marked activity, tremors, headache, diarrhea, dry mouth with foul odor, sweating, tachycardia, arrhythmia, dilated pupils	Amphetamines
Slow respirations, pinpoint pupils, euphoria, or coma	Opiates
Salivation, lacrimation, urination, defecation, miosis, and pulmonary congestion	Organic phosphates or poison mushrooms
Sleepiness, slurred speech, nystagmus, ataxia	Barbiturates or tranquilizers
Hypernea, fever, and vomiting	Salicylates
Oculogyric crisis, ataxia, and unusual posturing of head and neck	Phenothiazines
Nausea, vomiting, sweatiness, and pallor are early manifestations; late manifestations include stupor and signs of liver failure	Acetaminophen

The following list expands on signs and symptoms and the toxins with which they may be associated.

18

ATAXIA

Alcohol
Barbiturates
Bromides
Carbon monoxide
Diphenylhydantoin
Hallucinogens
Heavy metals
Organic solvents
Tranquilizers

CONVULSIONS AND MUSCLE TWITCHING

Alcohol
Amphetamines
Antihistamines
Boric acid
Camphor
Chlorinated hydrocarbon insecticides (DDT)
Cyanide
Lead
Organic phosphate insecticides
Plants (lily of the valley, azalea, iris, water hemlock)
Salicylates
Strychnine
Withdrawal from barbiturates, benzodiazepine (Valium, Librium), meprobamate

COMA AND DROWSINESS

Alcohol – ethyl
Antihistamines
Barbiturates and other hypnotics
Carbon monoxide
Narcotic depressants (opiates)
Salicylates
Tranquilizers

PARALYSIS

Botulism
Heavy metals
Plants (coniine in poison hemlock)
Triorthocresyl phosphate

PUPILS

Pinpoint
Mushrooms (muscarine type)
Narcotic depressants (opiates)
Organic phosphate insecticides

Dilated
Amphetamines
Antihistamines
Atropine
Barbiturates (coma)

Cocaine
Ephedrine
LSD
Methanol
Withdrawal-narcotic depressants

Nystagmus on Lateral Gaze
Barbiturates
Minor tranquilizers (meprobamate, benzodiazepine)

PULSE RATE

Slow
Digitalis
Lily of the valley
Narcotic depressants

Rapid
Alcohol
Amphetamines
Atropine
Ephedrine

RESPIRATORY ALTERATIONS

Rapid
Amphetamines
Barbiturates (early)
Carbon monoxide
Methanol
Petroleum distillates
Salicylates

Slow or Depressed
Alcohol
Barbiturates (late)
Narcotic depressants (opiates)
Tranquilizers

Wheezing and Pulmonary Edema
Mushrooms (muscarine type)
Narcotic depressants (opiates)
Organic phosphate insecticides
Petroleum distillates

Paralysis
Organic phosphate insecticides
Botulism

MOUTH

Salivation
Arsenic
Corrosive
Mercury
Mushrooms
Organic phosphate insecticides
Thallium

18

Dryness
   Atropine
   Amphetamines
   Antihistamines
   Narcotic depressants

BREATH ODOR

Acetone: acetone, alcohol (methyl, isopropyl), phenol, salicylates
Alcohol: alcohol (ethyl)
Bitter almonds: cyanide
Coal gas: carbon monoxide
Garlic: arsenic, phosphorus, organic phosphate insecticides, thallium
Oil of wintergreen: methyl salicylate
Petroleum: petroleum distillates
Violets: turpentine

SKIN COLOR

Jaundice (hepatic or hemolytic)
   Aniline
   Arsenic
   Carbon tetrachloride
   Castor bean
   Fava bean
   Mushroom
   Naphthalene
   Yellow phosphorus

Cyanosis
   Aniline dyes
   Carbon monoxide
   Cyanide
   Nitrites
   Strychnine

Red Flush
   Alcohol
   Antihistamines
   Atropine
   Boric acid
   Carbon monoxide
   Nitrites

VIOLENT EMESIS OFTEN WITH HEMATEMESIS

Acetaminophen
Aminophylline
Bacterial food poisoning
Boric acid
Corrosives
Fluoride
Heavy metals
Phenol
Salicylates

ABDOMINAL COLIC
Black widow spider bite
Heavy metals
Narcotic depressant withdrawal

OLIGURIA-ANURIA
Carbon tetrachloride
Ethylene glycol
Heavy metals
Hemolytic poisons (naphthalene, plants)
Methanol
Mushrooms
Oxalates
Petroleum distillates
Solvents

Reference: Mofenson, H.C., and Greensher, J.: Pediatrics, *54:*336, 1974.

18

DISEASES AND POISONINGS ASSOCIATED WITH UNUSUAL BREATH ODOR

The odor of a patient's breath may suggest a particular disease state or ingestion of a toxic substance. The table below lists these suspicious odors and their diagnostic significance.

ODOR	PRODUCT OR DISEASE STATE TO SUSPECT
Acrid (pear-like)	Paraldehyde
Alcohol (fruit-like)	Alcohol
Ammoniacal	Uremia
Bitter almonds	Cyanide (in chokecherry, apricot pits)
Coal gas (stove gas)	Carbon monoxide (odorless, but associated with coal gas)
Disinfectants	Phenol, creosote
Garlic	Phosphorus, tellurium, arsenic (breath and perspiration), parathion, malathion
Halitosis	Acute illness, poor oral hygiene
Musty fish (raw liver)	Hepatic failure
Pungent, aromatic	Ethchlorvynol (Placidyl)
Rotten eggs	Hydrogen sulfide mercaptans
Shoe polish	Nitrobenzene
Sweet acetone (russet apples)	Lacquer, alcohol, ketoacidosis, chloroform
Stale tobacco	Nicotine
Violets	Turpentine
Wintergreen	Methylsalicylate

Reference: Hospital Physician, March 1976, p. 12.

THE "DONE NOMOGRAM" FOR SALICYLATE INTOXICATION

The nomogram in Figure 18–3 has proved extremely useful as a rough guide to the severity of salicylate intoxication in previously well patients. In order to use the nomogram appropriately, you must know the approximate time of ingestion as well as make the assumption that the salicylate was all taken over a brief period. The nomogram helps to identify rapidly those patients who are not likely to recover with conventional treatment alone.

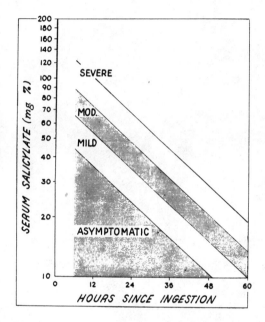

FIG. 18-3

Nomogram relating serum salicylate concentration and expected severity of intoxication at varying intervals following the ingestion of a single dose of salicylate.

Reference: Done, A.K.: Pediatrics, *26*:800, 1960.

18

ACETAMINOPHEN POISONING

As with aspirin poisoning, acetaminophen toxicity is determined by the plasma levels of this drug. The treatment with agents such as cysteamine should be dependent on the probability of significant toxicity. Figure 18–4 can be used in this assessment.

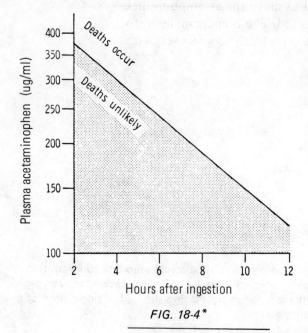

FIG. 18-4*

Reference: Prescott, L.F., et al.: Cysteamine, methionine, and penicillamine in the treatment of paracetamol poisoning. Lancet, *2:*109, 1976.

*From Dreisbach, R.H.: Handbook of Poisoning, 10th ed. Los Altos, CA, Lange Medical Publications, 1980.

TREATMENT OF COMMON POISONINGS

In many cases the ingestion of a toxic substance may be successfully treated pharmacologically. The following is a list of "antidotes" for frequently ingested poisons.

POISON	ANTIDOTE
Arsenic, bismuth, chromium, cobalt, copper, iron, lead, magnesium, radium, selenium and uranium	BAL (Dimercaprol) *Dose:* 3–4 mg/kg (0.3–0.4 ml/10 kg) every 4 hours for 2 days, then 3 mg/kg every 12 hours for a total of 10 days. If nausea and sweating develop, give ephedrine, 25 mg by mouth before each dose of BAL.
Lead, mercury, copper, nickel, zinc, cobalt, beryllium, and manganese	EDTA (calcium disodium edetate) *Dose:* 15–25 mg/kg (0.08–0.125 ml/kg of a 20% solution) intravenously in 250–500 ml of a 5% dextrose solution over 1–2 hours twice daily. Maximum dose 50 mg/kg/day. Give in 5-day courses with a rest period of 2 days between courses. Or: 12.5 mg/kg as a 20% solution intramuscularly every 4–6 hours. Dilute each dose with an equal volume of 1% procaine. Maximum dose 50 mg/kg/day.
Cyanide	Sodium nitrite *Dose:* 3% solution intravenously at 2.5–5 ml/minute. Stop administration if systolic blood pressure goes below 80 mm Hg. Methemoglobin should be measured and should not exceed 40%.
Narcotics	Naloxone (Narcan) *Dose:* 0.01 mg/kg intravenously
Warfarin, dicumerol	Vitamin K_1 *Dose:* 1–5 mg for mild overdosage; 20–40 mg if bleeding is severe.
Ferrous sulfate	Deferoxamine *Dose:* 0.5–1 gm intramuscularly followed by 0.25–0.5 gm every 4 hours for a total of 80 mg/kg in the first 24 hours. Or: Mix 0.5 gm in 2 ml sterile water and give 0.25–0.5 gm intravenously every 4–12 hours. Maximum daily dose should not exceed 80 mg/kg (see p. 360).

18

POISON	ANTIDOTE
Methanol	Ethanol (50% or 100 proof) *Dose:* 1–1.5 ml/kg orally initially diluted to not more than 5%, followed by 0.5–1.0 ml/kg every 2 hours orally or intravenously for 4 days. Blood ethanol level should equal 1–1.5 mg/ml.
Insecticides that are cholinesterase inhibitors	Atropine *Dose:* 2 mg intramuscularly and repeat every 3–8 minutes until signs of atropinization appear. As much as 12 mg of atropine may be needed in the first 12 hours. And: Pralidoxime *Dose:* 1 gm intravenously slowly in an aqueous solution. Repeat after 30 minutes if respirations do not improve. This dose may be repeated twice within each 24 hour period.
Amphetamines	Chloropromazine *Dose:* 0.5–1.0 mg/kg every 30 minutes as needed.
Phenothiazines	Diphenhydramine (Benadryl) *Dose:* 1–5 mg/kg intravenously.
Carbon monoxide	Oxygen
Nitrite induced methemoglobinemia	Methylene blue *Dose:* 0.1 ml/kg of 1% solution over 10 minutes.
Scopalamine	Physostigmine *Dose:* 1–5 ml intravenously of dilution of 1 mg in 5 ml of saline. May be repeated every 5 minutes up to a total dose of 2 mg in children and 6 mg in adults every 30 seconds. Atropine (1 mg) should be available if physostigmine causes bradycardia, convulsions, or severe bronchoconstriction.

"Alas! regardless of their doom,
The little victims play;
No sense have they of ills to come,
Nor care beyond today."

Gray

ACUTE IRON POISONING

Physicians caring for children spend a good deal of time making sure their patients are getting enough iron. Occasionally, an emergency arises when a child's life is threatened by the ingestion of too much iron. Procedures for determining the amount of iron ingested and for instituting treatment are discussed below.

Symptoms of acute iron toxicity include irritability, nausea, vomiting, and diarrhea. Shock and coma may occur with very large ingestions. The child who presents in shock or coma with a history of iron ingestion should receive deferoxamine mesylate therapy as below, regardless of the history of quantity of iron ingested.

Prompt treatment literally may mean the difference between life and death for children who have ingested toxic quantities of iron. Unfortunately, most patients, including those who may ultimately die, appear clinically well when first examined, so that a consistent and logical approach must be followed in every case of iron ingestion. Listed below are a series of sequential steps to be undertaken following the ingestion of iron. The major difference with this approach in comparison with previous approaches is the rather liberal use of deferoxamine. In recent years the wider availability of this drug has proved its efficacy and relatively wide margin of safety. This drug may cause falsely low levels of serum iron if colorimetric determinations are performed, unless special modifications of the assay are done. This should not be of much concern, anyway, since there is no good correlation between the magnitude of the rise in serum iron and the degree of toxicity observed. Vin rosé-colored urine indicates that deferoxamine is still removing excessive iron, and is an indication to continue treatment.

18

For All Patients with a History of Excessive Iron Ingestion

A. Perform the following

1. Give deferoxamine (2 gm IM, unless the patient is in shock)
2. Give ipecac (if patient is conscious and if gag reflex is present)
3. Lavage (after emesis) with deferoxamine (2 gm in 1 liter of water containing enough $NaHCO_3$ to alkalinize [pH >5] the gastric contents)
4. Leave in stomach (via lavage tube) deferoxamine (10 gm in 50 ml of water with sufficient $NaHCO_3$ to alkalinize [pH >5] the gastric contents
5. Provide IV fluids as necessary
6. Obtain a serum iron level, total iron binding capacity, CBC, electrolytes
7. Obtain an abdominal roentgenogram

B. Consider the following three conditions and initiate action as follows (C,D)

1. Signs or symptoms by history or observation
2. Vin rosé-colored urine with good urine output
3. Evidence of iron tablets by abdominal roentgenogram

C. If all three conditions are negative for six hours of observation, then discharge after six hours

D. If any of the three conditions is positive, admit for further treatment as follows

1. Give deferoxamine by continuous IV infusion (15 mg/kg/hr)
2. Monitor and support intravascular volume and tissue perfusion
3. Continue therapy until urine is clear of vin rosé color and patient is asymptomatic for at least 24 hr
4. Discharge patient
5. Perform follow-up examination

Reference: Robotham, J.L., and Lietman, P.S.: Acute iron poisoning. Am. J. Dis. Child., 134:875, 1980. Copyright 1980, American Medical Association.

IS THIS A POISONOUS SNAKE BITE?

This question is posed to physicians in offices and emergency rooms several thousand times a year in this country. A correct and prompt answer is essential for proper treatment. Failure to use antivenom early when indicated can be fatal; its inappropriate employment for a bite by a harmless snake may be hazardous due to severe reactions.

The problem has two parts. First, was the bite due to a harmless or a poisonous snake? Second, if the snake was venomous, is envenomation present or likely? The question may be resolved by examination of the snake so that it may be put in the category of either a venomous or nonvenomous variety and by examination of the patient to determine if venomation has occurred. Basic dependable guidelines for attaining both these goals will be outlined. They may be used by the amateur who has no knowledge of serpents at all. This discussion applies only to those snakes that are *native to the continental United States* and does not relate to foreign species introduced into this country as pets or exhibits.

Examination of the snake

One should not attempt to identify the exact species, since this is often a challenge for even the genuine expert due to pitfalls involving confusing color variante (albinism and melanism) and deceptive patterns (atypical or absent). Undue delay may result by waiting to locate an available herpetologist in a nearby zoo, museum, or zoology department. One should instead inspect the snake and, from the guidelines provided, assign it to the harmless or harmful group. The problem is somewhat simplified since in the mainland United States there are only two families of indigenous poisonous serpents.

Crotalidae. These are the pit vipers, which include all rattlesnakes, cottonmouths (water moccasin), and copperheads (highland moccasin). One or more of this family has been found in all states, with the exception of Maine, Alaska, and Hawaii. The head is large and triangular. The neck is relatively slender, so that it is readily distinguishable from the thick, heavy body. The pupil is vertically elliptical. Pit organs (loreal pits) are pathognomonic of all members of this group. A pit is present on each side of the head, and it resembles an extra nostril. The pits are deep, readily visible between the eye and the nostril, and located just below a line connecting these two structures. One or two fangs are found on the upper jaw of all pit vipers. They are specialized hollow or grooved teeth, which are recurved and longer than the other teeth. It is through these that the venom is injected. In this family the fangs are movable and when not in use are folded up against the palate. A white membrane may cover the fang down to the tip. Normally there are two fangs in the upper jaw — one on each side of the maxilla — so the classic bite pattern shows two fang punctures. However, one or both may be broken off or shed, in which instance there may be only a single fang mark present or none at all. *No envenomation is possible if fangs are absent.* Reserve fangs are always present, so the missing fang is replaced soon. Rarely, one or two reserve fangs may be functioning along with the customary complement of one or two fangs. In such a circumstance the bite pattern will be atypical, demonstrating three or four fang punctures.

Herpetologists identify species by meticulous scale counts of the head, neck, body, and tail. For practical purposes one may observe the scales (scutes, shields, plates) on the ventral surface of the body just posterior to the anus (subcaudal scales). In this family the subcaudal scales are usually arranged in a single row, but exceptions occur in which the rows are double. In the majority of harmless snakes the subcaudal scales are double, but this is not infallible either since exceptions are found. Rattles, of course, are specific for rattlesnakes and are not present in the copperhead, cottonmouth, other venomous species, or harmless snakes. They break off because of wear and tear, or during ecdysis (molting), so the number is inconstant regardless of the age of the reptile. If all rattles have been lost or if the specimen is a baby that has not yet developed rattles, there will be a slight enlargement at the tip of the tail known as the button. Other poisonous snakes do not show a button, nor do nonvenomous species. Also, the end of the tail of a rattlesnake that has lost its rattles is short and blunt, whereas the tip of the tail of a harmless snake is usually gradually tapered.

Elapidae. This family is represented in this country only by the coral snake. Unlike the pit vipers the coral snake is restricted to the southern states and is generally not found north of Arizona, Arkansas, or the Carolinas. Compared to the rattlesnakes and moccasins, the head is narrow and the neck and body are slender, giving a cylindrical configuration which is quite different from the shape of the pit vipers. The pupil is circular, thus resembling that of our indigenous harmless varieties. Pit organs are not present. Two fangs are present — one on each side of the maxilla (unless one or both have been shed). They are erect, fixed, and smaller than those of the pit vipers. Subcaudal scales tend to be in a double row similar to those of nonvenomous snakes, but rarely may be in a single row in the coral snake. Both rattles and tail button are absent. The coral snake is an exception to the general rule of not trying species identification, since there are confusing imitators that are harmless. Fortunately the nonvenomous mimics are easy to differentiate from the potent coral snake. The coral snake has a black snout and broad body rings of red and black that are separated by a narrower band of yellow. The mnemonic "red next to yellow kills a fellow" is helpful to keep in mind. The harmless look-alikes (scarlet snake, scarlet king snake) show a grey or red snout and red and yellow rings that are separated by a black band. Here the mnemonic to remember is "red against black is venom lack."

Summary of family characteristics — native harmless versus native venomous snakes in the continental United States

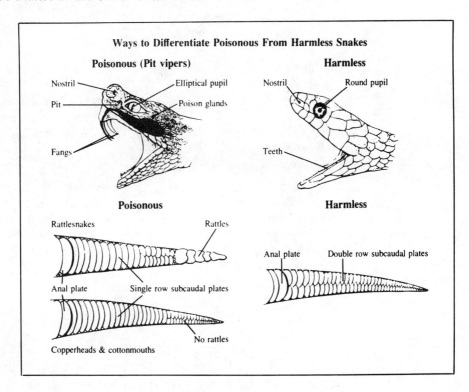

FIG. 18-5

NONVENOMOUS		VENOMOUS
Oval	Head	Large and triangular (pit vipers); small and narrow (coral snake)
Round	Pupils	Vertically elliptical (pit vipers); round (coral snake)
Absent	Pit organs	Present in all pit vipers (copperhead, cottonmouth, rattlesnakes); absent in coral snake
Absent	Fangs	Present in all venomous species. Large, long, recurved teeth. Long and movable in pit vipers. Short, erect, and fixed in coral snake. Usually 2 (1 on each side upper jaw) unless shed or reserve fangs also in use

18

NONVENOMOUS		VENOMOUS
Double row usually, but exceptions	Subcaudal scales (anus to tip of tail)	Single row in pit vipers, but with exceptions; double row in coral snake, but exceptions
Absent	Rattles	Present in all rattlesnakes unless lost or undeveloped in baby. If missing a button, present at tip of tail. No rattles in other venomous species or in harmless snakes
Usually ends in gradual taper	Tip of tail	Short and blunt in rattlesnake if rattles lost
	Bite pattern (seldom perfect)	
Total of 6 with no fang marks; four rows maxillary teeth and 2 rows mandibular teeth	Number of rows	Total of 4 with 1-2 fang marks (rarely 3-4 if reserve fangs functional). Two rows with fang marks from maxillary teeth. Two rows without fang marks from mandibular teeth
Series scratches or tiny punctures (1-2 mm deep); pattern of mandibular teeth often imperfect	Appearance	Series scratches or tiny punctures (1-2 mm deep) plus fang marks. Fang marks recognizable as larger and deeper punctures than those from nonfang teeth. Mandibular teeth often indistinct

Examination of the Patient

This is to determine if envenomation has taken place. If it has occurred, immediate vigorous therapy is required. If the snake was not captured, presence or absence of envenomation will be the sole criterion available for deciding if the snake was harmless or poisonous. Verbal descriptions of escaped snakes are generally unreliable. The bite pattern is helpful and may be diagnostic as indicated earlier, but it does not indicate if envenomation has in fact occurred. Even though the victim has been struck by a venomous serpent, envenomation may not ensue. This is the result of various circumstances that influence the flow of venom, the amount of venom injected, and the toxicity of the venom. Evaluation of envenomation depends on the development of local and systemic symptoms and signs. The following are the usual clinical effects which may appear after injection of a sufficient amount of a potent venom.

Local symptoms and signs. The two P's (puncture and pain) and the two E's (edema and erythema) constitute the classic local reaction to deposition of a potent venom in the tissues. At least two should be present to substantiate the diagnosis.

I. *Puncture:* One or two fang marks are present (rarely three or four if reserve fangs in use). These punctures are larger and deeper than those from the other teeth. A wheal or vesicle may develop at the site. If at least one fang mark is not present, then envenomation could not have taken place. Bleeding is usually brisk.

II. *Pain:* Usually develops within 5 to 10 minutes of the strike. It may be delayed up to an hour under certain conditions and may be lacking with a coral snake bite. In a classic case of moderate to severe envenomation involving a pit viper, the pain appears promptly and is severe and unremitting.

III. *Edema:* Typically obvious within 5 to 10 minutes. It also may be delayed up to an hour or absent with a coral snake bite. The swelling may progress up the limb during the next 36 hours and eventually reach the trunk. The overlying skin becomes tense and shiny. The extent of the edema is one of the criteria used in the clinical grading of the severity of envenomation for assessing the amount of antivenom required and for monitoring the progress of the case.

IV. *Erythema:* Redness is ordinarily visible within 5 to 10 minutes. It may not appear for an hour and may be absent after a bite by a coral snake. Later, other types of discoloration develop with pit viper bites as hemorrhages occur in the tissues. Eventually some blueness usually follows unlike the typical reaction to a severe insect bite.

NOTE: Exceptions in the time of appearance and number of these four cardinal signs occur in some pit viper bites owing to variability of potency and amount of venom injected. Also in the event of a fortuitous strike directly into a vessel, there may be absence of local manifestations along with the rapid appearance of systemic signs. Local signs may be missing with coral snake bites owing to the predominance of neurotoxin over hemotoxin.

V. *Hemorrhage:* Petechiae and ecchymoses commonly occur, particularly with pit viper bites. Oozing from fang marks often continues for several hours. This is in contradistinction to the wounds from nonfang teeth, which cease bleeding promptly with both poisonous and nonpoisonous species.

VI. *Paresthesias:* Numbness and/or tingling frequently are noted at the bite site and around the mouth.

VII. *Late local signs:* Tissue necrosis and thrombosis may develop, with sloughing of tissues and gangrene of the extremities. This type of response is common with pit vipers but less so with coral snakes due to the difference in the venoms. Localized lymphadenopathy is a feature in some.

Systemic symptoms and signs. These are produced by the hematogenous or lymphogenous dissemination of the venom. Some of the toxins have enzymatic activity. Owing to the multiplicity of the effects of these diverse protein molecules, the clinical manifestations are numerous and protean. A consistent clinical picture may not be present.

I. *General:* Lassitude, weakness, fatigue, nonwhirling dizziness, diaphoresis, sialorrhea, and the sensation of a "full" or "thick" tongue.

II. *Pulmonic:* Edema, respiratory failure, and death.

III. *Cardiac:* Hypotension, congestive failure, cardiac arrest, and death.

IV. *Renal:* Hematuria, proteinuria, azotemia, and renal failure with death.

V. *Gastrointestinal:* Nausea, emesis, hematemesis, and melena.

VI. *Hematologic:* Alterations of the coagulation system, with petechiae, ecchymoses, bleeding into subcutaneous and muscle tissues, hemorrhages into viscera, and bloody effusions into serous cavities. Laboratory determinations may demonstrate prolonged prothrombin time, thrombocytopenia, fibrinolysis, and prolonged bleeding and clotting times. Epistaxis, hematuria, hematemesis, and melena are common with severe envenomation.

VII. *Central nervous sytem:* Headache, blurred vision, paresthesias, slurred speech, bulbar palsies, generalized convulsions, and paralyses of the extremities. Deep tendon reflexes are variable. The sensorium typically remains intact, with a lucid and oriented patient. Sometimes somnolence may be a feature, and occasionally euphoria is present if the individual has been dosed with the traditional snake bite remedy, whiskey. Disorientation and states bordering on delirium and mania may occur in some victims owing to the hysteria and snake phobia seen in some adults following exposure to a serpent.

VIII. *Death:* Fatalities are due to respiratory failure, cardiac decompensation, renal shutdown, hemorrhage, or irreversible shock.

The physician who has no knowledge of snakes can render an intelligent decision about a snake bite by following the guidelines given regarding inspection of the snake, observation of the bite pattern, and examination of the patient. Irrefutable proof of the poisonous nature of a snake native to the continental United States includes the presence of fangs, pit organs, rattles, and a vertically elliptical pupil. All of these are present in the pit vipers (rattlesnakes, copperheads, and cottonmouth moccasins). The coral snake lacks the pit organs and rattles and has a circular pupil. Otherwise, all indigenous snakes with a round pupil are harmless. Fang marks are diagnostic of a venomous species and are larger and deeper than the scratches or superficial punctures produced by the nonfang teeth. If the patient shows pain, puncture, edema, and erythema, envenomation has taken place. These local signs appear within an hour of the bite, and systemic signs develop later. Local manifestations may be absent with coral snake bite, in which case generalized signs and symptoms develop rapidly.

Specially prepared by Dr. William D. Alsever, Syracuse, New York.

REFERENCES

1. Conant, R.: A Field Guide to Reptile and Amphibians of Eastern and Central North America. New York, Houghton-Mifflin, 1975.

2. Dept. of the Navy, Bureau of Medicine and Surgery; Poisonous Snakes of the World: A Manual for Use by the U.S. Amphibious Forces. Washington, D.C., U.S. Government Printing Office, 1968.

3. Stickel, W.H.: Venomous Snakes of the United States and Treatment of their Bites. Wildlife leaflet 339. Washington, D.C., U.S. Department of the Interior, Fish and Wildlife Service, 1952.

4. Pope, C.H., and Perkins, R.M.: Differences in the patterns of venomous and harmless snake bites. Arch. Surg., *49*:331, 1944.

5. Parrish, H.M., et al.: Snake bite: A pediatric problem. Clin. Pediatr., *4*:237, 1965.

6. Snyder, R.: Snake bite seminar. Am. J. Dis. Child., *103*:117, 1962.

7. Russell, F.E., et al.: Snake venom poisoning: Experiences with 550 cases. JAMA, *233*:341, 1975.

8. Glass, T.G., Jr,: Snake bite. Hosp. Med., Am. J. Dis. Child., July, 1971, p. 31.

9. Parrish, H.M., et al.: Snake bite: Poisonous until proven otherwise. Patient Care, May 30, 1971, p. 76.

10. Russell, F.E.: Injuries by Venomous Animals. National Clearinghouse for Poison Control Centers, Bulletin for Jan.-Feb., 1967. Washington, D.C., U.S. Department of Health Education and Welfare, 1967.

11. Arnold R.E.: What To Do about Bites and Stings of Venomous Animals. New York, Collier Books, 1973.

19
PATIENT CARE

HINTS IN CARING FOR THE HOSPITALIZED CHILD

Children are particularly susceptible to emotional trauma during hospitalization. Painful procedures and separation from home and family cannot be avoided, but the physician can do a great deal to diminish fear and gain the trust of patients. Some useful hints are listed below.

Inform parents of hospital mealtimes, and urge them to visit during that time.

Establish an area where several children may sit together during mealtime.

Provide opportunities for the parents and child to talk to the dietician so that the child's likes and dislikes may be noted. This is also the time to point out particular touches that the dietary department may provide to make meals more appealing; for instance, a straw for milk, extra ketchup, or smaller portions that do not overwhelm the child.

Permit parents to bring food to children, even if they are not on regular diets. Parents may be advised to tell the nurse what their child ate from home.

Encourage parents to provide a doll, blanket, or other favorite object from home in order to have some familiar object in the unfamiliar environment.

If the child is used to falling asleep with a bottle, this is no time to change that practice. The parents may be instructed about the danger of producing caries at the time of discharge.

Avoid performing procedures in the middle of the night. Children may fear night in a strange place, and fear of painful procedures may make relaxation and sleep impossible.

Whenever possible, the child's room and the playroom should be safe havens for the child. Procedures should be reserved for the treatment room.

If procedures must be performed within sight and sound of another child, they should be carefully explained to both children, and the observing child should be reassured that he will not be involved.

The patient should be asked what he knows about an impending procedure. Gaps in his understanding of what will be done should be filled in so that what is actually done will be no more or less than what is expected.

Keep pleasant, inexpensive trinkets with you to provide a surprise for the child.

Find some way to express interest in patients, such as brief participation in a game they were playing when you entered the room, before beginning a procedure or examination.

Encourage parents to visit at any time, even if this means writing special orders for unlimited visiting hours.

If a child is to be examined on the parent's lap, explain what is to be expected of the parent; that is, is the child to be restrained, comforted, or just supported?

Supply a roll-away cot for parents who wish to spend the night with a child who is under 5 years old or in pain.

Explain to parents the need for children to talk about the hospitalization and play out their strong feelings about it. Help them guide their children to draw pictures, pound clay, hammer nails, and engage in any activity that will help the child express emotion.

Excessively loud or long outbursts of crying, throwing objects, hurting others, and other frightening behavior are obvious calls for help. They should be responded to with comfort and explanation of what the child may expect during the rest of the hospital stay.

Reference: Azarnoff, P.: Resident and Staff Physician, May 1976, p. 153.

THE PRESCRIPTION

The sequence of events that starts with a decision to prescribe a medication and ends with the patient receiving the drug is fraught with many possible errors. Among these errors can be included:

1. Inappropriate drug selection. Never write for a medication whose mechanism of action is unknown to you; be familiar with indications, contra-indications, and common side-effects; remember that many drugs have multiple ingredients.
2. Errors in writing and illegible writing.
3. Failure to take prescription to be filled because of transportation or financial reasons.
4. Error in filling of prescription by pharmacist.
5. Noncompliance on part of the parent or patient because of misunderstanding directions for taking the medicine or because of stopping the medicine prematurely.

The important aspects of prescription writing include the following.

Name of drug	Generic names are preferred. Trade name may be added, although when trade name is specified a comment should be included as to whether a substitution can be made by the pharmacist if item is not in stock. For some multiple component medications, such as Lomotil, a trade name alone is adequate.
Form of drug	Always specify; e.g., 500 mg capsules, 125 mg/5 ml.
Amount of drug	Whenever possible, prescribe the precise amount of medication to treat the current illness. Always make a notation in your record as to the amount pre-scribed, thereby providing yourself with a convenient means of detecting compliance. If, for example, a child is seen after a ten-day course of treatment for otitis media, you may ask the mother casually, "How much medicine is left?" The response may vary from "Doctor, I just ran out" to "Doctor, I don't need any more because the bottle is half-full." When prescribing medications that may be abused, such as narcotics or tranquilizers, it is a good practice to write out the amount of drug, i.e., fifteen rather than 15. Numbers can be easily altered unless written in full.
Directions	Specify amount and time of dose, as well as route when appropriate. When writing for more than one drug, try to give them simultaneously. Do not merely write, "Take as directed." Specify the duration of treatment or state, "Until the bottle is empty." Remember that school children may have difficulty with medicines to be taken four times daily or every six hours.
Label notation	Always request that the pharmacist place the name of the drug on the label.

Refill notation	A statement concerning refills should always be provided, even if only to say "no refills."
Daily maximum	If a drug is to be taken "prn," always specify the indications for its use and the maximum quantity to be taken in a 24-hour period.
Signature	Make it legible.
BNDD number	Must be included where required.

To encourage compliance, verbal instructions should accompany the written prescription. Areas to discuss include the following.

1. An explanation of the purpose of the medicine. This explanation should include the name of the drug, the amount and duration of the treatment, and instructions about refills, if appropriate.

2. An explanation of side-effects. This should include those predictable side-effects that should cause no concern, e.g., darkening of stools with iron, as well as those side-effects that require notification of the physician, e.g., staggering or rash while taking phenytoin (Dilantin).

3. An explanation, when a child is receiving multiple drugs, of which drugs should or should not be taken together.

4. Suggestions on how best to give the drug. This is particularly useful for new mothers.

5. Instructions on where to store the medicine in terms of need for refrigeration. Warnings, when necessary, about the drug's potential dangers if ingested by other children.

6. Instructions not to use the medicine for illness in other children.

7. An inquiry as to whether the parents may have problems reaching a drugstore or paying for the medicine.

8. A request that you be called if the parents find it difficult to get or give the medication or have noted unanticipated side-effects.

THE PATIENT MANAGEMENT PLAN
(WRITING HOSPITAL ORDERS)

In order to facilitate nursing care and to insure against omissions in the management of your patients, it is important to develop a routine method of writing hospital orders. Each individual, or institution, should develop such a routine and use it continually. A suggested sequence and its components is described below.

AREA OF MANAGEMENT	DETAILS OF MANAGEMENT
Vital signs	Request the specific signs you wish monitored and the frequency of such measurements. Do not request more than is useful — it consumes a great amount of nursing time. Always specify what should be done when certain limits are exceeded. For example: Notify physician if pulse is greater than 160 or less than 80; notify physician if respirations are greater than 60 or less than 20; notify physician if temperature exceeds 39° C. These instructions should be tailor-made to the patient's disease and your therapeutic plans.
How frequently is the patient to be weighed?	All patients receiving intravenous fluids should be weighed at least daily. All patients under 2 years of age should be weighed daily. All hospitalized patients should be weighed at least weekly.
Are intake and output to be recorded?	All patients receiving intravenous fluids will require such measurements. All patients with diarrhea or vomiting require such information.
Patient's environment and activity	Items to be considered in this category include: croup tent, isolation precautions, crib, bed, bed with side rails, bathroom privileges, playroom privileges, bedtime hour, parents and friends' visiting privileges.
Diet	Specify caloric goals. Do not write "diet for age" in patients under 2 years of age. Specify type and frequency of feedings. Are fluids to be from bottle or cup? Any dietary exclusions.
Is calorie count required?	

AREA OF MANAGEMENT	DETAILS OF MANAGEMENT
Nutritional supplements	Patients receiving intravenous medications will require vitamin supplements. Patients receiving less than optimal diets will require supplements as well. Infants not receiving the equivalent of a reconstituted quart of a commercial formula are not receiving daily vitamin requirement.
Therapy	Intravenous fluids — composition, amount, rate. Medications — dose, route, frequency, duration.
Special treatments	Eye care, skin care, respiratory care, physical therapy, pulmonary toilet, occupational therapy, school teacher.
Diagnostic procedures and preparations for procedures	May include stools for occult blood, urine testing, and other ward procedures as well.
Special nursing	Observe mother-child interaction; child-to-child interactions; child's understanding of disease process.

When orders are written, they should be accompanied with both the date and the *time* the entry was made. Unfortunately, in some instances, hours may go by without the order being translated into action.

When changes in therapy are instituted, they should be accompanied by a progress note in the patient's record so that your colleagues, sharing in the care of the patient, will understand the reasons for change in the patient's management.

PAINLESS VENIPUNCTURE

Obtaining cooperation of children for procedures can be enhanced by making the procedure less uncomfortable. One simple but often neglected step is that of allowing the isopropyl alcohol on a venipuncture site to dry before puncturing the skin. Your patients will appreciate you for it.

Reference: Phillips, P.J., Pain, R.W., and Brooks, G.E.: N. Engl. J. Med., *294*:116, 1976.

19

A FLASHLIGHT CAN HELP YOU FIND A VEIN

A flashlight can assist you in finding a vein in the hand or the foot of one of your small patients. When attempting this maneuver, darken the room slightly and put the lighted flashlight against the patient's palm or sole. This should enable you to "see through" the extremity and find a vein that had previously escaped detection. (See Figure 19–1.)

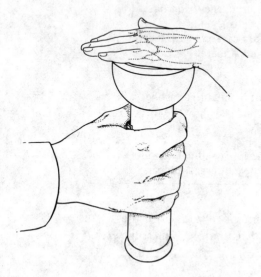

FIG. 19-1

mEq/liter and mg %

Confusion often exists in the conversion of mEq/liter to mg % (mg/100 ml). The table below is intended to minimize such confusion.

ION	IONIC WEIGHT (gm)	EQUIVALENT WEIGHT (gm)	CONVERSION FACTORS mEq/liter	CONVERSION FACTORS mg %
Na^+	23.0	23.0	mg % × 0.435	mEq/liter × 2.30
K^+	39.1	39.1	mg % × 0.256	mEq/liter × 3.91
Ca^{++}	40.1	20.0	mg % × 0.498	mEq/liter × 2.00
Mg^{++}	24.3	12.2	mg % × 0.823	mEq/liter × 1.21
Cl^-	35.5	35.5	mg % × 0.282	mEq/liter × 3.55
HCO_3^-	61.0	61.0	vol % (CO_2) × 0.45	mEq/liter × 2.22 (vol %)
HPO_4^{--}	96.0	48.0	mg % (P) × 0.580	mEq/liter × 1.72 (P)
SO_4^{--}	96.1	48.0	mg % (S) × 0.613	mEq/liter × 1.60 (S)

CONVERSION TABLES

TEMPERATURE °F	TEMPERATURE °C	TEMPERATURE °C	TEMPERATURE °F	WEIGHT lb	WEIGHT kg	WEIGHT kg	WEIGHT lb	LENGTH in	LENGTH cm	LENGTH cm	LENGTH in
0	−17.8	0	32.0	1	.5	1	2.2	1	2.5	1	.4
95	35.0	35.	95.0	2	.9	2	4.4	2	5.1	2	.8
96	35.6	35.5	95.9	4	1.8	3	6.6	4	10.2	3	1.2
97	36.1	36.	96.8	6	2.7	4	8.8	6	15.2	4	1.6
98	36.7	36.5	97.7	8	3.6	5	11.0	8	20.3	5	2.0
99	37.2	37.	98.6	10	4.5	6	13.2	12	30.5	6	2.4
100	37.8	37.5	99.5	20	9.1	8	17.6	18	46	8	3.1
101	38.3	38.	100.4	30	13.6	10	22	24	61	10	3.9
102	38.9	38.5	101.3	40	18.2	20	44	30	76	20	7.9
103	39.4	39.	102.2	50	22.7	30	66	36	91	30	11.8
104	40.0	39.5	103.1	60	27.3	40	88	42	107	40	15.7
105	40.6	40.	104.0	70	31.8	50	110	48	122	50	19.7
106	41.1	40.5	104.9	80	36.4	60	132	54	137	60	23.6
107	41.7	41.	105.8	90	40.9	70	154	60	152	70	27.6
108	42.2	41.5	106.7	100	45.4	80	176	66	168	80	31.5
109	42.8	42.	107.6	150	68.2	90	198	72	183	90	35.4
110	43.3	100	212	200	90.8	100	220	78	198	100	39.4

°F to °C: 5/9 (°F − 32)
°C to °F: (9/5 × °C) + 32

1 lb = 0.454 kg
1 kg = 2.204 lb

1 inch = 2.54 cm
1 cm = 0.3937 inch

19

REMOVAL OF A FOREIGN BODY IN THE EYE — ANOTHER USE FOR THE BAND-AID

An easy method for removing nonpenetrating foreign bodies from the eye — objects such as eyelashes, dust, or dirt — is illustrated in the accompanying figure. All you need is a clean band-aid. Simply touch the foreign body with the adhesive portion of the band-aid. You can even do this to yourself with the aid of a mirror when necessary.

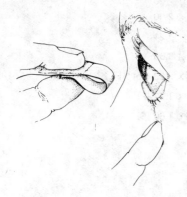

FIG. 19-2

Reference: Pryatel, W.: Resident & Staff Physician, January, 1977, p. 99.

TALKING WITH THE ADOLESCENT — 10 SUGGESTIONS

1. Listen carefully and ask questions that demonstrate your interest.
2. Avoid a moralizing attitude.
3. Don't unwittingly encourage sexual rebellion.
4. Demand accurate knowledge.
5. Become comfortable with the subject of sex and your own morals.
6. Don't be shocked.
7. Know what adolescents want to talk about.
8. Maintain confidentiality.
9. Don't vicariously enjoy an adolescent's sex life.
10. Don't joke about the body.

Courtesy of Dr. Stanford Friedman.

NONMEDICAL FACTORS INFLUENCING TREATMENT

Medicine alone often fails to produce the desired result. The physician should be aware of the extramedical factors that have a bearing on the outcome of any interaction between doctor and child. Some of these factors are described below.

Factors Promoting Optimal Care	Factors Complicating Care
ENCOURAGING A FLEXIBLE REALISTIC APPROACH TO THE CHILD'S PROBLEM	MAY RESULT IN LESS FLEXIBLE APPROACH TO THE CHILD'S PROBLEM

For the Physician

Well established in the community	New physician in the community
Excellent reputation as children's doctor	Not recognized as expert with children
Physician known to family, with good rapport	Physician unknown to family; no opportunity to establish rapport
Physician's personal life presently tranquil	Physician's personal life in unsettled state
Physician likes and enjoys the child	Physician has no rapport with child
Physician has adequate time	Physician is rushed

For the Child

No serious past illnesses	Many serious past illnesses
No chronic illness	Complicating chronic illness
Child enjoys contact with physician	Child seems to dislike or is afraid of physician
Child has had infrequent respiratory tract infections in the past	Child has recently had a large number of or prolonged respiratory tract infections

For the Parents

Intact family unit	Single parent
One parent able to stay home and nurse ill child	Parent(s) must work unless child is critically ill
Family life emotionally tranquil at this time	Family life under stress
No serious financial problems	Family under great financial pressure and this visit is expected to solve all problems
Parents feel that physician accepts and likes them	Parents feel the physician does not like or accept them
Parents selected the physician as their first choice	Parents accept physician because he is available
Parents have had no past experience with unexpected or catastrophic illness with another child	Parents have had a past experience with a sudden, unexpected, or catastrophic illness with another child

For the Parents (Continued)

Parents plan to remain in the city
Parents have no major events planned
   the next week

Parents about to leave on trip or
   vacation (with or without the child)
Parents involved in some major family
   event (wedding, party, etc.)
   within the next week

Reference: Lipow, H. W.: Respiratory tract infections. *In* Green, M., and Haggerty, R. J. (Eds.): Ambulatory Pediatrics II. Philadelphia, W. B. Saunders Company, 1977, p. 39.

THINGS TO REMEMBER IN CARING FOR A CHILD WITH A CHRONIC ILLNESS

1. Without an effective plan for continuity of care, the initial evaluation makes but a limited contribution.

2. Time and regularly scheduled visits are needed to clarify the illness and to permit a trusting relationship between patient and doctor.

3. While planning for the future, concentrate on the present.

4. Try to alleviate guilt, a feeling always present.

5. Include the father.

6. Be interested in how the mother and siblings are getting along.

7. Help the parents understand the identity of their child.

8. Understand that parents may initially feel overwhelmed and inadequate.

9. Promote communication.

10. Help the parents and child to avoid social isolation.

11. Encourage the early and active participation of the parents in the care of their child.

12. Increase parental competence in the care of the child.

13. Help the child understand his illness.

14. Enhance the child's sense of competence and his active role in management of his illness.

15. Prepare the child for what is going to happen.

16. Be comfortable in sharing the care of the child with others.

17. Work with the child's and parents' strengths and resources rather than exclusively with their problems and weaknesses.

18. For the child, be experienced as a long-time friend as well as a physician.

19. Make the family and the child feel that you are glad to see them.

20. If there is hope, be hopeful.

Reference: Haggerty, R. J. and Green, M.: Illness and problems. *In* Green, M. and Haggerty, R. J. (Eds.): Ambulatory Pediatrics II. W. B. Saunders Company, Philadelphia, 1977, p. 22.

BUGS IN THE BAND-AID BOX

Wide-eyed and frightened, they appear with white knuckles clutching the metal Band-Aid box. Their gaze is intense and expectant.

You suspect what is in the box without having them tell.

"Is it alive?" you ask phlegmatically.

Frequently, residents of the Band-Aid box include the following:

CRAB LICE *(Phthirus pubis)*

This small (1 mm), round, reddish-brown louse causes itching. Transmission is by close personal contact. On close examination, the crab louse is found in the pubic area with its head buried in a hair follicle or clutching two adjacent hairs. The dark nits are frequently difficult to find. Crabs may infest the chest and axillary hair *as well as the eyelashes. Treatment:* 25 per cent benzyl benzoate or gamma benzene hexachloride on two successive days. Infested eyelashes are treated with daily applications of yellow oxide of mercury.

Crab louse
(Phthirus pubis)

SCALP LICE *(Pediculus humanus* var. *capitis)*

This long (up to 4 mm), slender, white louse causes pruritus and excoriations with frequent secondary infection. The densest involvement is posteriorly, behind the ears. There may be tender occipital nodes as well as excoriated bites on the neck and shoulders. You may not find the adult louse, but the small white nits glued to hair shafts are obvious. Nits fluoresce under Wood's light. *Treatment:* Gamma benzene hexachloride shampoo for two days, repeated in a week. Comb out nits with a fine-toothed comb.

BODY LICE *(Pediculus humanus* var. *corporis)*

The adult louse is 1 to 4 mm long and lives, loves, and lays eggs (nits) in the seams of clothing. This louse feeds on the body, leaving an urticarial wheal with a hemorrhagic central punctum.

Examination of the skin reveals parallel linear excoriations that often are secondarily infected. *Treatment:* Thorough laundering of clothes and bedding. Iron all seams. Bedding and clothing may be dusted with 10 per cent DDT powder. 1 per cent gamma benzene hexachloride may be applied topically once.

19

Head or body louse
(Pediculus humanus
var. capitis or corporis)

PINWORMS *(Enterobius vermicularis)*

The patient may find small, white worms at the anal orifice in the early morning hours. Infestation produces intense perianal pruritus, which leads to excoriations, lichenification, and infection. Bruxism and nightmares are common. The diagnosis is usually made by identifying ova on transparent tape that has been pressed to perianal skin at bedtime. *Treatment:* The Medical Letter has recommended pyrantel pamoate (Banminth) (11 mg/kg) as a single oral dose. Mebendazole, 100 mg X one dose, regardless of weight, may also be used. The treatment should be repeated in two weeks.

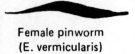

Female pinworm
(E. vermicularis)

MAGGOTS *(Fly Larvae)*

Rarely, maggots will be picked from an open sore, the nose, the ear canal, or from the stool.

Maggot

FISH TAPEWORM *(Diphyllobothrium latum)*

This is a very large cestode that produces enormous numbers of yellowish eggs. It has been an occupational disease of Jewish housewives who taste raw ground fish to check seasoning when making gefilte fish. Thus, its incidence may be decreasing (at least in this population). Immobile, white, flat segments may be found in the stool. Treatment is with niclosamide, 1 gm for children under 35 kg and 1.5 gm for children over 35 kg. The tablets should be chewed thoroughly.

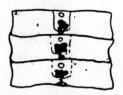

Fish tapeworm
(D. latum)

BEEF TAPEWORM *(Taenia saginata)*

Gravid, white, mobile segments of this worm may be passed in the stool. *Treatment:* Quinacrine, 200 mg every 5-10 min for four dosages, on an empty stomach, followed by a magnesium sulfate purge 2 to 4 hr later. Niclosamide may also be employed in the same dose as for fish tapeworm.

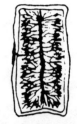

Beef tapeworm
(T. saginata)

ROUNDWORM *(Ascaris lumbricoides)*

Ascaris lumbricoides is characterized by an elongated, cylindric, nonsegmented, translucent, flesh-colored body 15-35 cm long. A cosmopolitan worm, ascaris infects 25 per cent of the world's population. One or more worms may be passed in the stool or, less frequently, vomited. Worms have been known to crawl out of the nose, ear, and umbilical fissures! *Treatment:* Piperazine citrate syrup 75 mg/kg daily X 2. Pyrantel pamoate may also be employed as a single-dose therapy (11 mg/kg with a 1-gm maximal dose).

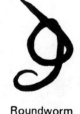

Roundworm
(A. lumbricoides)

DEBRIS

Vegetable particles, such as seeds (corn), stems, and celery, and other debris, like dirt, gravel, stringy fuzz, and cellophane, can be swollen and discolored by passage through the alimentary canal. Even a normal person would be alarmed, and the person with parasitophobia will be in panic. *Treatment:* Show the patient the characteristics of the debris by hand lens or dissecting microscope.

MISCELLANEOUS

Products of conception, menstrual blood clots thought to be products of conception, "grape-like bodies" of hydatidiform mole, fragments of tampons, and clotted mucus and blood from cystitis have all made it to the Band-Aid box.

Reference: Gottlieb, A.J., Zamkoff, K.W., Jastremski, M.S., Scalzo, A., and Imboden, K.J.: The Whole Internist Catalog. Philadelphia, W.B. Saunders Company, 1980, pp. 497–499.

20
POTPOURRI

RED HERRING

During hunts in the seventeenth century, the challenge to the hunting dogs was sometimes increased by dragging a red herring (i.e., a cured or smoked herring or other dead animal) across the quarry's track in an attempt to throw the dogs off the scent. Thus, the term has come to mean any subject that diverts attention from the question at hand.

Reference: Oxford English Dictionary. New York, Oxford University Press, 1971.

WHO INVENTED THE POPSICLE?

Frank Epperson was the inventor who made lemonade from a specially prepared powder that he sold at an Oakland, California, amusement park. While visiting friends in New Jersey, he prepared a batch of special lemonade and inadvertently left a glass of it on a windowsill with a spoon in it. The temperature went down below zero during the night, and in the morning Epperson saw the glass. He picked it up by the spoon handle and ran hot water over the glass, releasing the frozen mass. In his hand was the first Epsicle, later to be known as the Popsicle. Epperson saw immediately the potential of what he held in his hand and applied for a patent, which was granted in 1924. He was fortunate, because research conducted by *The Ice Cream Review*, in 1925 revealed that a major ice cream company was experimenting with "frozen suckers" at the time of the windowsill incident, and as far back as 1872 two men doing business as Ross and Robbins sold a frozen-fruit confection on a stick, which they called the Hokey-Pokey.

Reference: Dickson, P.: *In* The Great American Ice Cream Book. New York, Atheneum, 1973. (Reprinted in Pediatrics, 55:29, 1975.)

20

THE BEST FRISBEE

As a physician caring for children you should be prepared to give advice on many subjects. When the young adolescent inquires about which Frisbee to buy are you prepared to help him? If the answer is "no" perhaps this portion from the book "The Best Encore" by Peter Passell may save the day.

Not all frisbees are equal. For that matter, not all frisbees are Frisbees. The name is a trademark owned by the Wham-O Company of San Gabriel, California.

Your modern frisbee is a work of science and art, far from its humble origins before World War II as the container for Mr. Joseph P. Frisbie's commercial pies.

But enough history. Whatever their source, good frisbees are made of polyethylene and have a curved flight plate and tucked-in lip. All serious designs are based on the original Wham-O Pluto Platter, first produced in the mid-1950s.

Heavy frisbees (150 grams or more) work well in gusty winds but are a bear to catch. Large platters appear to have superior stability, but this is because they have proportionately more weight in the rim; the key is angular momentum. With few exceptions, light-to-medium-weight frisbees have an edge in distance contests.

Hence the best frisbee depends upon priorities. For all-around play, where distance, catchability, hover, stability, and accuracy count, we go with the Pro. Wham-O's Professional Sport model checks in at 108 grams and 22.5 centimeters across.

People with big hands generally prefer the Super Pro, with its extra weight and extra 5 centimeters in circumference.

For stability in wind, Wham-O's oversize, overweight disks, the Tournament and Master models, dominate. Given a choice, pick the 175-gram Tournament. For sheer distance, a strong player should opt for Concept Products' All Star model.

The fastest frisbee of them all is Wham-O's lithe Fastback; unfortunately the Fastback's profile renders it hopelessly unstable.

So much for serious frisbees. Perhaps you are ready for the Explorer II from the L. M. Cox Company. An ordinary frisbee does nothing but hover. Spin the Explorer II and centrifugal force automatically lights two tiny bulbs. Best for night play or during an eclipse of the sun.

Reference: Passell, P.: The Best Encore. New York, Farrar, Strauss and Gordon, 1977.

SUICIDE, A PROBLEM OF ADOLESCENCE

Suicide ranks high among the list of causes of death during adolescence and early childhood. Symptoms preceding an attempted suicide are similar to those of adults and basically are a reflection of depression. This may manifest itself as sleeping difficulties (especially early awakening), anorexia, decreased energy, feelings of worthlessness, difficulty in thinking or remembering, loss of interest, and preoccupation with death. Unfortunately, many of these symptoms are often seen in individuals who are merely adjusting to a variety of common adolescent problems, so that the warning signs are often overlooked.

In boys, successful suicides far exceed unsuccessful attempts. In adolescent girls under 14, suicides are successful in roughly half the attempts. Of all adolescent suicides, 80 per cent are committed by boys. Although death by self-inflicted gun shot wounds is the most common type of successful suicide in both girls and boys, girls are five times more likely to ingest pills. The spectrum of methods of suicides in adolescence may be seen in the following table. Adolescents are contrasted with the age group of 20 to 29, which has the highest incidence of suicides.

Suicides by Method, Age, and Sex

METHOD	AGE 10-19*		Age 20-29†	
	Male (%)	Female (%)	Male (%)	Female (%)
Poisoning by solid or liquid	5	24	9	32
Poisoning by gas	6	44	9	8
Suffocation (hanging, drowning, strangulation)	24	14	18	11
Firearms and explosives	62	55	60	44
Cutting or piercing instruments	< 1	< 1	1	< 1
Jumping from high places	2	3	3	5

*Constitutes 6.5 per cent of all suicides reported to the National Center for Health Statistics in 1975.
†Constitutes 22 per cent of all suicides.

Reference: Murphy, G. E.: Hosp. Pract., *12:*73, 1977.

20

WHAT IS MEANT BY "USUALLY"?

The lexicon of medicine is burdened by words such as "rarely," "frequently," "usually," "infrequently," "occasionally," or "almost never." What do you mean when you use them? What does your audience believe you mean?

A group of 51 individuals, highly skilled or professional workers, were asked to quantitate a number of inherently imprecise terms. Listed below are the words and what the readers believed to be the occurrence rate signified by the terms. The mean value as well as two standard deviations from the mean are provided so that you can appreciate how diverse are the interpretations of these commonly used words.

TERM	OCCURRENCE RATE	
	Mean	*± 2 S.D. (%)*
Always	100%	—
Almost always	89%	75–100
Usually	71%	35–100
Frequently	68%	42–93
Often	59%	28–92
Occasionally	20%	0–42
Infrequently	12%	0–28
Rarely	5%	0–17
Never	0%	—

Since nothing is ever "never" or "always" you can see the problems you create in interpretation every time you use these imprecise words.

Reference: Toogood, J.H.: Lancet, *1*:1094, 1980.

INCIDENCE OR PREVALENCE

"It has been said that the easiest way to distinguish a clinician from an epidemiologist is by the clinician's incorrect use of the term 'incidence.' " It is unfortunate, both for interpretation of facts and figures, as well as for personal expression, to be unaware of the difference between incidence and prevalence. The correct definitions are:

$$\text{Incidence rate} = \frac{\text{number of new cases of a disease}}{\text{total population at risk}} \quad \text{per unit of time}$$

$$\text{Prevalence rate} = \frac{\text{number of existing cases}}{\text{total population}}$$

Reference: Friedman, G.D.: Ann. Intern. Med., *84*:502, 1976.

20

WHAT DO ALL THOSE PERCENTILES MEAN?

Both percentiles and standard deviations indicate how far a measurement deviates from the mean of a set of measurements. For any particular set of measurements, percentiles can be converted into standard deviations and vice versa. Figure 20–1 shows these relationships; since most of us have fuzzy recall of what all of this exactly "means," a review never hurts.

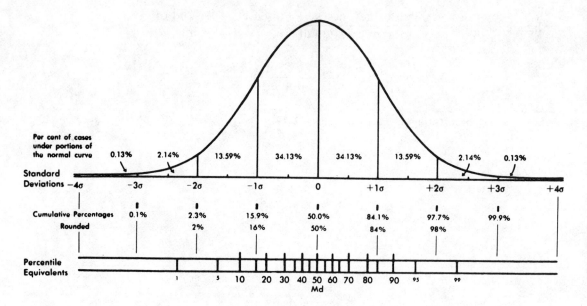

FIG. 20-1

Normal curve showing relationship between standard deviations and percentiles

Reference: Valadian, I., and Porter, D.: Physical Growth and Development. Boston, Little, Brown & Co., 1977, p. 15. Reproduced with permission from the Test Service Notebook of The Psychological Corporation.

METRIC SYSTEM PREFIXES
(Small Measurements)

Most health workers today are familiar with metric measurements. Many however, may be confused by prefixes used to measure very small increments. The following table may be of assistance.

k	kilo	10^3
c	centi	10^{-2}
m	milli	10^{-3}
μ	micro	10^{-6}
n	nano (formerly millimicro, mμ)	10^{-9}
p	pico (formerly micromicro, μμ)	10^{-12}
f	femto	10^{-15}

HOUSEHOLD MEASURES

Despite the fact that we are gradually adopting the metric system in the United States, pockets of resistance are bound to persist. Old ways die hard. You should be familiar with common household measures and what they signify in order to give appropriate instructions to parents. Some of the more common household measures are listed below.

120 drops of water	1 teaspoon	5 ml
2 teaspoons	1 dessert spoon	10 ml
3 teaspoons	1 tablespoon	15 ml
16 tablespoons	1 cup	240 ml
4 tablespoons	¼ cup	60 ml
2 tablespoons	1 ounce	30 ml
1 cup	½ pint	240 ml
4 cups	1 quart	960 ml
3 tablespoons of flour	1 ounce	30 gm

ON AN AVERAGE DAY IN AMERICA

10,930,000 cows are milked.
80 million people hear Muzak.
Schoolchildren ride 12,720,000 miles on school buses.
10,205 people give blood.
205 animals are buried in pet cemeteries.
$54,794 is spent to fight dandruff.
10,000 people take their first airplane ride.
68,493 teenagers come down with VD
3 million people go to the movies.

20

Someone is raped every 8 minutes, murdered every 27 minutes, and robbed every 78 seconds. A burglar strikes every 10 seconds, and a car is stolen every 33 seconds.

Amateurs take 19,178,000 snapshots.

9077 babies are born, including about 360 twins or triplets. 1282 of them are illegitimate. Between 16 and 27 of them were conceived through artificial insemination.

2466 children are bitten by dogs.

Eight children swallow toys and are taken to emergency rooms.

28 mailmen are bitten by dogs.

Industry generates nearly 1 lb of hazardous waste for every person in America.

1.1 million people are in the hospital.

3231 women have abortions.

Three bike riders are killed in accidents. Fifteen people drown.

1,885,000 people go to sleep in a hotel or motel.

679 million telephone conversations occur and 50 million of them are long distance.

5962 couples wed, and before the sun sets 2986 divorce.

Drunk drivers do $.18 million worth of damage.

U.S. rivers discharge 1.3 million tons of sediment.

The typical American spends two hours reading, if you count signboards, labels, the daily mail, and everything else.

41 million people go to school, kindergarten through graduate school.

People drink 90 million cans of beer.

Every one of us, on average, produces nearly 6 lb of garbage.

The snack bars at Chicago's O'Hare Airport sell 5479 hot dogs covered with 12 gallons of relish and 9 gallons of mustard, and washed down with 890 gallons of coffee.

56,000 animals are turned over to animal shelters. 36,986 dogs and cats are executed in these establishments.

$10 million is spent on advertising.

5041 people observe their 65th birthday.

2740 kids run away from home.

Motorists pay $4,036,000 in tolls.

1370 men undergo vasectomies.

176,810,950 eggs are laid.

Ten doctors are disciplined by state medical boards.

One of every three high-school students in Boston misses school.

88 million people watch prime-time TV programs.

2740 teenagers get pregnant.

1.3 million people commute more than 100 miles, round trip.

One American in eight has a beer.

63,288 cars crash, killing 129 people.

Reference: Feinsilber, M., and Mead, W.B.: American Way Magazine, July, 1980, pp. 64-67.

FIRST AID EQUIPMENT AND SUPPLIES

As a pediatrician you will frequently be asked to serve as a team physician or provide advice to a school or camp as to the appropriate composition of a First Aid Kit. The list below has been prepared by the American Academy of Pediatrics.

American Medical Association's First Aid Manual
American Academy of Pediatric Publications
    Accidents in Children
    Disaster and Emergency Medical Services for Children
    Handbook of Acute Poisonings in Children
    First Aid Chart
    First Aid Treatment for Poisoning Chart
Sterile first aid dressings in sealed envelope, 2 X 2 in, for small wounds and eye pads
Sterile first aid dressings in sealed envelope, 4 X 4 in, for large wounds and for compress to stop bleeding
Small, sterile compresses, with adhesive attached, in sealed envelopes
Roller bandage, 1 in. X 5 yd, finger bandage
Roller bandage, 2 in. X 5 yd, to hold dressings in place
Adhesive tape, roll containing assorted widths
Triangular bandages, for slings and as a covering over a larger dressing
Mild soap for cleaning wounds, scratches, and cuts
Absorbent cotton, sterilized to use as swabs or pledgets for cleaning wounds
Applicator sticks for making swabs
Tongue blades for splinting broken fingers and stirring solutions
Splints ¼ in thick, ½ in wide, and 12 to 15 in long. for splinting broken arms and legs
Scissors with blunt tips for cutting bandages or clothing
Tweezers to remove stingers from insect bites or to remove small splinters
Hemostats
Hot water bottle with cover
Ice bag for relief of pain and to reduce swelling
Eye dropper for rinsing eyes
Portable stretcher
Blankets, sheets, pillows, pillow cases (disposable covers suitable)
Cot and mattress with waterproof cover
Wash cloths, hand towels, small portable basin
Covered waste receptacle with disposable liners
Thermometer and covered container for storing thermometer in alcohol
Safety pins
Adjustable crutches
Flashlight
Airways

20

Elastic bandages, 3 in, 4 in, 6 in
Container for heating water
Assorted foam rubber and felt
Cervical collar
Spine board with neck traction unit or 5 lb sand bags
Heating unit
Paper drinking cups
Disposable tissues
Tourniquet
Self-filling bags, valve, portable oxygen, with child and adult sized masks
Oxygen cylinder and flow meter
Fluorescin eye strips
Emergency tags
Syringes and needles for subcutaneous, intramuscular, and intravenous injections
70 per cent isopropyl alcohol for use with thermometer
One 30 ml bottle of Ipecac Syrup
One can of activated charcoal (Darco)
Epinephrine, 1:1,000
Aromatic Spirits of Ammonia
Lidocaine, 0.05 per cent solution
Sodium bicarbonate solution

Reference: School Health: A Guide for Health Professionals. American Academy of Pediatrics Publication, Evanston, Illinois.

RELIGIOUS RITES

On occasion we may forget about our own religion, but we should never lose sight of its importance to our patients and their families. The table below provides some guidelines for the physician when dealing with the birth, death, and special dietary customs of the three major faiths.

OCCASION	JEWISH	PROTESTANT	ROMAN CATHOLIC
Birth			
General precepts	Jewish infants are not baptized. It is a basic ritual among all Jews that male babies be circumcised on the eighth day after birth. (Circumcision of an infant in poor health may be postponed.) There is no special rite for Jewish girl babies.	Emergency baptism should be performed on all Protestant infants in danger of death, with the exception of Baptists and Disciples of Christ. If possible, a baptized person should be present as sponsor. If none is available, anyone present may serve as a witness.	Emergency baptism must be conferred on every Catholic infant in probable danger of death; on every monstrosity; on every stillborn and aborted fetus, whatever its stage of development, unless it is certainly dead. *For purposes of baptism*, the only certain sign of death is noticeable corruption.
What to do	Nothing.	Call a minister. But if there is danger of death and the minister may not arrive in time, anyone may baptize. Pour water on the infant's head (not merely on the hair), saying simultaneously: "(Name), I baptize you in the name of the Father and of the Son and of the Holy Spirit. Amen." If the child has not yet been named, use the equivalent of "Baby Boy Smith." Excess water must be poured off onto the ground. If cotton was used to wipe baby's head, it must be burned. Later, report all available information about the infant to a clergyman of his denomination.	Call a priest. But if there is danger the infant will die before the priest arrives, anyone may and should baptize. Pour water on the infant's head (*not* merely on the hair), saying simultaneously: "I baptize you in the name of the Father and of the Son and of the Holy Spirit." Water must flow on the skin. Giving a name is not essential. If it is a medically dead fetus still enclosed in membranes, immerse it in a basin of water, break the membranes, and pronounce the words while moving the fetus about in the water. If the infant is likely to die in utero, a medically qualified person should attempt baptism in utero with a sterile syringe containing sterile water; the membranes must be pierced before the water is released; after delivery, the baptism should be repeated. Following such a baptism, report all available information about the infant to the priest. *Continued*

OCCASION	JEWISH	PROTESTANT	ROMAN CATHOLIC
Death			
General precepts	When a Jewish patient dies in the hospital, a rabbi, or some responsible member of the Jewish community, will make proper arrangements for burial. Since many Jews are opposed to autopsy for religious persons, a rabbi, or some responsible member of the Jewish community, should discuss the matter of autopsy with the deceased's family.	Most Protestant denominations do not observe last sacraments. Those that do administer them before death. There is no moral objection to autopsy among most Protestants.	Every Roman Catholic should receive the last sacraments (penance, Communion, and extreme unction) before death. But penance and extreme unction can be administered conditionally up to several hours after medical death has occurred. The patient's body should not be wrapped in a shroud until after the last rights have been administered. There is no moral objection to autopsy performed in accordance with the provision of civil law.
What to do	Notify a rabbi or some responsible member of the Jewish community. Follow routine care for the body after death.	Call a minister. Follow routine care for the body after death. Place arms at the sides, or fold them; close eyes.	Call a priest. When he's finished his ministrations, follow routine care for the body after death.
Dietary Rules	Observant Jews eat only kosher (permissible) meat, fish, and dairy products. These are prepared in utensils and served in dishes that have been cleaned and kept separate in a ritually prescribed manner; and they are eaten in a prescribed sequence. If the patient's medical diet requires him to have milk and meat products at the same meal, the milk products should be served *first*. During Passover, the observant Jews will not eat leavened products or drink liquids containing grain alcohol.	Many Protestants observe rules of fasting (only one full meal a day) and abstinence (no meat). It is wise to ask the patient about special dietary rules he prefers to follow.	On weekdays of Lent and on certain other days, Catholics between the ages of 21 and 59 are subject to the law of fasting. This law does not apply to the genuinely sick for whom fasting would be detrimental or exceptionally difficult.
How to Address Clergy	Rabbi	Mister or Doctor. When in doubt, Mister (never Reverend). Lutheran ministers are usually called Pastor. Many Episcopal priests are called Father.	Father.

Reference: Medical Economics, June 1959.

MEDICAL MURPHOLOGY

Six Principles for Patients

1. Just because your doctor has a name for your condition doesn't mean he knows what it is.
2. The more boring and out-of-date the magazines in the waiting room, the longer you will have to wait for your scheduled appointment.
3. Only adults have difficulty with child-proof bottles.
4. You never have the right number of pills left on the last day of a prescription.
5. The pills to be taken with meals will be the least appetizing ones.
   Corollary:
   Even water tastes bad when taken on doctor's orders.
6. If your condition seems to be getting better, it's probably your doctor getting sick.

Matz's Warning

Beware of the physician who is great at getting out of trouble.

Matz's Rule Regarding Medications

A drug is that substance which, when injected into a rat, will produce a scientific report.

Cochrane's Aphorism

Before ordering a test decide what you will do if it is (1) positive, or (2) negative. If both answers are the same, don't do the test.

Bernstein's Precept

The radiologist's national flower is the hedge.

Lord Cohen's Comment

The feasibility of an operation is not the best indication for its performance.

Telesco's Laws of Nursing

1. All the IVs are at the other end of the hall.
2. A physician's ability is inversely proportional to his availability.
3. There are two kinds of adhesive tape: that which won't stay on and that which won't come off.
4. Everybody wants a pain shot at the same time.
5. Everybody who didn't want a pain shot when you were passing out pain shots wants one when you are passing out sleeping pills.

20

Barach's Rule

An alcoholic is a person who drinks more than his own physician.

Finally, as Murphy's Law

If anything can go wrong, it will.

Corollaries

1. Nothing is as easy as it looks.
2. Everything takes longer than you think.
3. If there is a possibility of several things going wrong, the one that will cause the most damage will be the one to go wrong.
4. If you perceive that there are four possible ways in which a procedure can go wrong, and circumvent these, a fifth way will promptly develop.
5. Left to themselves, things tend to go from bad to worse.
6. Whenever you set out to do something, something else must be done first.
7. Every solution breeds new problems.
8. It is impossible to make anything foolproof because fools are so ingenious.
9. Nature always sides with the hidden flaw.
10. Mother Nature is a bitch.

References: Bloch, A.: Murphy's Law and Other Reasons Why Things Go Wrong! Los Angeles, Price/Stern/Sloan, 1979. Bloch, A.: Murphy's Law. Book 2. Los Angeles, Price/Stern/Sloan, 1980, pp. 62–64.

A MEMORANDUM FROM YOUR CHILD

1. Don't spoil me. I know quite well that I ought not to have all I ask for. I'm only testing you.
2. Don't be afraid to be firm with me. I prefer it. It lets me know where I stand.
3. Don't use force with me. It teaches me that power is all that counts. I will respond more readily to being led.
4. Don't be inconsistent. That confuses me and makes me try harder to get away with everything that I can.
5. Don't make promises; you may not be able to keep them. That will discourage my trust in you.
6. Don't fall for my provocations when I say and do things just to upset you. Then I'll try for other such "victories."
7. Don't be too upset when I say "I hate you." I don't mean it, but I want you to feel sorry for what you have done to me.
8. Don't make me feel smaller than I am. I will make up for it by behaving like a "Big Shot."

9. Don't do things for me that I can do for myself. It makes me feel like a baby, and I may continue to put you in my service.

10. Don't let my "Bad Habits" get me a lot of your attention. It may encourage me to continue them.

11. Don't correct me in front of people. I'll take much more notice if you talk quietly with me in private.

12. Don't try to discuss my behavior in the heat of a conflict. For some reason my hearing is not very good at this time and my cooperation is even worse. It is all right to take the action required, but let's not talk about it until later.

13. Don't try to preach to me. You'd be surprised how well I know what is right and wrong.

14. Don't make me feel that my mistakes are sins. I have to learn to make mistakes without feeling that I am no good.

15. Don't nag. If you do, I shall have to protect myself by appearing deaf.

16. Don't demand explanations for my wrong behavior. I really don't know why I did it.

17. Don't tax my honesty too much. I am easily frightened into telling lies.

18. Don't forget that I love and use to experiment. I learn from it, so please put up with it.

19. Don't protect me from consequences. I need to learn from my own experiences.

20. Don't take too much notice of my small ailments. I may learn to enjoy poor health if it gets me much attention.

21. Don't put me off when I ask HONEST QUESTIONS. If you do, you will find that I stop asking and seek my information elsewhere.

22. Don't answer "silly" or meaningless questions. I just want you to keep busy with me.

23. Don't ever think that it is beneath your dignity to apologize to me. An honest apology makes me feel surprisingly warm toward you.

24. Don't ever suggest that you are perfect or infallible. It gives me too much to live up to.

25. Don't worry about the little amount of time that we spend together, since it is *HOW* we spend it that counts.

26. Don't let my fears arouse your anxiety. Then I will become more afraid. Show me courage.

27. Don't forget that I can't thrive without lots of understanding and encouragement, but I don't need to tell you that, do I?

TREAT ME THE WAY YOU TREAT YOUR FRIENDS, THEN I WILL BE YOUR FRIEND, TOO. REMEMBER, I LEARN MORE FROM A MODEL THAN FROM A CRITIC.

Reference: Unknown.

20

HOW TO EAT LIKE A CHILD

Does this bring back memories? Share it with mothers who are frustrated and upset about their children's eating habits.

Peas: Mash and flatten into thin sheet on plate. Press the back of the fork into the peas. Hold fork vertically, prongs up, and lick off peas.

Mashed potatoes: Pat mashed potatoes flat on top. Dig several little depressions. Think of them as ponds or pools. Fill the pools with gravy. With your fork, sculpt rivers between pools and watch the gravy flow between them. Decorate with peas. Do not eat.

Alternate method: Make a large hole in center of mashed potatoes. Pour in ketchup. Stir until potatoes turn pink. Eat as you would peas.

Animal crackers: Eat each in this order — legs, head, body.

Sandwich: Leave the crusts. If your mother says you have to eat them because that's the best part, stuff the crusts into your pants pocket or between the cushions of the couch.

Spaghetti: Wind too many strands on the fork and make sure at least two strands dangle down. Open your mouth wide and stuff in spaghetti; suck noisily to inhale the dangling strands. Clean plate, ask for seconds, and eat only half. When carrying your plate to the kitchen, hold it tilted so that the remaining spaghetti slides off and onto the floor.

Ice-cream cone: Ask for a double scoop. Knock the top scoop off while walking out the door of the ice-cream parlor. Cry. Lick the remaining scoop slowly so that ice cream melts down and outside of the cone and over your hand. Stop licking when the ice cream is even with the top of the cone. Be sure it is absolutely even. Eat a hole in the bottom of the cone and suck the rest of the ice cream out the bottom. When only the cone remains with ice cream coating the inside, leave on car dashboard.

Ice cream in bowl: Grip spoon upright in fist. Stir ice cream vigorously to make soup. Take a large helping on a spoon, place spoon in mouth and slowly pull it out, sucking only the top layer of ice cream off. Wave spoon in air. Lick its back. Put in mouth again and suck off some more. Repeat until all ice cream is off spoon and begin again.

Spinach: Divide into little piles. Rearrange again into new piles. After five or six maneuvers, sit back and say you are full.

Fried egg: Eat either the white or the yolk.

Chocolate-chip cookies: Half-sit, half-lie on the bed, propped up by a pillow. Read a book. Place cookies next to you on the sheet so that crumbs get in the bed. As you eat the cookies, remove each chocolate chip and place it on your stomach. When all the cookies are consumed, eat the chips one by one, allowing two per page.

Milk shake: Bite off one end of the paper covering the straw. Blow through straw to shoot paper across table. Place straw in shake and suck. When the shake just reaches your mouth, place a finger over the top of the straw — the pressure will keep the shake in the straw. Lift straw out of shake, put bottom end in mouth, release finger and swallow.

Do this until the straw is squished so that you can't suck through it. Ask for another. Open it the same way, but this time shoot the paper at the waitress when she isn't looking. Sip your shake casually — you are just minding your own business — until there is about an inch of shake remaining. Then blow through the straw until bubbles rise to the top of the glass. When your father says he's had just about enough, get a stomach ache.

Baked apple: With your fingers, peel skin off baked apple. Tell your mother you changed your mind, you don't want it. Later, when she is harrassed and not paying attention to what she is doing, pick up the naked baked apple and hand it to her.

French fries: Wave one french fry in air for emphasis while you talk. Pretend to conduct orchestra. Then place four fries in your mouth at once and chew. Turn to your sister, open your mouth and stick out your tongue coated with potatoes. Close mouth and swallow. Smile.

Reference: From "How to Eat Like a Child" by Delia Ephron. Copyright ©1978 by Delia Ephron. Reprinted by permission of Viking Penguin, Inc.

AUTHOR INDEX

SUBJECT INDEX

Note: Page numbers in *italics* refer to illustrations.

561